New Directions in Interpreting the Millon™ Clinical Multiaxial Inventory-III (MCMI-III™)

New Directions in Interpreting the Millon™ Clinical Multiaxial Inventory-III (MCMI-III™)

Edited by

Robert J. Craig

WILEY

John Wiley & Sons, Inc.

Published by John Wiley & Sons, Inc., Hoboken, New Jersey.
Published simultaneously in Canada.

For general information on our other products and services please contact our Customer Care Department within the United States at (800) 762-2974, outside the United States at (317) 572-3993 or fax (317) 572-4002.

Wiley also publishes its books in a variety of electronic formats. Some content that appears in print may not be available in electronic books. For more information about Wiley products, visit our web site at www.wiley.com.

Library of Congress Cataloging-in-Publication Data:

New directions in interpreting the million clinical multiaxial : inventory-III (MCMI-III) / edited by Robert J. Craig.
    p.   cm.
  Includes bibliographical references.
  ISBN 978-0-471-69190-7 (cloth)
   1. Millon Clinical Multiaxial Inventory. I. Craig, Robert J., 1941–
RC473.M47N49   2005
616.89'075—dc22
                                            2004059092

Contents

Contributors

R. Michael Bagby, PhD
University of Toronto
Toronto, Ontario, Canada

James Choca, PhD
Roosevelt University
Chicago, Illinois

Robert J. Craig, PhD, ABPP
Jesse Brown VA Medical Center
Chicago, Illinois

Roger D. Davis, PhD
Digonex Technologies, Inc.
Miami, Florida

Cristian del Rio, PhD
Carlos Albizu University
Miami, Florida

Frank J. Dyer, PhD
Private Practice
Montclair, New Jersey

Patrick M. Flynn, PhD
Institute of Behavioral Research
Texas Christian University
Fort Worth, Texas

Paul Gibeau, PsyD
Argosy University
Chicago, Illinois

Seth D. Grossman, PsyD
Institute for Advanced Studies
    in Personology and
    Psychopathology, Florida
    International University
Miami, Florida

Louis Hsu, PhD
Fairleigh Dickinson University
Teaneck, New Jersey

Jeffrey J. Magnavita, PhD,
    ABPP, FAPA
Hartford Hospital
University of Hartford
Glastonbury, Connecticut

Margarita B. Marshall, PhD
University of Toronto
Toronto, Ontario, Canada

Ronald E. Olson, PhD
Oakland University
Rochester, Michigan

Michael J. Patterson, PhD
Digonex Technology
Miami, Florida

Gina Rossi, PhD
Vrije Universiteit Brussels
Brussels, Belgium

Andrew G. Ryder, PhD
Concordia University
Montréal, QC, Canada

Hedwig Sloore, PhD
Vrije Universiteit Brussels
Brussels, Belgium

Stephen Strack, PhD
U.S. Department of Veterans
    Affairs Ambulatory Care Center
Los Angeles, California

Scott Wetzler, PhD
Albert Einstein College of
    Medicine Montefiore Medical
    Center
Bronx, New York

Introduction

THE MILLON™ Clinical Multiaxial Inventory (as revised)–III™ (MCMI-III™) has become a mainstay in clinical assessment and is used in a multiplicity of settings and for a variety of assessment and treatment planning purposes. Research cited throughout this book documents its frequent use in clinical, counseling, medical, and forensic services in both public and private practice venues. Only the MMPI and the Rorschach have enjoyed such widespread application.

Clinicians value this test because of its clinical utility. And yet, science does not stand still. New discoveries, new conceptualizations, new research, and critical analysis continue to refine the way we assess and the way we frame these assessments. The same is true for personality assessment in general and for the MCMI-III in particular. Millon continues to refine his bioevolutionary model, on which the test is based, and his prototype personality disorders have evolved toward greater specificity with the theorized personality disorder subtypes. With the introduction of the third edition of the MCMI, researchers are determining how well this latest revision compares with its MCMI predecessors, as well as evaluating the test in light of some continuing controversies. Much of this new way of thinking about and understanding the MCMI are presented in this book. Contemporary research issues relating to the MCMI are also discussed.

This book is divided into three main sections. Part I addresses some new directions in interpreting the MCMI. Part II highlights some newer applications of the MCMI-III. Finally, Part III addresses some of the continuing controversies with the MCMI-III. The critical analyses on which these chapters are based actually appeared in relation to the MCMI-I and -II, and it remains to be seen whether or not these criticisms will remain applicable to the MCMI-III.

The MCMI is a theory-derived instrument for measuring Millon's taxonomy of personality classification. He initially used a biopsychosocial model for his theoretical notions, but this was eventually superseded by a bioevolutionary model that generated, *from theory*, basic personality styles for nonclinical populations as well as personality disorders that were consistent with but not isomorphic with diagnostic classification systems (i.e., *DSM, ICD*). He also invoked a domain model, consisting of structural and functional criteria, with which to characterize and describe each of the personality disorders in his classification system. The MCMI was designed to assess whether or not a given patient had the traits, characteristics, and behaviors associated with a given disorder *at the diagnostic level.* If so, the psychologist could use Millon's domain model to describe the prototypical patient with this disorder.

Millon was quite insistent in arguing that (1) there are no pure cases; (2) few, if any, patients would have every essential detail contained in the prototype characterization; and (3) real-world personalities would appear as variants and admixtures of the basic type. His next step was to suggest some basic subtypes or variants around the main type. Each subtype would have the essential features that define the disorder but would also have salient traits and behaviors that give a unique color or shading to this basic type. For example, although all patients with a Borderline Personality Disorder have common features, a borderline with dependent features appears quite different from a borderline with antisocial features. Millon suggested that each prototype has four or five subtypes (maybe more) and devised MCMI code types to reflect these variations.

In Chapter 1 ("The MCMI-III Facet Subscales"), Grossman and del Rio discuss the development of new content scales for the MCMI-III. The development of additional scales after a test has been published is not a new idea. The MMPI began with a basic set of validity and clinical scales but has evolved to the point where there are now more special scales for the MMPI than there are individual items (Dahlstrom, Welsh, & Dahlstrom, 1979). Gough's Adjective Check List (Gough & Heilbrun, 1983) began as a test with validity and basic need scales and has evolved to include more than a score of topical (i.e., special) scales. The same can be said for the Rorschach, 16 Personality Factor Test, and the California Psychological Inventory, Revised.

The MCMI has also seen the development of special content scales from the basic test. Retzlaff (1993) developed special scales for the MCMI-I, but his efforts were an attempt to "purify" the MCMI with psychometric and statistical applications to the MCMI item pool. In contrast, Grossman and del Rio have developed *facet subscales* to the basic MCMI-III Personality Disorder scales. These were anchored to Millon's bioevolutionary theory and began with a rational review of the test's basic scales and their structural and functional domains. Their chapter reviews the development of these facet subscales for each of the MCMI-III Personality Disorder parent scales and demonstrates their utility for personality assessment, treatment planning, and intervention.

In Chapter 2 ("Diagnosing Personality Disorder Subtypes with the MCMI-III"), Davis and Patterson begin by referencing some of the problems inherent in the assessment of personality disorders. These include the currently high comorbidity among personality disorder diagnoses based on current criteria sets, the lack of complete agreement among personality theorists as to the exact number of personality disorder diagnoses that should be referenced in official diagnostic nomenclature, and multiple theories of personality, each deriving a different set of personality construct measurements. Millon's theory, they argue, fixes the actual number of personality disorders that exist in nature, though Millon and Davis (1996), in an earlier publication, developed an initial list of possible personality disorder subtypes that may exist but that are not fixed in nature. These personality disorder subtypes are presented in Davis and Patterson's chapter, along with the interpretive logic to assess them with the MCMI-III. Finally, they discuss how Millon's theoretical model could be used, with some modification, to explain the derivation of the personality disorder subtypes themselves.

In Chapter 3 ("Alternative Interpretations for the Histrionic, Narcissistic, and Compulsive Personality Disorder Scales of the MCMI-III"), Craig marshals empirical research over the past 20 years that suggests that the MCMI Compulsive scale is measuring a compulsive style and not a Compulsive Personality Disorder, and the MCMI Histrionic and Narcissistic scales each may be measuring a style or a disorder. He offers interpretive guidelines and descriptors when the test is measuring either the style or the disorder.

In Chapter 4 ("Combined Use of the PACL and MCMI-III to Assess Normal Range Personality Styles"), Strack discusses the developmental history of both the MCMI and the Personality Adjective Checklist, a test designed to assess Millon's hypothesized personality styles in nonclinical populations using adjectives rather than questionnaire methodology. He then demonstrates how these two tests can be used in combination to refine personality assessments in nonclinical populations. Two case histories are provided as examples of this process. Strack's methodology provides the clinician with a way to use the MCMI in settings where the likelihood of the manifestation of a personality disorder is low, yet the strengths of the MCMI can be applied in a nontraditional manner.

When assessing substance abusers, clinicians have to consider issues that often are not present when assessing other populations. How much does substance abuse affect the test results? Is the resulting profile a manifestation of the person's personality, or is it a drug-induced characterization? Can we assess someone while in detoxification, or should we wait until the detoxification has been completed? How long should we wait before beginning the assessment? Testing clients early in treatment might capture their personality but could interact with withdrawal states, and testing clients later in treatment could interact with possible treatment effects. In Chapter 5 ("Issues in the Assessment of Personality Disorders and Substance Abusers with the MCMI"), Flynn highlights five key issues in assessing this population with the MCMI.

Most experts on personality agree with the experts on culture who argue that our personality tests were developed from a Eurocentric, Western frame of reference. All major (objective, self-report) personality tests have been translated into other languages, yet this, in itself, does not resolve the question of whether or not the test can be validly applied outside the culture on which the test was based. Although such understandings certainly apply to the MCMI, this test has an additional complication. Because personality disorders are not normally distributed in the general population, Millon persuasively argued that it is inappropriate to use normal scale distributions (such as T-Scores, or standard scores) with which to transform raw scores. Instead, he developed a base rate distribution and a base rate (BR) score. This distribution is based on that point in the distribution of scores where the patient has all the defining features of the disorder at the diagnostic level. BR scores are also dependent on the prevalence rate of the disorder within the standardization sample. This means that, in atypical settings, where the prevalence rate of a disorder is different from that observed in the standardization sample, the resulting BR score could be inaccurate. This is not much of a problem in the United States, but what about cross-culturally?

It is well known that culture does play a role in the manifestation of psychopathology. The *DSM-IV* Appendix B lists many culture-bound syndromes typically not found in Western culture. Most of the empirical research on psychological tests has focused on race, exploring possible differences in test scores among African Americans, Hispanics, and Caucasians, and debating whether any differences are manifestations of actual psychopathology or merely evidence of test bias against a given group. Rarely is the variable of *culture* considered apart from race, except at a theoretical level. I have not found any empirical study demonstrating that culture affects test scores.

In Chapter 6 ("International Uses of the MCMI: Does Interpretation Change?"), Rossi and Sloore, working in Belgium, look at the issue of culture and its effects on MCMI-III interpretation. (The MCMI is also in frequent use in the Scandinavian countries.) They discuss how culture can influence psychopathology and personality taxonomies. They argue that it cannot be presumed that the base rates of different syndromes and disorders are equivalent in different cultures or countries, even though U.S.-

developed personality instruments are in frequent use across Europe. In this chapter, Sloore and Rossi take up the question of whether BR scores from the MCMI-III manual are interpretively applicable in Belgium. Remember that the BR score is based, in part, on the prevalence rate of the disorder in the standardization sample. To the extent that prevalence rates of these disorders may differ, say, in Europe, this may result in diagnostic error unless the BR score itself is adjusted for those differences in prevalence rates. Using a large sample size of 524 patients, the authors compared the diagnostic efficiency of using base rates compared to receiver operating characteristics (ROC) for a Belgian sample. They compared sensitivity and specificity levels between both methodologies. They conclude that BR scores, derived from the ROC approach, performed better than BR scores based on prevalence rates. Their data are provocative, but one cannot argue with their conclusion: When using a diagnostic test, clinicians should have all possible diagnostic validity statistics available to them.

In an address to the Society for Personality Assessment, which was later published in the *Journal of Personality Assessment* (2002), Millon titled his talk (and, later, his publication) "Assessment Is Not Enough." He argued that personality-guided assessment should lead to personality-guided therapy and offered some ideas as to how this can be accomplished. These ideas were later expanded in his book on therapy (Millon, Grossman, Meagher, Millon, & Everly, 1999). In Chapter 7 ("Using the MCMI-III for Treatment Planning and to Enhance Clinical Efficacy"), Magnavita discusses the utility of the MCMI-III in a variety of practice settings (psychiatric and medical hospital practice, community mental health centers, private practice, forensic settings) and stresses the importance of accurate clinical assessment for treatment planning. He introduces the concept of *treatment packages,* an individualized, comprehensive, and holistic approach to intervention that has targeted assessments at its base. He relies on Millon's theoretical formulations as a foundation for assessment, understanding, and strategizing interventions. He provides a case example of marital dysfunction with spousal abuse to illustrate his seminal approach.

The MCMI-III can be used as a stand-alone test or as part of a psychological test battery. Many psychologists prefer to evaluate clients with a test battery because of issues that could result in convergent validity. That is, to the extent that the same psychological issues appear in more than one test, those issues are likely to be salient for a given respondent. Historically, psychologists have been trained to use a battery of both objective and projective tests in their clinical assessment. Examples of this abound in books and journals, but there have been few reports on using more than one objective test in an objective test battery. In Chapter 8 ("Use of the MCMI-III with Other Personality Inventories"), Craig uses a case example to illustrate how the MCMI can be integrated into other objective tests for further refinement.

In Chapter 9 ("Forensic Application of the MCMI-III in Light of Current Controversies"), Dyer discusses the forensic applications of the MCMI-III in the light of recent criticisms of the test. Dyer notes that most of these criticisms are based on misconceptions and presents arguments with data and case law findings to counter conclusions by a few authors who allege that use of the MCMI is problematic in forensic settings. For example, Dyer refutes the argument that the MCMI-III cannot be used in forensic assessments because it was standardized using clinical but not normal populations. He argues that these criticisms are based on flawed logic and cites persuasive counterarguments. Another criticism of the MCMI is that it uses BR scores instead of more common standardized scores such as the T-score. Dyer points out that the BR score is a kind of criterion-referencing score rather than a deviation score. Finally, he contests the argument that MCMI scales do not meet the legal standards for the admissibility of scientific evidence. He argues that there is ample evidence for the convergent validity of the MCMI scales and the manual provides a detailed summary of the test's content validity vis-à-vis *DSM-IV* criteria. Dyer's chapter provides rebuttal arguments for potential challenges on these issues in court.

Millon had earlier argued that a "deliberate or random misrepresentation on clinical inventories is much less frequent than is commonly thought . . . the role of response styles seems to be a minor factor when compared to the substantive content of [the] scales" (1987, p. 115). Yet, there are clinical settings where the context of testing can affect how a respondent answers a questionnaire. For the first time in the published literature, the research on the MCMI validity scales (termed *modifer indices*) is presented cogently and tersely by Bagby and Marshall in Chapter 10 ("Assessing Response Bias with the MCMI Modifying Indices"). They focus on the Disclosure Index, the Desirability Score, and the Debasement Index, but they also address the Validity Index (unlikely statements that, if endorsed, bring into question the validity of the respondents' answers) and the Weight Factor, designed to raise or lower BR scores on certain scales affected by high scores on these modifier scales. They summarize how well these scales work for their intended purpose. It is unfortunate that, despite the MCMI's popularity, research on the test's validity scales remains in its infancy.

The MCMI was designed as a diagnostic tool that provides an assessment of both personality disorders and major clinical syndromes. This allows the clinician to understand how basic personality affects clinical syndrome development and vice versa. In Chapter 11 ("Validity of the MCMI-III in the Description and Diagnosis of Psychopathology"), Ryder and Wetzler discuss the validity of the MCMI Personality Disorder and Clinical Syndrome scales, focusing on content, construct, structural, and diagnostic validity and profile analysis, given the state-trait controversy and the possible effects of mood, anxiety (trauma and PTSD manifestations), and psychotic disorders on the Personality Disorder scales and vice versa. They offer their conclusions on the diagnostic strengths of the various scales. They present two case histories, both patients presenting with depression, yet each having a different underlying personality structure. In their examples, the MCMI-III was able to detect these differences, which would require differential interventions.

The MCMI-III has the advantage of an ability to provide diagnoses for both Axis I and Axis II disorders. While the preponderance of research on the MCMI has been related to its use as a diagnostic instrument for personality disorders, there also has been some attention paid to the validity of the MCMI in diagnosing major clinical syndromes. In Chapter 12 ("The Diagnostic Efficiency of the MCMI-III in the Detection of Axis I Disorders"), Gibeau and Choca present original research on the accuracy of the MCMI-III to diagnose Axis I disorders under common clinical conditions. They report data from 371 clinical patients in which they compared clinician-generated diagnoses to those suggested by MCMI-III test results. They conclude that the MCMI-III has good specificity and negative predictive power, but has a range of sensitivity levels and positive predictive power. They offer their opinion as to which scales are particularly strong in this regard.

In Chapter 13 ("On the Decline of MCMI-Based Research"), Craig and Olson report on a literature search for all research articles appearing in published journals over the past 20 years. They found a statistically systematic decline, peaking in 1990 and ebbing thereafter. They offer some possible reasons for this disturbing trend that may apply to other personality tests as well. Perhaps their final comment is most prescient: "We need to improve our advocacy of well-validated instruments among those we train who will use those instruments in their career and among those who influence public policy. Only then will succeeding generations receive the full benefit from our competence."

In Chapter 14 ("Using Critiques of the MCMI to Improve MCMI Research and Interpretations"), Hsu discusses some of the major criticisms of previous versions of the MCMI (its alleged pathology bias, the psychometric problem of item overlap, the interpretation and data analysis issues and consequences of the BR score, the issue of response sets, problems in diagnostic efficiency statistics), determines whether or not these issues are applicable to the MCMI-III, and suggests future research to address remaining concerns. His chapter provides a thoughtful tool for clinicians, a kind of forewarning to forensic psychologists when testifying in court, and a road map for researchers.

Another way to consider using the MCMI-III as a diagnostic tool is to use an actuarial approach. Here, an individual case is compared to similar patients with the same diagnosis previously reported in the literature. To the extent that a patient has the same MCMI code type as similar patients with this same diagnosis, it is probable that this patient will also have that diagnosis.

In Appendix A ("Diagnoses Associated with MCMI Code Types"), Craig presents MCMI modal code types by diagnoses based on linear and also cluster analytic methodologies from various diagnostic groups that have appeared in the published literature since the test's inception. In this way, an individual clinician can look up a diagnosis and see what MCMI codes have appeared in the literature. Appendix A may be used as a reference chapter to help supplement a more empirical approach to the computer diagnosis of the MCMI.

Finally, Appendix B presents all of the published research on the MCMI from U.S. and Canadian journals.

REFERENCES

Dahlstrom, W. G., Welsh, G. S., & Dahlstrom, L. E. (1979). *An MMPI Handbook: Vol. II. Handbook of research applications.* Minneapolis, MN: University of Minnesota Press.

Gough, H. C., & Heilbrun, A. B., Jr. (1983). *The Adjective Check List manual.* Palo Alto, CA: Consulting Psychologists Press.

Millon, T. (1987). *Millon Clinical Multiaxial Inventory-II: Manual for the MCMI-II.* Minneapolis: Pearson Assessments.

Millon, T. (2002). Assessment is not enough: The SPA should participate in constructing a comprehensive clinical science of personality. *Journal of Personality Assessment, 78,* 209–218.

Millon, T., & Davis, R. (1996). *Disorders of personality: DSM-IV and beyond.* New York: Wiley.

Millon, T., Grossman, S., Meagher, S., Millon, C., & Everly, G. (1999). *Personality-guided psychotherapy.* New York: Wiley.

Retzlaff, P. D. (1993). Special scales for the MCMI: Theory, development, and utility. In R. J. Craig (Ed.), *The Millon Clinical Multiaxial Inventory: A clinical and research information synthesis* (pp. 237–252).

PART I

New Directions in MCMI Interpretation

CHAPTER 1

The MCMI-III
Facet Subscales

SETH D. GROSSMAN AND CRISTIAN DEL RIO

THE MILLON Clinical Multiaxial Inventory-III (MCMI-III) possesses multiple levels of information regarding the structure of personality that is accessible via rational and empirical means. A recent study by the first author (Grossman, 2004) examined the MCMI-III for its potential to support facet subscales intrinsically tied to Millon's (1990) evolutionary theory, the guiding framework for the development of the original instrument. Rational examination of the 14 personality scale item pools sought a reflection of the theory's specifications regarding eight functional and structural domains of personality. Each personality pattern, according to the theory, is predicted to present most saliently with two to three of the eight personologic domains; the aforementioned analysis proposes 35 facet subscales for the MCMI-III that coincide with personologic domains predicted by the theory and demonstrate sufficient internal consistency to be applied as supportive, clinical hypothesis-building subscales for the MCMI-III. This chapter examines the proposed facet subscales to be published in an upcoming MCMI-III revision and discusses implications for their utilization in personality assessment, treatment planning, and intervention.

Psychologists and other mental health professionals carry a burden never before seen in their treatment settings. Since the advent of managed care, clinicians have become overloaded with short-term patients, rapid turnover, and less clock time in which to assess and interact with a given patient. While the merits of such trends are dubious at best, it is clear that for some time to come, this unprecedented onus on practitioners will continue. Further, accountability for clinical time has moved to the forefront as a result of third-party insurers' interest in controlling health care costs. What may be useful is a methodology that affords the practitioner greater power and efficiency in assessing multiple facets of a patient's need, without a concurrent sacrifice in quality of care. In short, the need for economical clinical specificity has never been greater.

The MCMI-III's primary measurement scales may be described as multifaceted psychological constructs adhering to principles of Millon's (1990) evolutionary theory, demonstrating both construct and content validity consonant not only with the overarching theory, but with *DSM-IV-TR* (American Psychiatric Association, 2000) diagnostic categories as well. In itself, the test is quite parsimonious and pragmatic, but there are even finer distinctions that can be made that hierarchically fit under its constructs. This chapter examines the theoretical underpinnings of the proposed Grossman Facet Subscales of the MCMI-III, to be published in the upcoming revision of the instrument.

Millon and Davis (1997), in commenting on historical and future developments of the MCMI and other Millon instruments, encouraged researchers and clinicians using the MCMI-III to view the instrument as a constantly evolving entity that will continue to undergo revisions and development as the field's knowledge base expands and modifies. Further, they lament that although the instrument is, in fact, capable of discriminating subtypes (admixtures of personality styles), the current categorical approach of the *DSM* limits its ability to do this in a clean manner, often yielding a confusing array of elevated scales. It is their hope that future *DSMs* will yield a more dimensional approach congruent with the intent of Millon's evolutionary theory and that future incarnations of the MCMI will further reflect this. Congruent with their call to further explore the instrument's more molecular elements, the new facet subscales seek to reflect fundamental facets of personality that may be clinically useful.

Indeed, working on a more molecular level than the instrument's original scales (which, in most cases, are construct scales), content subscales allow test administrators to examine underlying dimensions and latent facets at a level of detail beyond the scope of the original test design. Also, content scales are developed from the original test's item pool in a post hoc manner; as a consequence, the development of content scales presents a substantial opportunity for clinical gain without detracting in any manner from the original instrument's design.

THE MCMI AND MILLON'S EVOLUTIONARY THEORY

Millon's evolutionary theory of personality was first defined as a biosocial-learning theory (Millon, 1969); it has since evolved into the more comprehensive ecological-motivational theory closely related to evolutionary biology, and it now shares parallel constructs with the physical sciences as a whole (Millon, 1990; Millon & Davis, 1996). The theory has, at its core, three polarity structures believed to be universal motivating aims shared in the animal and plant kingdoms and connected to principles found in studies of particle physics, chemistry, and cosmogony, among other natural sciences. These include a *pain—pleasure (survival)* polarity, an *active—passive (adaptation)* polarity, and a *self—other (replication)* polarity. These structures form the basis for this categorical and dimensional approach to personality assessment.

From these dimensions, a further deduction may be made into functional (F) and structural (S) domains of personality (Millon & Davis, 1996), each of which is represented in the individual personality styles or disorders. These eight dimensions are *Expressive Acts* (F), *Interpersonal Conduct* (F), *Cognitive Style* (F), *Self-Image* (S), *Object Representations* (S), *Regulatory Mechanisms* (S), *Morphologic Organization* (S), and *Mood/Temperament* (S). From here, *prototypal* constructs of the basic personality disorders are deduced (Choca, 1999), with prototypical features along these domains, although in reality, admixtures of several personality styles are likely to occur (e.g., antisocial personality with schizoid features). These *subtypes* contain an admixture of dimensional features of both prototypical constructs. From here, it is possible, after assessment, to deduce the subtype structure of the personality and address salient therapeutic concerns from a personality-oriented conceptualization of the individual (Davis, 1999; Dorr, 1999; Millon, Grossman, Meagher, Millon, & Ramnath, 2004). Items on the MCMI are derived based on the polarity scheme and expressed via the prototypical functional and structural domains.

DEFINITION OF CONTENT SCALES

Operationally, content scales are particularly challenging to define due to the lack of clear demarcation between the terms *content* and *construct.* In actual practice, these ideas overlap considerably, and their fine distinction may lack usefulness beyond basic pedagogical purposes. However, their direct comparison, at specific points, may help delineate differences that are essential to an understanding of the need for content subscales of a particular instrument.

The primary scales of any given psychological inventory are generally *construct* scales. By definition, constructs are based on a specific psychological theory (Cronbach & Meehl, 1955). Because they represent a man-made concept, they must be held to greater scientific rigor because they must demonstrate both content and construct validity. Constructs generally contain elements that may seem unrelated to each other at first glance but, according to the particular framework in question, bind together via correlation, criterion grouping, theoretical deduction, or other methodology. As such, the elements that constitute a construct scale may not be immediately apparent to nonpsychologists who are unfamiliar with the given framework from which the construct is derived. For example, the MMPI-2's scale 4, Psychopathic Deviate, contains subject matter dealing with family dysfunction, directed by an assumed concordance between strained family relations and the overarching construct of deviance. This MMPI-2 scale must demonstrate construct validity, delineating the relationship between these two subject areas. Constructs, thus, must be consonant with the framework and methodology of the scale's construction, but they do not necessarily demonstrate face validity, or the ability of the layperson to recognize these connections.

This example reveals the need for a more rudimentary breakdown in assessment. While constructs are certainly useful in generating hypotheses regarding the nature of presenting clinical phenomena in relation to what has been established in psychology and mental health, it is also necessary to gain a more elucidated, contextual picture of the patient and his or her multifaceted presentation. It is not enough, for example, for the clinician to note that an individual presents with a particular, established personality "label" and is showing signs of an Axis I condition such as clinical depression. It is much more useful to inspect the many elements of this individual's multifaceted personality style, noting the different presentation from what may be surmised based on "typical" diagnostic presentation.

Additionally, as in the previous case, it is possible that specific elements may be shared between separate theoretical constructs. Nowhere is this more evident than in the systemic, intricate area of personality and its assessment. While this polythetic quality is consonant with basic assumptions about personality (Millon, Davis, & Millon, 1997), the astute clinician must be able to make these important distinctions between disparate contents, a function that would be made more consistent with the use of content scales. In the example, family dysfunction is not an element unique to the construct measured by "psychopathic deviate" because it is certainly possible that an individual whose profile falls outside that description may acknowledge such an item. It would be safer to note this response as a member of a content scale, as represented under the subscale known as Family Discord (Harris & Lingoes, 1955, 1968).

HISTORY OF CONTENT SCALE DEVELOPMENT IN RELATED INSTRUMENTS

Content scales are rooted in a desire to make more specific and finite distinctions than are possible with an extant instrument. The most famous and historic example of this endeavor lies with the original MMPI scales (Hathaway & McKinley, 1943), designed to predict group membership. This method frustrated clinicians, who found the underlying dimensions of each scale inconsistent, and many scale elevations and profiles seen in practice remained mysterious and ill-defined (Graham, 2000). Fortunately, the large and diverse item pool inherent in that instrument served well in the development of a number of content scales, the most famous of which are those developed by Harris and Lingoes (1955, 1968). The widely used and comprehensive Harris-Lingoes subscales represent the first major effort to systematically analyze the heterogeneous content of many of the major MMPI scales. Six of the 10 standard clinical scales considered to be most heterogeneous underwent factor analysis, yielding between three and six underlying factors for each of these six scales.

The MMPI has been investigated for its factorial structure many times over the past half century. Several other content scales have achieved widespread use for this instrument, including those developed by Wiggins (1966, 1969), as well as those developed as part of the MMPI-2 restandardization project, known as the Content scales (Butcher, Graham, Williams, & Ben-Porath, 1990) and the MMPI-2 Content Component scales (Ben-Porath & Sherwood, 1993). Many supplementary scales have been developed, perhaps most notably Morey, Waugh, and Blashfield's (1985) MMPI *DSM-III* Personality Disorder scales. Other supplementary scales (e.g., the MacAndrew Alcoholism [MAC] scale; MacAndrew, 1965) tend to focus on a single construct, whereas the scales by Morey, Waugh, and Blashfield seem to capture more of the underlying content of the overall instrument.

The various MMPI content scales and subscales have demonstrated significant clinical contribution beyond the scope of the original instruments' design. In a study of the MMPI-2 content scales in an outpatient mental health environment, Barthlow, Graham, Ben-Porath, and McNulty (1999) found that many of these scales demonstrated incremental validity in predicting therapists' ratings of clients' behavior and personality characteristics, with seven scales for men and three scales for women adding to the information and interpretive power provided by the instrument's primary clinical scales. Similar results were also found in an earlier study examining incremental validity with the MMPI-2 content scales in a psychiatric sample (Archer, Aiduk, Griffin, & Elkins, 1996).

Analysis of particular content areas and specific mental health problems further reveal the clinical utility of examining personality dimensions on a more molecular level than allotted by the principal scales. Interpretation of the MMPI-2 content scales has been found particularly valuable in identifying distressing symptomatology among patients with traumatic brain injury in rehabilitation settings (Palav, Ortega, & McCaffrey, 2001) and providing significant discriminant identification of particular aspects of subjective distress in a population of chronic pain patients (Strassberg & Russell, 2000). In more traditional mental health settings, these factorially derived scales have been instrumental in identifying serious pathology and patient risk factors. Specific content scales and Harris-Lingoes subscales of the MMPI-A have been shown to predict suicide probability differentially in boys and girls to an extent beyond what is provided by the clinical scales (Kopper, Osman, Osman, & Hoffman, 1998). In the adult measure, Kopper, Osman, and Barrios (2001) found that two of the content scales, Anger (for women) and Type A (for men), contributed significantly to the predictability of suicidal behavior. In other studies, the MMPI-2 content scales, namely the Depression (DEP) and Bizarre Mentation (BIZ) scales, have contributed significantly to differential diagnosis and predictive utility beyond that afforded by the primary clinical scale 2 (Depression) in the affective and psychotic spectra. Boone (1994) noted that in a group of 62 psychiatric inpatients with diagnoses ranging from Adjustment Reaction with Depressed Mood to Schizophrenia, the DEP content scale not only correctly identified *DSM-IV* aspects of depression, but was a significant suicidal behavior predictor as well. In differentiating the often confusing realm of schizophrenic-spectrum disorders with their frequently comorbid affective features against affective-spectrum disorders with their sometimes comorbid psychoses, the two aforementioned content scales (in conjunction with the primary clinical scales) have demonstrated incremental contribution to meting out these clinical phenomena (Ben-Porath, Butcher, & Graham, 1991), a finding replicated in similar studies (e.g., Munley, Busby, & Jaynes, 1997).

FACTORIAL EXPLORATIONS OF THE
MILLON INSTRUMENTS

Several investigators have explored the factorial structure of Millon's theory and how it is measured utilizing the instruments derived from it. However, few studies have been carried out that explore subsets of factors within-scale, that is, attempts to identify the latent composition of individual personality construct scales of the MCMI-III. One study (Choca, Retzlaff, Strack, & Mouton, 1996) attempted to demonstrate the factorial structure of test items for each of the personality scales. A primary consideration for determining the number of factors was concurrence with what was theoretically expected. Five of the eight domains specified by the theory emerged in the analysis of the factors' content, with the three domains not represented in the factor structure belonging to those domains concerned with intrapsychic and psychodynamically oriented constructs. Another study (Petrocelli, Glaser, Calhoun, & Campbell, 2001) was more successful in demonstrating convergence with all eight domains of personality. This study identified the eight domains, plus one "core belief" composite, as relating directly to a cluster analysis of the instrument's scales identifying five cognitive schemas.

Although several unpublished attempts at subscales were carried out with the MCMI (Millon, 1977) and MCMI-II (Millon, 1983), there have been none whose principal focus was to uncover underlying "facets" within construct scales specifically for use as content subscales of the MCMI-III. A related undertaking was accomplished, however, by Davis (1993), who constructed content scales for the MCMI's sister inventory, the Millon Adolescent Clinical Inventory (MACI; Millon, 1993), a test derived via the same methodology as the MCMI and structured in the same manner but used with a younger, adolescent population. This instrument features personality construct scales parallel to its sister inventory, and Davis's study yielded content scales that hierarchically fit under each of the primary scales in a manner similar to the Harris-Lingoes subscales of the MMPI (Harris & Lingoes, 1955, 1968) but with more sound psychometric qualities.

SCALE CONSTRUCTION: METHODOLOGICAL TRADITIONS

One final question bears cause for exploration before commencing the current study: What is the most appropriate paradigm in which to develop content scales? Traditionally, content scales have been derived in a manner compatible with the primary personality scales of a given instrument. Burisch (1984) describes three prototypical methods historically used for personality scale construction: (1) external (criterion group), (2) inductive (internal consistency or itemic), and (3) deductive (rational, theoretical). These three methods are reviewed briefly here to help elucidate choices for the current study.

The MMPI, its revision, and its sister adolescent instrument, in large measure a result of their external criterion method of construction but not overlooking the popularity and longitudinal history of the instruments, stand as the sole outstanding examples of the need for content scales. Congruent with the external methodology of "dust bowl empiricism" (Meehl, 1945), the original MMPI items were retained solely on their ability to distinguish criterion groups from normal subjects. This was accomplished without regard to several important clinical and statistical concerns, such as internal consistency or item content.

To externalists, who consider themselves scientific realists, the world exists in categories (such as diagnoses), with groups such as narcissists, borderlines, and depressives composing the palette of human existence. The exact means by which an individual is classified, according to externalist thought, is a matter for other researchers to uncover. In this form of scale construction, a very large item pool is developed and given to a large number of diagnosed subjects and normal controls. These items need not demonstrate theoretical grounding or any other particular quality, aside from the ability to discriminate between groups. The resulting scales contain highly disparate sources of variation, a generally low Cronbach's alpha measure, and little to no insight concerning how or why an individual belongs to a category. Such questions of causality or context, in general, have been left to those subscribing to a more inductive approach (e.g., those who have developed factor or content scales for the MMPI instruments). These investigators have constructed several principal scales of their own.

Inductivists, as opposed to externalists, represent a second tradition in scientific instrumentation. Those subscribing to this paradigm believe that personality has some latent dimensional structure that is accessible primarily via statistical measures, such as factor analysis. The inductivist, like the externalist, does not approach scientific problems with any preconceived notions regarding overarching theory; for this reason, the inductive approach relies heavily on a representative sampling of the content domain. This methodology's most famous example is the Cattell, Eber, and Tatsuoka Sixteen Personality Factor Inventory (16PF; 1970). It is also represented contemporarily by the NEO-Five Factor inventories representing the five-factor model of personality (Costa & McCrae, 1992; Costa & Widiger, 1994), Goldberg's Big Five lexical model (1990) and models for personality disorders proposed by Livesley, Jackson, and Schroeder (1989) and Clark (1993).

Although the inductive approach yields the most internally consistent, statistically sound measures of personality based on ostensibly real traits, there is a real danger in that the methodology and sampling procedure may serve as a magnifying lens that distorts appearances. In other words, the results may be biased by the procedure itself. Davis and Millon (1993) present an important argument that calls into question the validity of the inductivists' claim that their methodology is a true reflection of underlying personality structure. These approaches are based in a lexical tradition, yet new constructs are introduced as latent theoretical, as opposed to surface, manifest constructs. By definition, however, the lexical approach begins with words based in the natural lexicon. This begs the question of whether the distillation of terms in the natural language can serve as the basis of a science. Such a methodology seems prone to distortion by virtue of this lexical assumption. As Davis and Millon state, inductive methods of theory building

> achieve simplicity mechanically, essentially by projecting data into some geometric space. If one is willing to go to the next step, to assume that the axes of this geometric space drive behavior, then one has only to name the axes to feel that something of fundamental importance has been discovered . . . far from selecting and discarding on some theoretical basis, the claim of [such] models rests on the representative sampling of content domains. (p. 107)

The third tradition, the deductive or rational approach, seeks to answer many of the shortcomings found in the expression of the previous two methods. In contrast with inductivists, deductivists believe that the structure of personality may be accessed most pragmatically via theoretical grounds. An inventory is prepared, which incorporates core constructs selected by the theorist in accordance with his or her theory, and items are written to represent operational definitions of those chosen constructs. After construction, the theory or inventory is statistically and psychometrically evaluated. This methodology, of the three discussed, is the one most congruent with the decisive, now historic discussion by Cronbach and Meehl (1955) regarding construct validity, in which they explicitly call for a theoretical basis for any given construct. Rather than make the often quantum leap from observation to theory (e.g., content to construct validity), as is seen with the inductive approach, the deductive theoretician begins his or her study with theory. The MCMI-III, as with all Millon instruments, is derived deductively via theoretical means. So, too, may the entire *DSM* taxonomy of personality disorders be derived, and this overlap of the objective, empirical standard of the *DSM* with the theoretically deduced instrument and taxonomy demonstrates convergent validity highly pragmatic for the purposes of achieving clinical economy and accuracy. The weakness, however, in this or any deductive approach, is simply that of theories in general. Virtually any theory is possible (if not plausible), and some are simply better than others.

DEVELOPMENT SCHEME FOR MCMI-III FACET SUBSCALES

A schema that addresses the development of content scales or, more specifically, post hoc scales for an established instrument, may illuminate the choices facing an investigator seeking to develop scales from an already fixed item pool (that is, the items composing the established instrument). Burisch's (1984) taxonomy, discussed earlier, applies primarily to original scale development wherein the item pool has not been written or the boundaries of constructs are extremely fluid; such a taxonomy, while a good guideline for overarching theoretical orientation to the development of content scales, does not fully define specific methodology for the task. A schema that is specific to post hoc scales, in addition to the obvious task of helping structure choices to be made by the scale developer, should ideally serve two additional roles: (1) It should possess some logical basis allowing it to serve as a means of categorizing sets of content scales that have already been developed. (2) It should be generative with respect to ways that content scales might be developed in the future. In constructing the MACI content scales, Davis (1993) suggested a model that serves this purpose. His schema involved two elemental choices to be made by content scale developers, each represented in a bipolar axis. The first axis involves the method of scale development—rationally initiated and statistically refined versus statistically initiated and rationally defined. The second involves the level at which the post hoc scales are designed—using the entire inventory as an item pool versus using some logical subset of the inventory's scales.

The researcher's first choice is whether to construct the candidate content scales with rational or statistical means as the initial consideration. An investigator choosing a rational route will most likely have in mind a functional need the scale will serve. The methodology here invariably fits existing items to some set of concepts. The researcher choosing a statistically initiated route will develop content scales by some multivariate technique, such as factor or cluster analysis, to identify domains of communality or clusters of items. These investigators typically believe that the statistical methodology is sufficient to have latent dimensions emerge from an existing item pool. Here, the definition of candidate content scales is left to methodological formalities rather than the researcher's theoretical orientation or utilitarian desire. Functionality is generally determined after the construction has taken place.

The second decision in this schema is whether the established inventory's entire item pool may serve as the raw material for the candidate content scales, or whether some extant logical boundary exists that may be retained in the development process. Advantages and liabilities exist with either choice, as they do with the first choice regarding methodological initiation. In a multiaxial inventory, this decision is further divided into subset decisions; that is, some items represent Axis I constructs, and others represent Axis II constructs (although some overlap is common). In this case, a first consideration is whether the focus is on classic psychiatric symptomology or personality characteristics.

In constructing the MCMI-III subscales, further questions resided in what sublevel of inquiry would be most meaningful and desirable in terms of clinical efficacy and consonance with the parent instrument. Several possible delineations existed within the theory. One possibility was Millon's (1990; Millon & Davis,1996) four distinctions between groups of personalities: the Pleasure-Deficient, the Interpersonally Imbalanced, the Intrapsychically Conflicted, and the Structurally Defective (the last representing a deeper level of pathology than the first three). Items from these scales could be pooled in an effort to seek out organizational and structural elements of personality. A second possibility was to organize an analysis to explore the three polarities (Existence, Adaptation, Replication) in an attempt to illuminate motivational patterns from the core of the theory.

The most molecular choice was the possibility of utilizing the items of each principal scale as its own separate, small item pool. At this level of analysis, the size of the pools is minimized, and the logical meaningfulness of potential content scales, by virtue of the theory that deduces these personalities, is maximized. Each set of content scales, which might aptly be termed *facet subscales*, may be taken as representations of the larger scale-level polythetic construct. A further utilitarian purpose to such a design is the ability to examine dissociations between elevations within the primary scales and their associated subscales for purposes of treatment planning. Knowing from a clinical interview that the person is likely to be diagnosed with a Histrionic Personality Disorder, for example, the clinician would be in a position to determine what *subtype,* or admixture of personality prototypes, of histrionic expression this individual may present.

PROCEDURAL CONSIDERATIONS
FOR THE CURRENT STUDY

The theoretical grounding of the original instrument, and the nature of what the researcher sought to accomplish, suggested that the most empirically sound, theoretically logical, and clinically effective framework for development of MCMI-III content scales, stated in terms of Davis's (1993) model, was to develop subscales for each prototypical personality pattern of the MCMI-III (working within logical boundaries of the extant scales) utilizing a combined rational-empirical approach, with the initial generation of the subscales grounded in the MCMI-III's guiding theory (initiating via rational means).

It was necessary, first, to identify a pragmatic level of the overarching theory on which to base predictions. One simple choice was between the evolutionary-dimension level (i.e., survival, modification, adaptation) and the functional-structural personologic-domain level (e.g., behavioral acts, intrapsychic mechanisms). However, neither of these bore much theoretical or empirical promise for facet subscales. The former represented the derivation of personality styles *across* logical domains and would have been more appropriate for an analysis that had as its goal the construction of content scales utilizing the instrument's entire item pool across constructs. The latter would attempt to extract precisely eight factors for each individual, small item pool. This would be unwieldy, at best, in terms of clinical utility and highly unlikely to be psychometrically sound, given properties of available statistical procedures. There were two other logical possibilities for this breakdown, however, that have been described by the theory.

Millon and Davis (1996) describe two logical means of organization for the presentation of the personality styles. First, the eight personologic domains may be further broken down into four logical levels, as follows:

1. *Behavioral* (subsuming Expressive Behaviors and Interpersonal Conduct)
2. *Phenomenologic* (subsuming Cognitive Style, Self-Image, and Object Representations)
3. *Intrapsychic* (subsuming Regulatory Mechanisms and Morphologic Organization)
4. *Biophysical* (subsuming Mood/Temperament)

These categories appeared highly convenient in terms of clinical use because they correspond to contemporary treatment modalities, and four similar subscales for each personality scale certainly would have proven useful. However, this represents the basic prototypal structure of each personality style on which the primary scales are based, but each prototypal pattern presents different domains in its primary presentation, while other domains may be quite subtle. The MCMI-III, then, does not equally represent all eight domains for each personality. Instead, it concentrates items as the theory predicts for prototypical presentation.

The second possibility is represented by the theory as the *salience of personologic domains*. For each personality style, Millon (1990; Millon & Davis, 1996) posits that two or three of the personologic domains will be most salient for a given prototype, one to three others will likely be of moderate (supportive) importance, and the remaining domains will be present but subtle. Which domain presents as the most salient, according to prototypal structure, varies among personality styles. For example, the prototypal histrionic is primarily identified by interpersonal conduct and mood/temperament, with expressive behavior and cognitive style features playing a secondary but important role. In contrast, the depressive prototype, whose cognitive style and mood/temperament are the most salient features, has three other domains presenting as significant but more moderate. Statistical analyses conducted within each item pool would further support these theoretical notions and would be consistent with the ultimate objective: the construction of subscales under each primary scale.

This level of the theory appeared to be the most congruent and stable starting point to guide examination of the items contained in each of the 14 item pools. The investigation began with predictions as to the most salient domains contained in each primary scale, most of which should match the most salient domains of the theory. It should be noted, however, that in some cases, secondary domains were better represented in the MCMI-III. Preliminary choices at this stage determined which and how many domains would best capture extant item content, guided by salience predictions of the overarching theory as well as rational examination of each item pool. Table 1.1 delineates the functional and structural domains of each of the prototypical personality patterns.

The next stage involved a choice of statistical methodology to support these predictions. The data pool to be used consisted of item responses from the original MCMI-III standardization sample. Subjects 600 individuals used for the development of the clinical scales and 393 individuals used for cross-validation purposes, who were administered an MCMI research form. As has been the case with most content scales or subscales in the past, the most logical choices for empirical substantiation of the subscales would be those found in factor analytic methods. However, because of the enigmatic scale construction using single items on multiple primary scales, the brevity of each item pool, and the high covariance expected due to the polythetic nature of the theory, most statistical methods would not be expected to yield highly parsimonious results (Choca, 1998).

Given the theoretical nature of the task, we might argue that a sound choice would be to employ confirmatory factor analytic (CFA) methods now available (Goldberg & Digman, 1994). However, CFA, by its nature, assumes a normal distribution of the data under consideration. The MCMI-III does not follow this assumption. Rather, its normative data are based on estimates of prevalence rates of clinical patterns known to not be normally distributed (Millon et al., 1997). Hence, as other researchers considering CFA in analyzing Millon instrumentation have noted (e.g., Derksen & Sloore, in press), CFA is inappropriate for applications involving the MCMI-III, while exploratory factor analysis (EFA) options remain viable.

Alpha method factoring was chosen for this purpose because it maximizes internal consistency of the extracted factors; it differs from principal components analysis, a more widely utilized method, in that it extracts factors specifically with this end in mind. This affords a degree of freedom to the researcher to concentrate on distal concerns, such as the rational

Table 1.1

Personality Pattern Attributes by Functional/Structural Domain

	Behavioral Acts	Interpersonal Conduct	Cognitive Style	Self-Image	Object Representation	Regulatory Mechanisms	Morphologic Organization	Mood/ Temperament
Schizoid	Impassive	Unengage	Impoverished	Complacent	Meager	Intellectualization	Undifferentiated	Apathetic
Avoidant	Fretful	Aversive	Distracted	Alienated	Vexatious	Fantasy	Fragile	Anguished
Depressive	Disconsolate	Defenseless	Pessimistic	Worthless	Forsaken	Asceticism	Depleted	Melancholic
Dependent	Incompetent	Submissive	Naive	Inept	Immature	Introjection	Inchoate	Pacific
Histrionic	Dramatic	Attention-Seeking	Flighty	Gregarious	Shallow	Dissociation	Disjointed	Fickle
Narcissistic	Haughty	Exploitive	Expansive	Admirable	Contrived	Rationalization	Spurious	Insouciant
Antisocial	Impulsive	Irresponsible	Deviant	Autonomous	Debased	Acting-out	Unruly	Callous
Sadistic	Precipitate	Abrasive	Dogmatic	Combative	Pernicious	Isolation	Eruptive	Hostile
Compulsive	Disciplined	Respectful	Constricted	Conscientious	Concealed	Reaction Formation	Compartmentalized	Solemn
Negativistic	Resentful	Contrary	Skeptical	Discontented	Vacillating	Displacement	Divergent	Irritable
Masochistic	Abstinent	Deferential	Diffident	Undeserving	Discredited	Exaggeration	Inverted	Dysphoric
Schizotypal	Eccentric	Secretive	Autistic	Estranged	Chaotic	Undoing	Fragmented	Distraught or Insentient
Borderline	Spasmodic	Paradoxical	Capricious	Uncertain	Incompatible	Regression	Split	Labile
Paranoid	Defensive	Provocative	Suspicious	Inviolable	Unalterable	Projection	Inelastic	Irascible

Source: Disorders of Personality: DSM-IV & Beyond, 2nd Ed., by Theodore Millon. Copyright 1996, Wiley. Reprinted with permission of John Wiley & Sons, Inc.

refinement of the resultant factors without as much concomitant concern with deleting items manually to maximize coefficient alphas (Davis, 1993). Additionally, an oblique rotation method was employed, allowing for correlated factors consonant with the polythetic model that undergirds the *DSM* personality disorders. Of the available choices for oblique rotations, promax rotation was the best choice, given the large size of the data set and its endorsement by previous investigators of polythetic personality attributes (e.g., Goldberg & Digman, 1994).

Owing to the first rational step, a factor analysis procedure to help substantiate theoretical predictions required some rationale for extracting the appropriate number of factors likely to differ from common approaches, such as Kaiser's (1960) stopping rule related to eigenvectors over 1 or Cattell's (1966) graphical scree test procedure. Hair, Anderson, Tatham, and Black (1992) suggest an alternative, a priori criterion, useful for researchers motivated by a predetermined theory that specifies an appropriate number of factors. This procedure was followed, using the first stage predictions as a guide for specifying factor solutions.

Following the aforementioned factor analytic stage, the emerged factors were subjected to a final rational refinement stage. Results of the factor analysis were scrutinized for their concordance with the predicted personologic domains, and adjustments were made based on content and relative factor loadings. The next stage involved calculating alphas for the proposed subscales. Given the predicted brevity of many of the subscales and the polythetic nature of personality constructs, a moderate alpha of .50 was deemed acceptable, and those scales falling under this level were discarded.

The final preparation stage, incorporation of the proposed facet subscales as a supplementary MCMI-III interpretive tool, is now in process in collaboration with the MCMI-III's primary author, Theodore Millon. This final stage involves further scrutiny of various elements of the emerged factor structure. Intercorrelations, as predicted by the polythetic model, are anticipated to be moderately high; those scales demonstrating more orthogonal qualities will be scrutinized closely for their concordance with the theory. Also, personality measures demonstrating an unacceptably high level of skewness may lack appropriate sensitivity at the higher end of the scale, where clinical distinction is most important; those scales demonstrating unacceptably high skewness will also be scrutinized. Finally, several additional facet subscales derived from the theory may be added in order to add robustness and clinical utility to the final set. When these procedures are complete, base rate scores for the final facet subscales will be calculated, and the facet subscales will be adopted for use in conjunction with the established inventory.

Table 1.2

Stages in the Development of the MCMI-III Facet Subscales

Stage 1: Identification of salient personologic domains in the MCMI-III

Examination of all personologic domains of Millon's evolutionary theory
Examination of each MCMI-III personality construct item pool
Determination of salient domains represented by MCMI-III items; tentative scale naming based on most salient domains
Determination of appropriate factor structure for each item pool

Stage 2: Factor analytic procedure

Alpha method factor analysis procedure for each personality construct item pool using a priori approach for number of factors extracted (determined by stage 1)
Promax rotation
Initial examination of resultant factors
Determination of factor-to-domain relationship

Stage 3: Rational refinement

Adjustment of individual items based on content and relative factor loading
Final review of facet subscale labels based on comparison with item content

Stage 4: Statistical substantiation

Calculation of internal consistency (alpha) coefficients for each facet subscale
Acceptance of subscales achieving a = 0.50 for final incorporation scale

Stage 5: Proposed incorporation stage (following current investigation)

Final review of subscale intercorrelations
Final review of skewness for each subscale
Calculation of base rate scores for MCMI-III facet subscales
Incorporation in MCMI-III

Table 1.2 details and summarizes all five stages of development for the MCMI-III facet subscales.

Thirty-five of the 36 personality components tested for use as personality facet subscales survived the rational/statistical procedure, with several modest modifications. One scale, originally hypothesized as a component of the MCMI-III Compulsive scale, Conscientious Self-Image, failed to meet internal consistency criteria and was tentatively excluded from the overall set pending further analysis. Also, Worthless Self-Image replaced Pessimistic Cognitive Style in the rational refinement stage of the Depressive pattern, although this change did not bring about the exclusion of items or changes in the hypothesized factor structure. It may be useful to present an overview of general trends found in these results.

The first consideration for component identification was rational examination of each of the 14 item pools for concurrence with the most salient domains of each prototypal pattern as specified by Millon's theory. For each primary scale, individual items were assessed for their congruence with the personologic domains as described for that primary personality pattern. In concert with the current study's hypothesis, most items could be identified as operationalized constructs of the two to three most salient domains for that primary personality pattern. In only a few cases, domains predicted by the theory to have more moderate salience in prototypical construction appeared to have better item representation than those predicted to be most salient. It was also typical to have several outlier items match best with secondary or even tertiary domains; these items were reviewed for their possible use as a contextual, supportive member of a better represented domain. Although definitive assignments to domains were not made at this time, this process served as the guiding influence to identify latent structure and confirm representation of predicted domains.

The second stage, factor analysis of each item pool, supported most of the initial hypotheses in terms of giving further support to item response trends from the original normative sample. Generally, the factor solutions imposed via a priori criteria from stage 1 yielded strong trends that gave credence to the theoretical predictions. In some instances, results were initially unclear, which gave partial impetus for the third planned stage, rational refinement. The facets most affected by this consideration were found in the Depressive, Narcissistic, and Paranoid subscales. Further detail will follow in the explication of each analysis.

Taking into consideration item content and relative loadings from each factor analysis, the subscales entered the third stage of development, rational refinement. Some items were reassigned to make the scales more cohesive and better aligned with the hypothesized domain. Although not all items within each resultant subscale were entirely face valid, specific wording of the item and suggestiveness in the context of the domain allowed their inclusion as part of the component being measured. It should also be noted that the eight domains specified by each of Millon's prototypal patterns are highly related to one another and that the original test was designed to reflect more than the resultant factors; at the same time, almost all of the items from each pool were used, excepting those appearing only in one discarded Compulsive subscale. This apparent inconsistency is clarified by the fact that many items, theoretically, may be suggestive of more than one facet, as measured in these analyses. This issue was predictable, based on the discovery of outlying items from stage 1. However, there was no item overlap within each of the 14 discrete item pools. Instead, items were carefully considered for use in terms of which facet they appeared to best represent. Items not meeting empirical standards but retained for rational/clinical grounds are presented in each table in italics; however, these items, as proposed for inclusion, are included in stage 3 alpha calculations.

After these final patterns were identified, internal consistency was established for the proposed subscales. Alpha coefficients were calculated for each facet; all but one scale met the minimum established criterion of .50. Overall results of the alpha criterion were impressive, given the brevity of many scales, some of which comprise only four items. For the 35 surviving scales, five scales exceeded an alpha of .80. These included Melancholic Mood/Temperament (Depressive), Inept Self-Image (Dependent), Admirable Self-Image (Narcissistic), Estranged Self-Image (Schizotypal), and Labile Mood/Temperament (Borderline). Twenty-one of the remaining scales achieved an alpha between .70 and .80, with four achieving a level of .60 to .70 and five attaining levels lower than .60. Although this last group only marginally survived, each of the facets represented was considered to be central to the parent construct and did not merit deletion based on statistical grounds alone. Overall, with a mean alpha across all accepted scales of .72, the alpha coefficients were satisfactory, especially in light of the brevity of many scales and the polythetic nature of clinical personality constructs.

It is anticipated that in the final preparatory stage, the scales will adopt base rate conversions reflective of each of the parent scales but will not retain the weighted point system. It is also anticipated, due to the MCMI-III system of shared items between primary scales, that a threshold for interpretability will be established for the facet scales. This consideration is in light of the shared items between primary scales and the small number of items on some subscales and is consistent with the tradition set by the Harris-Lingoes subscales of the MMPI (Harris & Lingoes, 1955, 1968). Although it may be useful to interpret some facet subscales without a clinically significant elevation on the corresponding primary scale, limits must be set to increase clarity and decrease the number of false positives on less relevant facets. This threshold may take the form of an assigned cut-off value on a primary scale (e.g., BR 65) or via a cutting rule (e.g., interpretability on the highest two to three primary scales only).

The proposed MCMI-III facet subscales are presented in Table 1.3.

DISCUSSION

The proposed MCMI-III Grossman Facet Subscales demonstrate a more finite breakdown of attributes contributing to the MCMI-III personality scales, in concert with the original theory that generated the primary scales. A natural question evolves from this development: How might this

Table 1.3

The MCMI-III Grossman Facet Subscales

Schizoid
1: Apathetic mood/temperament (a = .65)
2: Unengaged interpersonal conduct (a = .74)
3: Impassive expressive behavior (a = .56)

Avoidant
1: Aversive interpersonal conduct (a = .78)
2: Alienated self-image (a = .78)
3: Vexatious object representations (a = .78)

Depressive
1: Melancholic mood/temperament (a = .86)
2: Worthless self-image (a = .75)

Dependent
1: Inept self-image (a = .83)
2: Submissive interpersonal conduct (a = .72)

Histrionic
1: Gregarious self-image (a = .77)
2: Attention-seeking interpersonal conduct (a = .70)
3: Dramatic expressive behavior (a = .64)

Narcissistic
1: Admirable self-image (a = .86)
2: Expansive cognitive style (a = .52)
3: Exploitive interpersonal conduct (a = .52)

Antisocial
1: Impulsive expressive behavior (a = .71)
2: Acting-out regulatory mechanism (a = .71)

Sadistic
1: Hostile mood/temperament (a = .74)
2: Eruptive morphologic organization (a = .62)
3: Pernicious object representations (a = .55)

Compulsive
1: Constricted cognitive style (a = .73)
2: Disciplined interpersonal behavior (a = .57)

Negativistic
1: Irritable mood/temperament (a = .79)
2: Resentful expressive behavior (a = .75)

Masochistic
1: Discredited object representations (a = .76)
2: Diffident cognitive style (a = .73)
3: Undeserving self-image (a = .76)

(continued)

Table 1.3 Continued

Schizotypal
1: Estranged self-image (a = .83)
2: Disorganized cognitive style   (a = .76)

Borderline
1: Labile mood/temperament (a = .83)
2: Paradoxical interpersonal conduct   (a = .71)

Paranoid
1: Suspicious cognitive style (a = .73)
2: Defensive expressive behavior   (a = .69)

new system be incorporated into the existing MCMI-III paradigm for personality testing? This inquiry speaks directly to personality assessment. Additionally, both research tradition and demand for greater specificity and accuracy in personality testing invoke two vital questions following a demonstration of enhanced utility of an established psychometric instrument. The first is an extension of the prior inquiry and involves the explication of what is now available that was not readily accessible prior to the current research. This is suggestive of treatment planning and intervention options that may be generated via the proposed facet subscales. The other question involves what shortcomings could be inherent in this new protocol and what, in an ideal sense, could still be developed.

INCORPORATION OF FACET SUBSCALES INTO THE MCMI-III PARADIGM

Recall that in the polythetic model, personality disorders are a covariant attribute structure. As such, they are composed of facets that, taken individually, are conditions neither necessary nor sufficient for a diagnosis of the personality syndrome. Both Millon's evolutionary theory (Millon, 1990; Millon & Davis, 1996) and the *DSM-IV-TR* (American Psychiatric Association, 2000) demonstrate this concept. For example, the *DSM* specifies nine criteria for the Narcissistic Personality Disorder, but only five are required for a diagnosis. In Millon's evolutionary theory, eight domains are listed as core components of the prototypical Narcissistic personality pattern (as is the case with all prototypical patterns derived from this theory), but, as stated previously, there are very few prototypal narcissists, antisocials, avoidants, schizoids, and so on. Instead, most clinical presentations involve admixtures of personality patterns, likely involving parallel domains from other prototypes in the spectrum of personologic patterns. In other words, two people equally diagnosed according to *DSM* Axis II are almost guaranteed to differ in their clinical presentation, and this divergence is very likely to be clinically significant. Regardless of whether an assessment clinician is oriented toward one or the other or possibly both of these paradigms, simply stating that a person falls under one (or more) of the established diagnostic categories is not sufficient for real clinical utility. The real world demonstrates that divergence between the diagnosis and possession of its defining features is the norm, not the exception, and considerable heterogeneity is probable in the established diagnostic system.

The facet scales address these assessment shortcomings on several levels. The first level speaks to distinctions that are now illuminated in each primary scale, a consideration obviously consistent with the polythetic model. Two individuals diagnosed with the same Axis II syndrome are highly unlikely to present identically. Rather, they may be expected to demonstrate markedly different problematic domains within that diagnostic category. The addition of these facet scales allows for a more molecular view of the primary diagnosis, highlighting important dimensions of personologic function at a more discriminating level than can be achieved via categorical labels. In other words, clinicians may now note the most important functional and structural domains of a person's Axis II diagnosis.

Another level of consideration relates to individuals who present with problematic personality features not reaching the level of an Axis II diagnosis. Indeed, the *DSM* multiaxial system allows personality features to be noted on Axis II to allow clinicians to conceptualize how personality traits may be affecting an Axis I presentation. However, this system does not allow for specificity beyond a notation that an individual presents with "histrionic traits," "antisocial traits," and so on. The personality facet scales do not require a full elevation of a primary MCMI-III scale to hold interpretive value; rather, they will likely adhere to a cut-off rule to be established in the final incorporation stage during base rate assignment. In this capacity, the clinician may then make note of specific problematic functional and structural domains with a greater degree of specificity.

A final gain as a result of the current research goes well beyond within-category distinctions, to a level that may not be as obvious on initial examination of the facet subscales. Whether or not a clinically significant elevation occurs on one or more primary MCMI-III scales, the facet subscales will be able to detect specific elevations between primary scales. Millon's evolutionary theory predicts that most personality presentations, as mentioned previously, are not prototypical in nature. Rather, they are admixtures of two or more personality patterns that form a subtype (e.g., Narcissistic with Antisocial features, Dependent with Avoidant features). Sixty-one subtype patterns are identified in Millon's writings of the past decade or so (Millon, 1999; Millon & Davis, 1996; Millon et al., 2004); further combinations appear regularly in clinical presentation. The facet subscales utilize a level of the theory that specifies eight functional and structural domains that are consistent across all primary patterns. Therefore, it is possible that a subtype pattern may be detected by the primary scales, and specific comparable facets may be identified by the corresponding subscales. For example, it is now possible to note that an individual presents as Antisocial with Histrionic features (identified by the theory as a Risk-Taking Antisocial) via relative elevations on the primary scales, while the subscales identify problematic domains such as Impulsive Expressive Behavior (from the Antisocial facets) and Attention-Seeking Interpersonal Conduct (from the Histrionic facets). A clearer, more detailed clinical picture emerges with this greater level of specificity.

BEYOND ASSESSMENT: IMPLICATIONS FOR TREATMENT PLANNING AND INTERVENTION

In a mature science, a theory is posited that serves as the generative source for a system of classifying the phenomena found within the domain of the subject matter at hand, as well as a method for measuring and substantiating the content of the classification system. What makes such a science clinical in nature is the additional ability to manipulate and modify those phenomena (Millon, 1990). Clinical psychology, of course, is no exception to this rule; the definitive function that makes this subject domain a clinical science is the ability to intervene in a manner most consonant with beneficial change. The ultimate goal of the MCMI-III facet subscales is aligned with this basic premise.

Perhaps the most parsimonious and cohesive, albeit the most obvious, example of the subscale's utility may be found in the personologic intervention methods (i.e., Personality-Guided Therapy; Millon, Grossman, Meagher, Millon, & Everly, 2000) that are a direct outgrowth of the same guiding theory from which the subscales are generated. This paradigm is integrative in nature, recognizing the eight personologic domains employed by the subscales as key guides to appropriate therapeutic strategies. As explained earlier, each domain, viewed as a separate entity, is aligned with one of the principal schools of thought in modern psychotherapy (e.g., cognitive, psychodynamic, pharmacologic). Taken together, however, they constitute the complex, interwoven spectrum of the individual's personality, which may be viewed as the *psychic immune system*. Any given personality pattern will have certain vulnerabilities that may, given environmental and constitutional conditions, allow for problematic psychological functioning. By intervening pragmatically at the personality level (i.e., choosing strategies from the various available therapeutic modalities to match the personologic domains), while tactically orienting treatment toward balancing the *motivating aims* of evolutionary polarities (i.e., pain—pleasure, passive—active, self—other), this system of psychotherapy works to bolster the individual's personologic functioning, rather than treating the symptom alone and out of context. By aiding in identifying these problematic personologic domains, the MCMI-III facet subscales serve as a catalyst to efficient synergistic psychotherapeutic treatment planning and intervention.

Although the facet subscales are allied with but one of many theories found in the subject domain of clinical psychology, their use is in no way limited to this one paradigm. While purists and strict adherents to the various unilateral schools of psychotherapy are not likely to accept the myriad choices from competing therapeutic paradigms, there are a growing number of integrative and eclectic approaches to treatment in both traditional and short-term modalities that will benefit from the current research. For example, combinatorial cognitive and pharmacologic and cognitive-behavioral modalities (e.g., Beck, Freeman, Davis, 2004; Young, 1990) are now widely used strategies for the treatment of personality and mood disorders. Generally speaking, these models not only seek to ascertain an individual's cognitive schema (relating to subscales oriented to Cognitive Style and Self-Image), but also seek to understand and modify mood difficulties and behavioral tendencies (relating to subscales oriented to Mood/Temperament, Expressive Behavior, and Interpersonal Conduct). In these and other contemporary examples, the greater specificity afforded by the addition of personality facet subscales will enhance their aims at efficient and pragmatic intervention.

LIMITATIONS AND FUTURE DIRECTIONS

Clinical psychology in general, and personality assessment in particular, are mature but imperfect sciences. Because no current clinical methodology or assessment technology can be expected to approximate ideal conditions, research efforts in these areas are constrained to a system of probabilities. In an experimental laboratory setting, investigators may be able to limit measurement error to a minute potential, but clinical settings are, by their very nature, much less predictable. Nowhere is this more true than in the polythetic realm of personality constructs, and the subscales, further constrained by specific choices made by the authors of the established MCMI-III inventory, are no exception.

The first concern relates to the nature of personality constructs themselves. In contrast with many sister sciences now more fully investigated than any domain of psychology (e.g., biology, physics), most explored elements are well understood in terms of their composition, function, and interaction with other members of the natural world. Clinical syndromes of Axis I, being more homogeneous and readily identifiable when contrasted with personality concepts, are rapidly gaining status similar to elements of other natural sciences. Not so with personality constructs; the clinical science of personology features a core expression not found in adjacent sciences that inhibits modern investigation methods from reliably or validly capturing all aspects of personologic functioning. Millon's (1990) evolutionary theory describes this core expression as *abstraction,* a function found only in higher mammalian entities and confirmed only in human personality. A full discourse on this area of study is outside the parameters of this chapter; suffice it to say that there are data inherent in personology that are virtually unobservable that account for much of human functioning. A small sampling of this data is reasonably accessible via the most observable related phenomena: personologic dysfunction. The MCMI-III, being a theoretically derived, deductively constructed instrument, does attempt to capture the complex interrelationships and interactions that stem partially from this abstract expression, but it is limited to scientifically valid, established methodology. Indeed, this may account, in part, for obtained results that are, by and large, significantly greater than chance but fall short of currently held methodological ideals.

Directly related to the complexity inherent in personologic measurement, the MCMI-III, like the entire family of Millon instruments, utilizes methods oriented toward capturing as much personologic content as possible within a tolerable assessment framework. As noted previously, there is a complex system of item overlap that is reflective of the intricately intertwined covariance both within and between personality constructs. To adequately assess the personality variables alone without item overlap, it would be necessary to increase the personality item pool to 3 to 4 times its current size. This takes into account only the 14 personality scales; there are another 10 clinical syndrome scales that would need similar augmentation. The final "ideal" instrument could well exceed 1,000 items, a protocol virtually intolerable for any individual and highly subject to test-taking error due to subject fatigue. Instead, the instrument is reasonably brief, at 175 items, and captures a wide variety of personality content via shared items representing different meanings in different personality contexts.

As a result of these considerations, the proposed subscales are often re-markably short, sometimes containing as few as four items. Their distri-butional characteristics appear to be quite satisfactory but could be improved in some circumstances to demonstrate more discriminating power at the upper end of scoring, where finite distinctions are most needed. Furthermore, the initial intercorrelation patterns between con-structs of the same parent scale, though seemingly demonstrating good composite representation of the personality patterns, may be occasionally overwhelmingly correlated, causing doubt in the discriminating quality of one within-construct scale from another.

A major statistical concern for many users may be related to the facet scales' internal consistency characteristics. Although adequate for their intended use as supportive detail for the established primary scales, they may have been improved considerably were there more items available. However, these concerns are abated, in part, when comparing them to the Harris-Lingoes subscales, the most established and widely used MMPI subscales. It is notable that none of these well-established subscales achieves a coefficient alpha of .80. In fact, several subscales achieve only high .20s, and one (Hy5) only in the .10 to .20 range. The vast majority range from .50 to .80 (Graham, 2000). In comparison, the proposed MCMI-III facet subscales range from .51 to .86, with the majority of the scales in the .70 to .80 range. To the credit of both sets of subscales, traditional methods tend to underestimate internal consistency values, especially for short scales (Davis, Wagner, & Patty, 1994). Additional methods of internal consistency testing may be considered in subsequent research.

In terms of the available exploratory analytic options, the specific op-tion of alpha factoring combined with an oblique (promax) rotation was chosen for several reasons. First, this particular method of factor analysis was the most consistent with the polythetic nature of the constructs in-herent in the MCMI-III and, indeed, produced largely positively corre-lated results. Second, this method allowed for a means of approaching the data in the most consistent way with the task at hand (identifying a hy-pothesized number of factors in an a priori manner). Some may argue that cluster analysis, which constrains the variables to positive-only cor-relations, may have been a choice more consonant with the polythetic model. However, cluster analysis makes no assumptions that findings have relevance beyond a given data set (Goldberg & Digman, 1994); there-fore, this method lacks full usefulness for the matter at hand.

A final statistical question may be posed regarding the selection of op-timal numbers of factors per primary scale. The a priori approach utilized in the current research differed somewhat from more traditional stopping rules (e.g., eigenvalue threshold, scree plot). It is also true that using more traditional methods may have produced stronger alpha coefficients and better explanation of variance in the data, among other considerations. However, two arguments for the a priori approach eclipsed these other possibilities. First, there was validated guiding theory to initially predict the latent structure. Second, traditional methods were likely to produce some factors too short for consideration as content scales, yielding more unused items and less flexibility for the factors to be incorporated as measurement instruments. Regardless of method chosen, Goldberg and Digman (1994) note that the standard for viability lies in replicability. Future studies using different data sets should be able to yield factors similar to the ones now produced.

Although results of the current study indicate that the resultant subscales are acceptable as a supportive clinical tool, they might be most adequately used in assisting the clinician in terms of hypothesis building. As with any psychometric measure, no single instrument should stand alone, and the subscales are no exception. Fortunately, although subscales respecting logical boundaries at the personality construct level (i.e., MCMI-III primary personality scales) retain the disadvantages of their parent scale, they also inherit their advantages. As content areas reflective of the parent construct, they retain qualities such as validity and theoretical consonance and may be substantiated beyond their own internal consistency by virtue of this overarching theory and its primary personality patterns. However, they must be taken in context with the presenting clinical picture, and their measures can be sustained only insofar as the evidence external to the measure itself (inclusive of MCMI-III primary scales, other assessment data, and ongoing clinical observation) remains consistent with its findings. Although this is a caveat for all assessment inventories, given the level of specificity and its reliance on corroborating measures external to the subscales themselves, it is most true for factorially generated content subscales.

REFERENCES

American Psychiatric Association. (2000). *Diagnostic and Statistical Manual of Mental Disorders—4th Edition, Text Revision (DSM-IV-TR)*. Washington, DC: Author.

Archer, R. P., Aiduk, R., Griffin, R., & Elkins, D. E. (1996). Incremental validity of the MMPI-2 Content Scales in a psychiatric sample. *Assessment, 3,* 79–90.

Barthlow, D. L., Graham, J. R., Ben-Porath, Y. S., & McNulty, J. L. (1999). Incremental validity of the MMPI-2 Content Scales in an outpatient mental heath setting. *Psychological Assessment, 11,* 39–47.

Beck, A. T., Freeman, A., & Davis, D. D. (2004). *Cognitive therapy of personality disorders* (2nd ed.). New York: Guilford Press.

Ben-Porath, Y. S., Butcher, J. N., & Graham, J. R. (1991). Contribution of the MMPI-2 Content Scales to the differential diagnosis of schizophrenia and major depression. *Psychological Assessment, 3,* 634–640.

Ben-Porath, Y. S., & Sherwood, N. E. (1993). *The MMPI-2 Content Component Scales: Development, psychometric characteristics, and clinical application.* Minneapolis, MN: University of Minnesota Press.

Boone, D. E. (1994). Validity of the MMPI-2 Depression content scale with psychiatric inpatients. *Psychological Reports, 74,* 159–162.

Burisch, M. (1984). Approaches to personality inventory construction. *American Psychologist, 39,* 214–227.

Butcher, J. N., Graham, J. R., Williams, C. L., & Ben-Porath, Y. S. (1990). *Development and use of the MMPI-2 content scales.* Minneapolis: University of Minnesota Press.

Cattell, R. B. (1966). The meaning and strategic use of factor analysis. In R. B. Cattell (Ed.), *Handbook of multivariate experimental psychology* (pp. 174–243). Chicago: Rand McNally.

Cattell, R. B., Eber, H. W., & Tatsuoka, M. M. (1970). *Handbook for the Sixteen Personality Factor Questionnaire (16PF).* Champaign, IL: Institute for Personality and Ability Testing.

Choca, J. (1998). Review of the Millon Index of Personality Styles. In J. C. Impara & B. S. Plake (Eds.), *The thirteenth mental measurements yearbook.* Lincoln, NE: Buros Institute of Mental Measurements.

Choca, J. P. (1999). Evolution of Millon's personality prototypes. *Journal of Personality Assessment, 72,* 353–365.

Choca, J., Retzlaff, P., Strack, S., & Mouton, A. (1996). Factorial elements in Millon's personality theory. *Journal of Personality Disorders, 10,* 377–383.

Clark, L. A. (1993). *Schedule for Nonadaptive and Adaptive Personality (SNAP) manual.* Minneapolis, MN: University of Minnesota Press.

Costa, P. T., & McCrae, R. R. (1992). *Revised NEO Personality Inventory (NEO-PI-R) and NEO Five Factor Inventory (NEO-FFI) professional manual.* Odessa, FL: Psychological Assessment Resources.

Costa, P. T., & Widiger, T. A. (Eds.). (1994). *Personality disorders and the five-factor model of personality.* Washington, DC: American Psychological Association.

Cronbach, L. J., & Meehl, P. E. (1955). Construct validity in psychological tests. *Psychological Bulletin, 52,* 281–302.

Davis, R. D. (1993). *Development of content scales for the Millon Adolescent Clinical Inventory.* Unpublished masters thesis, University of Miami, Coral Gables, FL.

Davis, R. D. (1999). Millon: Essentials of his science, theory, classification, assessment, and therapy. *Journal of Personality Assessment, 72,* 330–353.

Davis, R. D., & Millon, T. (1993). The five-factor model for personality disorders: Apt or misguided? *Psychological Inquiry, 4,* 104–109.

Davis, R. D., Wagner, E. E., & Patty, C. C. (1994). Maximized split-half reliabilities for Harris-Lingoes subscales: A follow-up with larger Ns. *Perceptual and Motor Skills, 78,* 881–882.

Derksen, J., & Sloore, H. (in press). Issues in the international use of psychological tests. In S. Strack (Ed.), *Handbook of personology and psychopathology: Essays in honor of Theodore Millon*. New York: Wiley.

Dorr, D. (1999). Approaching psychotherapy of the personality disorders from the Millon perspective. *Journal of Personality Assessment, 72,* 407–426.

Goldberg, L. R. (1990). An alternative "description of personality": The Big-Five factor structure. *Journal of Personality and Social Psychology, 59,* 1216–1229.

Goldberg, L. R., & Digman, J. M. (1994). Revealing structure in the data: Principles of exploratory factor analysis. In S. Strack (Ed.), *Differentiating normal and abnormal personality* (pp. 216–242). New York: Springer.

Graham, J. R. (2000). *MMPI-2: Assessing personality and psychopathology* (3rd ed.). New York: Oxford University Press.

Grossman, S. D. (2004). *Facets of personality: A proposal for the development of MCMI-III content scales.* Unpublished doctoral dissertation, Carlos Albizu University, Miami, FL.

Hair, J. F., Anderson, R. E., Tatham, R. L., & Black, W. C. (1992). *Multivariate data analysis with readings* (3rd ed.). New York: Macmillan.

Harris, R., & Lingoes, J. (1955). *Subscales for the Minnesota Multiphasic Personality Inventory.* (Mimeographed materials). The Langley Porter Clinic, San Francisco, CA.

Harris, R., & Lingoes, J. (1968). *Subscales for the Minnesota Multiphasic Personality Inventory.* (Mimeographed materials). The Langley Porter Clinic, San Francisco, CA.

Hathaway, S. R., & McKinley, J. C. (1943). *Minnesota Multiphasic Personality Inventory (MMPI).* Minneapolis: University of Minnesota Press.

Kaiser, H. F. (1960). The application of electronic computers to factor analysis. *Educational and Psychological Measurement, 20,* 141–151.

Kopper, B. A., Osman, A., & Barrios, F. X. (2001). Assessment of suicidal ideation in young men and women: The incremental validity of the MMPI-2 content scales. *Death Studies, 25,* 593–607.

Kopper, B. A., Osman, A., Osman, J. R., & Hoffman, J. (1998). Clinical utility of the MMPI-A content scales and Harris-Lingoes subscales in the assessment of suicidal risk factors in psychiatric adolescents. *Journal of Clinical Psychology, 54,* 191–200.

Livesley, W. J., Jackson, D. N., & Schroeder, M. L. (1989). A study of the factorial structure of personality pathology. *Journal of Personality Disorders, 3,* 292–306.

MacAndrew, C. (1965). The differentiation of male alcoholic out-patients from nonalcoholic psychiatric patients by means of the MMPI. *Quarterly Journal of Studies on Alcohol, 26,* 238–246.

Meehl, P. E. (1945). The dynamics of "structured" personality tests. *Journal of Clinical Psychology, 1,* 296–303.

Millon, T. (1969). *Modern psychopathology: A biosocial approach to maladaptive learning and functioning.* Philadelphia: Saunders.

Millon, T. (1977). *Millon Clinical Multiaxial Inventory (MCMI) Manual.* Minneapolis, MN: National Computer Systems.

Millon, T. (1983). *Millon Clinical Multiaxial Inventory-II (MCMI-II) Manual.* Minneapolis, MN: National Computer Systems.

Millon, T. (1990). *Toward a new personology: An evolutionary model.* New York: Wiley.

Millon, T. (1993). *Millon Adolescent Clinical Inventory (MACI) manual.* Minneapolis, MN: National Computer Systems.

Millon, T. (1999). Reflections on psychosynergy: A model for integrating science, theory, classification, assessment, and therapy. *Journal of Personality Assessment, 72,* 437–457.

Millon, T., & Davis, R. D. (1996). *Disorders of personality:* DSM-IV *and beyond.* New York: Wiley.

Millon, T., & Davis, R. D. (1997). The MCMI-III: Present and future directions. *Journal of Personality Assessment, 68,* 69–85.

Millon, T., Grossman, S., Meagher, S., Millon, C., & Everly, G. (2000). *Personality-guided therapy.* New York: Wiley.

Millon, T., Grossman, S., Meagher, S., Millon, C., & Ramnath, R. (2004). *Personality disorders in modern life* (2nd ed.). New York: Wiley.

Millon, T., Millon, C., & Davis, R. (1997). *Millon Clinical Multiaxial Inventory-III (MCMI-III) manual* (2nd ed.). Minneapolis, MN: Pearson Assessments.

Morey, L. C., Waugh, M. H., & Blashfield, R. K. (1985). MMPI scales for *DSM-III* personality disorders: Their derivation and correlates. *Journal of Personality Assessment, 49,* 245–256.

Munley, P. H., Busby, R. M., & Jaynes, G. (1997). MMPI-2 findings in schizophrenia and depression. *Psychological Assessment, 9,* 508–511.

Palav, A., Ortega, A., & McCaffrey, R. J. (2001). Incremental validity of the MMPI-2 content scales: A preliminary study with brain-injured patients. *Journal of Head Trauma Rehabilitation, 16,* 275–283.

Petrocelli, J. V., Glaser, B. A., Calhoun, G. B., & Campbell, L. F. (2001). Early maladaptive schemas of personality disorder subtypes. *Journal of Personality Disorders, 15,* 546–559.

Strassberg, D. S., & Russell, S. W. (2000). MMPI-2 content scale validity within a sample of chronic pain patients. *Journal of Psychopathology and Behavioral Assessment, 22,* 47–60.

Wiggins, J. S. (1966). Substantive dimensions of self-report in the MMPI item pool. *Psychological Monographs, 80* (22 Whole No. 630).

Wiggins, J. S. (1969). Content dimensions in the MMPI. In J. N. Butcher (Ed.), *MMPI: Research developments and clinical applications* (pp. 127–180). New York: McGraw-Hill.

Young, J. E. (1990). *Cognitive therapy for personality disorders: A schema-focused approach.* Sarasota, FL: Professional Resource Exchange.

CHAPTER 2

Diagnosing Personality Disorder Subtypes with the MCMI-III™

Roger D. Davis and Michael J. Patterson

PROBABLY THE goal of every psychodiagnostician is to be as specific as possible, while also being accurate. Rather than simply conclude that the patient is depressed or anxious, we ask "What kind of depression is it?" or "What kind of anxiety is it?" Framing the issue in this way naturally leads to hierarchical models of diagnostic classification and seems well-suited to solving problems in psychiatric diagnosis. Indeed, the means by which human beings classify the world seems naturally hierarchical, with general categories composed of more specific categories, composed of still more specific categories. We might even speculate that as knowledge about a subject domain advances, the language of common sense gives way to technical jargon (Hempel, 1965), which then becomes ever more refined and hierarchical. In general, as professional terminology evolves, categories seem to become ever more narrow as students of the field repeatedly ask, "What kind is it?" Ultimately, whole tiers of generality arise, and in the final result, both "splitters" and "lumpers" may ultimately find their place in the taxonomic scheme. This is largely the history of the *DSMs* (American Psychiatric Association, 1980, 1987, 1994), and given their success and widespread acceptance, we should naturally want to extend the same ideal to the personality disorders.

But there are problems (e.g., Livesley, Schroeder, Jackson, & Jang, 1994). First, numerous studies point to high comorbidity of the personality disorder diagnoses (Westen & Muderrisoglu, 2003). Certainly there's nothing wrong with a degree of comorbidity: Expectations that every patient receive one and only one diagnosis are too reductionistic to be clinically useful. But how much comorbidity is enough, and how would we validate a taxonomic scheme so that the amount of comorbidity is "just right"?

The first problem dovetails with the second: The members of the *DSM* committees do not agree among themselves just exactly what personality disorders exist (e.g., Spitzer, Feister, Gay, & Pfohl, 1991). Thus, the Sadistic and Masochistic (i.e., Self-Defeating personality; Kass, Spitzer, Williams, & Widiger, 1989) constructs listed in the *DSM-III-R* do not appear in *DSM-IV* or *DSM-IV-TR*. Presumably, their constituent characteristics have been portioned out to various other constructs. Sadistic traits could be ascribed to Antisocial, Paranoid, Negativistic, Narcissistic, Borderline, Compulsive, Histrionic, and perhaps even some Avoidant personalities. Are these individuals for whom sadistic behaviors represent a secondary theme, or might there also exist persons for whom sadistic forms of relating represent their "core nature," being interwoven into the fabric not only of their interpersonal behavior, but also their defensive structure, fantasies, and social cognition (Fromm, 1973; Millon & Davis, 1996)? Are there individuals for whom the potential to inflict abuse, largely with impunity, is the primary metric of their own self-worth? Perhaps the answer depends on local base rates: Sadistic personalities can be expected to flourish in substance abuse and forensic settings (Spitzer et al., 1991). Work in such a setting, observe such individuals every day, and you'll probably favor that they be broken out into their own diagnostic category. What other disorders might flourish in other settings? Taxonomic issues with the Sadistic personality are, of course, only one example. Many examples could be given, including studies generally supporting the addition of the Depressive personality to *DSM-IV* (e.g., McDermut, Zimmerman, & Chelminski, 2003).

Third, there are a variety of theories of personality disorders, and they derive different higher-order personality constructs. That is, while Millon regards a certain set of personality constructs to be fundamental because they are derived from a theoretical framework (e.g., Millon, 1969, 1981, 1990), there are other theoretical frameworks that derive other sets of constructs (e.g., Cloninger, 1986, 1987) or develop dimensions of personality using other organizing principles. Some of these approach personality from a particular perspective, such as psychoanalytic (Kernberg, 1984, 1996; Lenzenweger, Clarkin, Kernberg, & Foelsch, 2001), interpersonal (e.g., Benjamin, 1974, 1986, 1993; Kiesler, 1982; Pincus, 1994), or cognitive (e.g., Beck & Freeman, 1990), and others are more methodologically driven (Clark, 1990, 1993; Clark & Watson, 1990; Livesley, Jackson, & Schroeder, 1989; Livesley & Jang, 2000). Of the latter, some advocate supplementing (Costa & McCrae, 1992; Widiger & Costa, 2002) or even abandoning the Axis II constructs completely (McCrae et al., 2001) in favor of

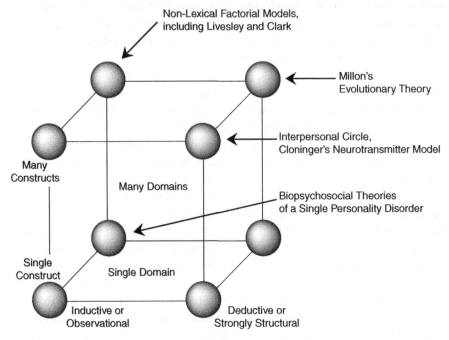

Figure 2.1
A three-dimensional framework organizing
various approaches to personality.

factor analytic models that at least appear to have impressive content validity (Reynolds & Clark, 2001) due to their foundation in the lexical approach (Allport & Odbert, 1936), which draws personality trait terms
from the common language. Davis and Millon (1999) argued that various
approaches to personality pathology could be organized into a three-
dimensional framework, depending on (1) whether they attempt to describe one personality construct versus many personality constructs, (2)
whether they are primarily inductive or methodological versus theoretical, and (3) whether they are concerned with a single content domain of
personality versus many domains (see Figure 2.1). Although there are
many inductive-factor models and many theoretical-domain models, according to these authors, Millon's (1990) evolutionary theory is unique in
being the only standing example that is simultaneously theoretical yet focused on integrating content across all major perspectives on personality,
while also describing an interrelated and differentiated schema of personality constructs. This point cannot be overemphasized.

Where do the personality disorder subtypes fit in this discussion? At
some point, it would be nice if theory and treatment in clinical psychology

had the same kind of close coupling that physical principles and equations have in physics and engineering. Otherwise, psychologists are merely doing what works (or worse, what doesn't work) without understanding exactly why, even though we may well have strong intuitions of why, and thus may in fact choose the best therapeutic course much of the time (Albeniz & Holmes, 1996). In general, eclectic psychotherapy may be seen as an attempt to adapt psychotherapy to a world in which human nature is far too complex to be completely modeled by a single theory (Millon, Everly, & Davis, 1993). Probably no one knows with certainty to what extent the subtypes might advance taxonomic and therapeutic understanding, even though—given the evolution of psychiatric nosology—subtypes are probably inevitable by about *DSM-VI* or *DSM-VII.* Their existence at least tells us that personality is inherently complex, with different kinds of narcissists, different kinds of avoidants, and so on. As such, the subtypes provide a rich set of clinical reference points by which different patients can be understood. A descriptively rich classification system is to be preferred over one that is descriptively impoverished, though it is certainly true that as a diagnostic system grows more complex, judgment and experience become more important as a precondition for effective clinical work, particularly where the decision rules (e.g., number of diagnostic criteria necessary to achieve threshold, level of elevation necessary before one personality diagnosis obviates other comorbid diagnoses) are difficult to explicate concretely, even for so-called experts.

In this chapter, we try to figure out how to make it work with the MCMI-III. As there is almost no published empirical research devoted specifically to diagnosing personality disorder subtypes with the MCMI-III, we tend to eschew hard and fast decision rules and instead give preference to general diagnostic principles. Because there is, as yet, no real substantive research in this area, we treat every aspect of the Millon system, from theory to taxonomy to instrumentation to intervention, as raw material that might be molded toward the goal of greater understanding of the construct of personality subtype and the specific content of the subtypes themselves. Because some have argued that the MCMI-III validity indices possess limited usefulness (see Charter & Lopez, 2002; Schoenberg, Dorr, & Morgan, 2003), we assume the existence of a valid profile to simplify our task.

ASSESSING SUBTYPES IN CLINICAL PRACTICE

Where do personality subtypes come from? The history of every science may be said to include a prescientific, natural history phase, where the main questions are What are the essential phenomena of the field? and

How can we know them? (Hempel, 1965; Kuhn, 1970; Pepper, 1942). Ideally, as more and more data are gathered through increasingly sophisticated methodologies, common sense gives way to theoretical accounts that not only integrate and unify disparate observations, but also actively suggest directions for future research. Every scientific model naturally rejects the incidental characteristics of its subject domain, exposing for intellectual consumption only those aspects deemed most relevant. In formulating such models, we naturally tend to retain the objective and reproducible, while rejecting that which is contingent and temporal. Indeed, probably the most beautiful, and most ambitious, aspect of the evolutionary model is that it attempts to tell us why this particular constellation of 14 personality disorders constructs exists, rather than some other set of constructs. The theory provides the promissory note that ensures that we are not at the mercy of some remote committee whose political ambitions and ultimate decisions might be susceptible to extrascientific influences. Rather than memorize an official list of uncertain length, we *know* that the constellation of disorders given to us by the theory will *never* change. Certainly their base rates may change, or the sensitivity of clinicians to certain constructs may change, but the theory nevertheless provides us with a final set of personality constructs that glues taxonomy and treatment firmly together.

In *Disorders of Personality: DSM-IV and Beyond,* Millon and Davis (1996) describe a variety of personality disorder subtypes. At this point, however, it is important to understand that the major constructs derived from the theoretical model and the personality disorder subtypes are on a different ontological footing. Whereas the theory is explicitly designed to provide the last word on personality taxonomy, the subtypes are not. Although a few subtypes do represent pure expressions, for the most part, there is no single narcissist, no single avoidant, and so on; instead, each disorder "contains" numerous variegated descendants. Some of these have their foundation mainly in the theoretical model and exist as amalgrams of the basic constructs. Others represent the confluence of the evolutionary model with various perspectives on personality, or "part functions" (Millon, 1990). The compensatory narcissist, for example, is primarily a psychoanalytically based formulation. Such persons build up a superior self-image as a defense against lasting wounds to self-esteem suffered during early development (Millon & Davis, 1996). Because these wounds are covered over by illusions of grandiosity, the individual is hypersensitive to slights and tends to interpret objectively neutral comments as criticism.

There is no necessary reason the compensatory narcissist should exist, however, and if such individuals were never to have existed at all, there would be no psychologists left gaping in astonishment, wondering why theory predicts the existence of a psychological phenomenon that can't be found, the way a particle physicist might be gaping in astonishment if a particular muon or quark did not exist even though theory predicts it should. Accordingly, the subtypes should be viewed as existing with one foot firmly grounded in the evolutionary model, and one foot loosely grounded in historical contingency, meaning that they must be understood inductively: We literally go to the world and ask, "What does the world have in it," and then develop generalizations based on a presumably thorough and rigorous review. In this way, the subtypes may be seen as a bridge from the "abstract and eternal realm of theoretical necessary," which is the evolutionary model, and the particular, transient, and temporal "realm of historical accident and contingency," which constitutes the individual human life. For better or worse, psychology exists at a level of organization that places it firmly between art and science, and its construct systems possess a literary or hermaneutic element that can be minimized but that cannot (and perhaps should not) be entirely eliminated.

What is the importance of contrasting the ontological status of the personality subtypes with that of the major constructs? First, there may be additional subtypes beyond those listed by Millon and Davis (1996) that have not been described. In fact, there could well be dozens of such subtypes because there are no real theoretical stopping rules that prevent their existence. We might further speculate that these subtypes are likely to flourish in settings where the base rates of the major constructs are substantially different from those on which the MCMI-III was normed, though there is, of course, no research that proves that this is the case. Whereas adding to the major personality types is largely impossible, the existence of personality subtypes provides an open invitation for researchers in the field to develop and publish richly detailed clinical descriptions that could take hold, or not, with clinicians elsewhere. Second, it is important to recognize that the personality subtypes given by Millon and Davis were not operationalized in terms of the eight domains of personality discussed by Millon (1990). Thus, the subtypes cannot be said to possess the descriptive precision of the major personality constructs. Doing so would involve writing up the subtypes with an eye toward their convergent and discriminant characteristics, ultimately producing a book-length manuscript.

Table 2.1 gives a complete list of the personality disorder subtypes and their expected MCMI code types (Millon & Davis, 1996). Table 2.2 on page 39 provides a brief summary of the psychometrics of the MCMI-III personality disorder scales. Ideally, application of the code types in a clinical setting would be straightforward: Determine the MCMI code type, look up the associated personality description in *Disorders of Personality*

Table 2.1
Personality Disorders, Their Subtypes, and Their
Associated MCMI-III 2-Point and 3-Point Profiles

Schizoid	Avoidant	Dependent	Depressive
Affectless 1-7	Hypersensitive 2A-P	Immature Pure 3	Restive 2B-2A
Remote 1-2A/S	Self-Deserting 2A-2B	Ineffectual 3-1	Self-Derogating 2B-3
Languid 1-2B	Phobic 2A-3	Disquieted 3-2A	Voguish 2B-4/5
Depersonalized 1-s	Conflicted 2A-8A	Accommodating 3-4	Ill-Humored 2B-8A
		Selfless 3-8A	Morbid 2B-8B
		Depressive	

Histrionic	Narcissistic	Antisocial	Sadistic
Theatrical Pure 4	Elitist Pure 5	Covetous 6A	Explosive Pure 6B
Appeasing 4-3	Amorous 5-4	Nomadic 6A-1/2A	Spineless 6B-2A
Vivacious 4-5	Unprincipled 5-6A	Risk-Taking 6A-4	Enforcing 6B-7
Disingenuous 4-6A	Compensatory 5-8A/2A	Reputation-Defending 6A-5	Tyrannical 6B-8A/P
Tempestuous 4-8A		Malevolent 6A-6B/P	
Infantile 4-C			

Compulsive	Negativistic	Masochistic
Conscientious Pure 7	Circuitous 8A-3	Self-Undoing 8B-3
Parsimonious 7-1	Vacillating 8A-C	Oppressed 8B-2B
Bureaucratic 7-5	Discontented 8A-2B	Virtuous 8B-4
Bedeviled 7-8A	Abrasive 8A-6B	Possessive 8B-8A
Puritanical 7-P		

Schizotypal	Borderline	Paranoid
Insipid S-1/2B/3	Discouraged C-2A/2B/3	Insular P-2A
Timorous S-2A/8A	Self-Destructive C-2B/8B	Malignant P-6B
	Impulsive C-4/6A	Obdurate P-7
	Petulant C-8A	Querulous P-8A
		Fanatic P-5

(Millon & Davis, 1996), and adapt the description as necessary for the clinical report, integrating and supplementing it with additional data and descriptors derived from all sources of information, including other objective and projective tests, the clinical interview, developmental data, and testimony from other sources. Obviously, the integration of all available information is potentially ambiguous and highly dependent on clinical judgment. Applying the code type, however, is just a matter of scoring

Table 2.2

Diagnostic Efficiency of the Axis II Scales for Three Versions of the MCMI

	Items	Alpha	Test-Retest	SENS	PPP
SCH	16	0.81	0.89	68	72
AVD	16	0.89	0.89	62	63
DPR	15	0.89	0.93	75	61
DEP	16	0.85	0.89	56	78
HST	17	0.81	0.91	75	79
NAR	24	0.67	0.89	72	77
ANT	17	0.77	0.93	81	76
SAD	20	0.79	0.88	74	81
CMP	17	0.66	0.92	74	76
NEG	16	0.83	0.89	59	67
MAS	15	0.87	0.91	85	73
SZT	16	0.85	0.87	73	67
BRD	16	0.85	0.93	79	81
PAR	17	0.84	0.85	89	65

SENS is sensitivity, PPP is positive predictive power. Test-retest intervals are from 5 to 14 days.

the MCMI-III correctly and consulting the appropriate description, amplifying this aspect of the narrative and attenuating that one, as the clinical evidence suggests. If only it were so easy.

RELIABILITY AND VALIDITY AT A SCALE LEVEL

As the old saying goes, the devil is in the details. Recall that the goal of any classification system is to be highly specific and highly accurate at the same time. In practice, this is difficult to achieve. Cronbach and Gleser (1965) referred to this as bandwidth versus fidelity: Statements that are accurate also tend to be highly general, whereas statements that are very precise also tend to be very specific, to lack adequate scope. In a seminal article about the "slow progress of soft psychology," Meehl (1978) provided a list of problems for clinical assessment and the field generally, none of which has ever been adequately addressed, much less solved. In another seminal paper, on the influence of method variance, Campbell and Fiske (1959) described reliability and validity as existing on a continuum. Self-report measures tend to correlate with each other more highly than do self-report measures and clinical rating scales simply because self-report measures share similar information biases. In fact, correlations between self-reports and clinical rating scales are quite often pathetic. The personality disorders literature is sprinkled with such findings. Kennedy et al.

(1995) found correlations generally around .40 between the SCID-II scales and those of the MCMI-II in eating disorder patients. Because shared variance is the square of the correlation coefficient, the respective scales share about 16% of their variance. Blackburn, Donnelly, Logan, and Renwick (2004) examined the convergent and discriminant validity of interview and self-report measures in an offender sample using the MCMI-II. Among other findings, these authors report that the Avoidant, Schizoid, and Schizotypal disorders were not clearly distinguishable and that error variance was substantial across instruments and disorders. In general, because the social cognition of Axis II patients is by definition disordered (e.g., Dreessen, Arntz, Hendriks, Keune, & van den Hout, 1999; Waldeck & Miller, 2000), some will interpret test items in unusual ways and produce unusual profiles. Others complete the instrument with a hidden, but not necessarily conscious, agenda. Some will become more introspective and aware, simply as a result of administration (Blount, Evans, Birch, Warren, & Norton, 2002). In an ideal world, clinical ratings would correlate perfectly with self-report, no presentational biases would exist, and there would be a deterministic relationship between personality profile patterns and the clinical report, a formula that could be applied to yield a narrative of perfect accuracy. Unfortunately, this will never exist.

Nevertheless, we can still ensure that our instruments do as well as possible within the constraints of the diagnostic process. First, does our instrument have an adequate level of reliability and validity? Interpreting the numbers in Table 2.2 requires some background in psychometrics, because higher is not necessarily better. Higher alphas are generally desired, but beyond a certain level, a high alpha could indicate that most of the items on a particular scale are simply rephrasings of other items. Ask a set of very similar questions, and you're likely to get a set of very similar answers, thus raising the aggregate intercorrelation of the items. Content validity could become an issue, as personality disorders can be viewed as highly, but not perfectly, correlated sets of personality traits. Moreover, false items tend to raise alpha, and some of the MCMI-III scales have numerous falsely keyed items, particularly the Compulsive personality (see Rossi, Van den Brande, Tobac, Sloore, & Hauben, 2003). Based on past experience more than anything else, most test authors probably regard alphas of .70 as acceptable, .80 as desirable, and .90 as pushing the envelope. Ten of 14 MCMI-III scales fall into the desirable range. Two more are acceptable but nearly desirable, and two fall below .70 (the Narcissistic and Compulsive personalities).

The test-retest reliabilities also look good: All are .85 or better at intervals of 5 days to 2 weeks. Unlike Cronbach's alpha, which can indeed be too high where the construct measured is assumed to have some intrinsic heterogeneity, better test-retest numbers are always better when it comes to the measurement of personality disorder constructs, because personality, by definition, is assumed to be stable across time and situations (the notable exception here being retesting conducted at intervals during or after psychotherapy, for which a decline of scores indicates a successful therapeutic course). The values for the MCMI-III are all .85 or better, which is excellent.

What these numbers don't tell us, however, is the extent to which various code types repeat and the extent to which they do not repeat. The problem is that high internal consistencies and high test-retest reliabilities should, but don't necessarily, indicate profile stability. Profile patterns and correlations are fundamentally different. Test-retest correlations are based on the relative movement of scores across time, not on the absolute level of the scores. Thus, in a sample receiving psychotherapy, all scores might move from greater than BR 100 before therapy to below BR 75 after therapy for all members of the sample. But, if the rank order of the scores is the same at both time points, the correlation remains high.

Moreover, even where test-retest correlations are high, the scales on the MCMI-III are short enough that the difference of several points can make the difference between BR 75 and BR 85. On the positive side, however, personality items on the MCMI-III use a weighting scheme in which the prototypical items, which are viewed as being core to their respective constructs, receive a weight of 2 points, whereas items more peripheral to the construct receive a weight of 1 point. Item overlap may increase profile stability. In general, we would expect the pattern of item overlap to mirror the way the personality constructs are derived from the polarity model. Thus, we would expect the Antisocial and Narcissistic personality scales to share numerous items. Although this is not always the case, the point is that we can expect the repeatability of personality profiles to be higher than what the alpha and test-retest reliabilities might indicate simply because overlapping scales share both common variance predicted by the theory and error variance intrinsic to each shared item. We thus arrive at the following conclusion: Although there is no strong empirical evidence to support the repeatability of code type patterns, there is also no reason to believe that the code type patterns lack enough repeatability to be clinically useful.

VALIDITY OF CODE TYPE PATTERNS

Because this chapter is concerned with personality subtypes, and because these subtypes are operationalized mainly as code type patterns, we might ask about the validity of various code types. Because the validity of any particular code type is dependent on the validity of its constituent scales, it definitely pays to know the strengths and weaknesses of the inventory. In other words, every strength and weakness of the MCMI-III is also a strength and weakness when assessing personality disorder subtypes. We can evaluate the potential for code type validity by looking at the sensitivity and positive predictive power of the MCMI-III scales. The numbers presented in Table 2.2 were derived from a study (Davis & Wenger, 1997) involving individuals who were both knowledgeable about the theory and knowledgeable about the test. The numbers compare favorably to the MCMI-I and MCMI-II and represent an incremental improvement in validity achieved from the two previous generations of research (see Hsu, 2002, for comments on diagnostic validity studies of various generations of the MCMI). Against this historical backdrop, the diagnostic efficiency statistics achieved by the MCMI-III are quite remarkable. What clinical pearls can be gleaned from Table 2.2? Using clinical judgment as the gold standard, the MCMI-III is not an especially sensitive measure of the Dependent or Negativistic personality patterns. Sensitivity scores for the Schizoid and Avoidant are similarly not especially remarkable. Accordingly, if the clinician suspects one of these disorders, and if one of these disorders does not appear prominently in the 2-point code, we might say that although the MCMI-III does not see the patient as being disordered in this way, a very substantial minority of clinicians might nevertheless believe this to be the correct diagnosis. In fact, because the diagnostic efficiency study validating the MCMI-III was not blind, clinicians frequently chose to overrule the instrument where these constructs were involved, awarding a Dependent, Negativistic, Schizoid, or Avoidant diagnosis even though the MCMI-III said no. Should you do the same? Maybe, but remember that these were clinicians who knew their subjects well enough to nominate them for a national validity study in which their ratings would be used as a gold standard. If compelling evidence exists, then certainly there is no reason not to assign any particular personality diagnosis; none of the sensitivity statistics for the MCMI scales is perfect. However, such decisions must be made on a case-by-case basis. Determining when this should be done or what specific diagnoses should be awarded involves consideration of extratest information, which varies considerably from patient to patient. Our goal is to set forth an interpretive logic for the personality subtypes based on the MCMI-III, and from that perspective, all we can do is look at the diagnostic efficiency statistics and suggest certain guidelines. Thus, we might point out, for example, that the sensitivity results for the Paranoid, Antisocial, Masochistic, Borderline, Histrionic, and Depressive are all above .75. Where the disorder exists, the MCMI-III tends to find it. Accordingly, if the clinician is tempted to add a diagnosis over and above what the profile suggests, it probably isn't one of these. Or perhaps it would be better to say that, in general, where the clinician is tempted to add a diagnosis, the evidence for adding one of these disorders needs to be stronger than for the Dependent, Negativistic, Schizoid, or Avoidant.

We can treat the positive predictive power (PPP) statistics the same way. Where the test identifies a Sadistic, Antisocial, Histrionic, Narcissistic, Compulsive, or Dependent personality, it tends to be highly accurate. If a disorder is to be eliminated from the profile, then it probably isn't one of these. If the clinician is faced with a 3-point or 4-point profile and needs to eliminate one of the scales from consideration to make the amount of information in the assessment more manageable, then, according to the PPP statistics, the scale to eliminate is the Avoidant, Depressive, Negativistic, Schizotypal, or Paranoid. All have PPP values in the .60 to .70 range.

In general, the numbers show that the Borderline, Antisocial, and Narcissistic scales are the strongest personality scales on the entire instrument, each having sensitivity and positive predictive power in excess of .75. The Negativistic is the weakest scale, having the lowest combination of sensitivity and positive predictive power in the test. And this makes sense: The Negativistic resides in the *DSM* appendix and clinicians may not be well enough acquainted with the construct to provide reliable and valid ratings (but see Sinha & Watson, 2001, who found that, at least for the MCMI-II, the Passive-Aggressive and Schizotypal had the highest convergent correlations with the MMPI and CATI).

RELIABILITY AND VALIDITY AT A CODE TYPE LEVEL

While the numbers indicate that the sensitivity and positive predictive power of the MCMI-III scales is quite good when each personality scale is considered singly against the respective clinical ratings of expert clinicians, the degree to which a self-report code type and a clinician-rated code type correspond can be made as poor as desired by developing stricter and stricter criteria for what constitutes code type agreement. For example, if a clinician diagnoses a subject as Paranoid Narcissist, and the instrument shows a Narcissistic Paranoid, do the test and instrument agree? From the perspective of measurement in the hard sciences, where precision is paramount, the answer is no. From a practical standpoint, however, the answer is probably yes. Until clinical psychology experiences a measurement revolution that elevates agreement between self-report and clinical ratings by several orders of magnitude, we can probably expect a potential for massive disagreements between self-report instruments and clinical judges at a code type level.

When, then, can we expect a code type to be valid? There are rules of thumb, most of which are based on common sense. Obviously, a personality subtype diagnosis should most likely be considered when the personality pattern is dominated by two and only two scales and when these two scales correspond to the clinician's prior expectations. To the extent that a 2-point pattern dominates the profile, a subtype diagnosis should be considered. As the obtained profile becomes more ambiguous, the issues involved become more ambiguous. If both base rate scores of a 2-point pattern are above 85, a personality subtype diagnosis should certainly be considered. But what happens where the highest personality base rate score is 115, and the second highest is exactly 85, and all other personality scales are 75 or below? In this case, we can still consider a personality subtype diagnosis, but the difference between the magnitude of the highest scales argues that in many situations and circumstances, the individual will operate more as a "pure prototype" than as a mixed subtype. We can hope that enough biographical information will be available to at least make a prediction about what these situations might be. Alternatively, the clinician can consider discussing the MCMI with the patient, reviewing the prototypical items of the second-highest scale, and asking the patient when that particular statement would be most true.

What if only one personality scale dominates the code type? At first glance, we might believe that no mixed-personality subtype diagnosis is warranted, the subject concerned being a relatively pure case. Certainly, if the base rate of the highest scale is 115, and no other scales are even above 75, then the possibility that a mixed subtype would be appropriate seems remote. But what if the highest scale is BR 80, and the next highest is BR 74? Would we reject the possibility that a description based on the personality subtype would describe the subject's behavior? The answer is no, simply because cutting scores, while necessary as interpretive guidelines, should not be applied rigorously. We can expect that most false negatives will cluster within a few points of the cutting score for any assessment instrument.

4-POINT AND 5-POINT PATTERNS

If even a relatively pure code type doesn't rule out the presence of a subtype, then what to do when the subject achieves a 4-point or 5-point code, where all the scales are approximately equal and above the threshold of BR 75, which indicates problematic traits, and 85, which indicates the presence of a personality disorder? This is the most difficult interpretive situation that a clinician can face, so it makes sense to develop our interpretive logic most fully here. Consider: If we assume that each personality construct is a cluster of five or six traits—perhaps a gross underestimate, because in the Millon (1990) theory, each personality construct is operationalized across eight domains, any one of which might contribute several distinctive traits—then a 3-point code type suggests extreme scores on some 15 to 18 traits, maybe more. The problem when faced with multiple but approximately equally elevated scales is too much information. One possibility is simply a massively disordered personality pattern. Sadly, some individuals do possess a developmental history that is so extreme, in so many ways, that they elevate numerous scales and resist any singular diagnosis. But it would be an error to assume that this is always the case. Instead, it is probably best to examine the entire profile, attempting to discard any elevations that are considered false positives.

Consider the interpretive logic advanced in Figure 2.2. As shown, the easiest situation occurs in the leftmost column, where there exists a direct and clearcut correspondence between the resulting MCMI-III code type and a personality subtype from *Disorders of Personality* (Millon & Davis, 1996). The clinician identifies the code type and follows four essential interpretive steps. First, the subtype narrative is checked against all available information and rewritten as necessary to change the content and emphasis in whatever way is consistent with the clinical data. For example, the Nomadic Antisocial manifests on the MCMI as a synthesis of the Schizoid and Antisocial patterns. Such individuals have largely withdrawn from life, existing at the margins of society as outcasts, scavengers, and migrants who violate social norms in connection with their own immediate needs. However, in the prototypical Nomadic Antisocial, the Antisocial scale is most highly elevated and, as such, contributes most of the trait content ("nomadic" is an adjective modifying Antisocial). In a pattern where the two scales are about equally elevated, the narrative should be modified to intensify the isolative characteristics of the Schizoid. Exactly how this should be done requires looking at not only the prototypical items endorsed by the subject, but also additional clinical data that might be available. Each of the prototypical items can be matched, to some degree, to descriptors and trait terms from the eight clinical domains, and these can be integrated into the interpretive report. On the other hand, where a particular prototypical item is not endorsed, the available clinical data evidence needs to be especially strong if the descriptors or traits referenced by the prototypical item are to be included.

What happens if the Schizoid scale is highest and the Antisocial is second highest in a 2-point profile, their two base rate scores being rather close together? Does the fact that the Schizoid is highest rule out the Nomadic Antisocial? The answer is no, for the reason we discussed earlier: Lack of perfect reliability and validity creates a "fudge factor" in the score of *every* psychological test. Many instruments use profiles as a visual guide to the interpretive process. If every scale score was displayed as being bounded by a 95% confidence interval, the resulting profiles would suddenly look much

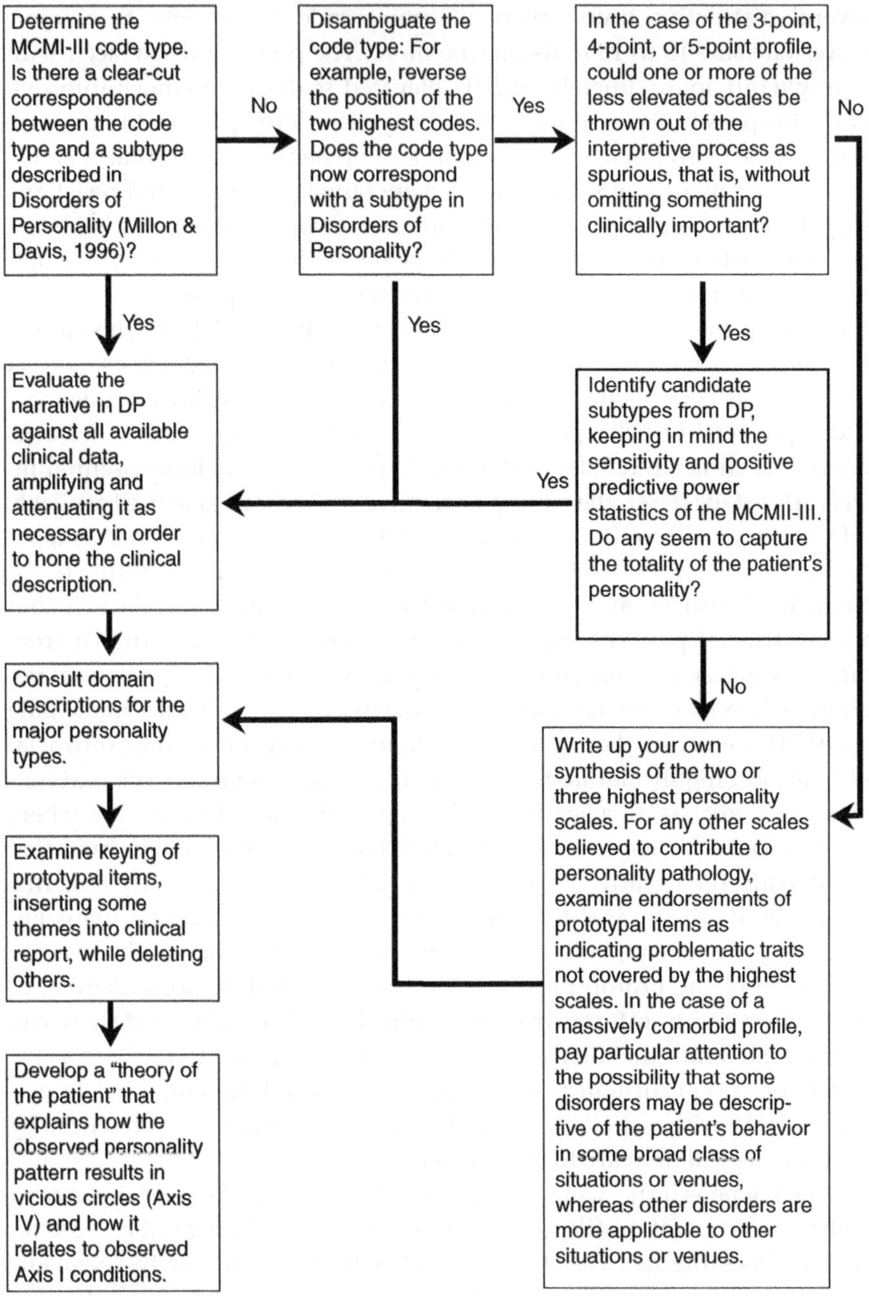

Determine the MCMI-III code type. Is there a clear-cut correspondence between the code type and a subtype described in Disorders of Personality (Millon & Davis, 1996)?

→ No →

Disambiguate the code type: For example, reverse the position of the two highest codes. Does the code type now correspond with a subtype in Disorders of Personality?

→ Yes →

In the case of the 3-point, 4-point, or 5-point profile, could one or more of the less elevated scales be thrown out of the interpretive process as spurious, that is, without omitting something clinically important?

→ No →

↓ Yes

↓ Yes

↓ Yes

Evaluate the narrative in DP against all available clinical data, amplifying and attenuating it as necessary in order to hone the clinical description.

← Yes ←

Identify candidate subtypes from DP, keeping in mind the sensitivity and positive predictive power statistics of the MCMII-III. Do any seem to capture the totality of the patient's personality?

↓

↓ No

Consult domain descriptions for the major personality types.

Write up your own synthesis of the two or three highest personality scales. For any other scales believed to contribute to personality pathology, examine endorsements of prototypal items as indicating problematic traits not covered by the highest scales. In the case of a massively comorbid profile, pay particular attention to the possibility that some disorders may be descriptive of the patient's behavior in some broad class of situations or venues, whereas other disorders are more applicable to other situations or venues.

↓

Examine keying of prototypal items, inserting some themes into clinical report, while deleting others.

↓

Develop a "theory of the patient" that explains how the observed personality pattern results in vicious circles (Axis IV) and how it relates to observed Axis I conditions.

Figure 2.2
Interpretive logic for MCMI-III personality subtypes.

more ambiguous. This is why so much of the clinician's job is concerned with ruling out possibilities. Indeed, very few clinical indictors are definitive. In this sense, subtypes are like shoes: It's important to try them on and see how they fit. Sometimes a shoe that isn't tailor-made fits just fine (is consistent with all available information), and one that nearly fits can be adapted with a little ingenuity. From this perspective, the personality subtypes are best approached as a rich source of generative clinical hypotheses, each providing a prefabricated synthesis that illustrates how the major personality constructs combine as we move down from the lofty level of what is, from the perspective of the evolutionary model, abstract, eternal, and idealized, to what is, from the perspective of the clinician, the concrete, present, and particular reality of the individual patient.

Considering the confidence interval that might be placed around scale scores, the interpretive situation begins to look much more like the right column of Figure 2.2. Here, there are few or no absolutes, and the clinician must use his or her best judgment in conjunction with all available information. Ultimately, the clinician should probably try to identify the two or three personality scales that are most relevant to the goals of the assessment, the prototypical items of other scales being examined as a means of getting this information into the interpretive report. If it proves impossible to rule out certain personality elevations, then it may be possible to sort various disorders, at or least traits from various disorders, to different settings. At first, this might seem counterintuitive, or even paradoxical. Isn't personality, by definition, required to be stable across time and situations? But, in fact, the construct of personality is itself a conceptual prototype, so that certain aspects of the construct may not apply to any particular person. Better, perhaps, to say that people vary in terms of the consistency of their behavior, and they vary in terms of the degree to which any particular trait is (in the language of genetics) penetrant across situations.

DERIVING SCALES FOR PERSONALITY SUBTYPES

In the previous section, the interpretive process was mainly inferential in nature: Given a personality profile, an interpretive process was put forward that would culminate in a theory-of-the-person and its associated clinical narrative. We noted that on every instrument, because of limitations largely inherent in psychological measurement itself, there exists a fudge factor that complicates the interpretive process, making it necessary, in our situation, to try various subtypes on the person to see if they fit.

Might there exist, however, some methodology whereby we could assess the personality disorder subtypes directly? Might we construct scales for each subtype, or at least for those subtypes having the highest base rates across most clinical settings? There is a trend toward increased efficiency in psychology in general, of which brief assessments and brief therapy (e.g., Marks, 2002; Shapiro et al., 2003) constitute prime examples. We know that there is only so much a brief instrument can do. In a series of "psychometric expeditions," Davis (1996) sought to develop abbreviated forms of the MCMI-III personality scales. Because these scales are heavily saturated with trait neuroticism, it was reasoned that high item-scale intercorrelations would facilitate the creation of "super-abbreviated scales." Several methods were pursued. The most successful involved selecting, for each scale, the item with the highest item-scale correlation, then selecting the item correlating most highly with remaining items but with the variance of the already selected items partialled out. The adventure was successful from a correlational point of view. From a clinical perspective, however, it was believed that the resulting scales would be highly limited, and in fact, they were so short that the difference of a single item endorsement could, in some cases, move the resulting base rate score from normal to pathological, or back again. The lesson, valuable for every practioner in every psychological assessment, is to be naturally suspicious when applying short scales in psychological assessment, particularly where some cutting score results in a diagnostic label.

Fortunately, however, most of the personality disorder subtypes advanced by Millon and Davis (1996) are amalgams, or 2-point combinations. As such, for any particular subtype, probably between 10 and 20 items could be portioned out as strong candidates for any particular subtype scale. In addition, as with the major scales of the MCMI-III, an item weighting scheme could be employed, with items considered prototypical of each subtype given a weight of 2 or 3 points, and more peripheral items a weight of 2 or 1 point. Would it be possible to create subscales for each personality disorder subtype? Probably not. The MCMI-III just doesn't have enough items. Would it be possible to create scales for some subset of personality disorder subtypes? Probably so, particularly if we view the resulting scales, not as the final word, but simply as a source of clinical hypotheses to be sustained by auxiliary evidence. Paying special attention to diagnostic efficiency, we might find, for example, that whereas a low score on any particular subscale might have only limited meaning, high scores on certain subscales might have high positive predictive power. When you see it, you can be absolutely sure it's there! This would be a genuine addition to the armamentarium of any psychodiagnostician.

As an example, consider the 10 subtypes of psychopathy advanced by Millon and Davis (1996, see Table 2.3), which are essentially psychopathic analogues of code type combinations that frequently occur with the MCMI-III Antisocial scale (some of these subtypes have scales other than the Antisocial as highest in their code type). Because of the importance of antisocial traits across nearly every venue of psychological assessment, because of its relatively high base rate across many of these venues, and because a substantial literature has accumulated regarding the use of the MCMI in forensic settings (Craig, 1999; McCann & Dyer, 1996; Retzlaff, Stoner, & Kleinsasser, 2002), development of subtype scales optimized for

Table 2.3
Essential Characteristics of 10 Subtypes of Psychopathy

The Unprincipled Psychopath

Activities kept near or at the boundaries of the law; stereotyped social roles: con man, charlatan, fast-talking used-car salesman.

Expansive fantasies and exaggerated sense of self-importance.

Willing to take advantage of and humiliate those who leave themselves open to deceit.

May cultivate persuasiveness or charm as a means of getting others to lower their guard, but sees all prosocial behavior as ultimately self-serving.

Contemptuous of "the system"; working "the system" to avoid punishment seen as just "part of the game."

The Covetous Psychopath

Sees self as wrongfully deprived of life's necessities, leading to envy and resentment.

Compensates by taking what he or she is entitled to as a means of revenging wrong and restoring "karmic balance" in life.

Sees self as victim of external forces, misunderstood by others and by society.

Manipulates others as a means of proving own superiority, as well as avenging attributions of worthlessness.

Smug and contemptuous toward victims, who may be viewed as pawns in the larger game.

Prone to ostentatious displays of conspicuous consumption.

The Risk-Taking Psychopath

Chronic underarousal leads to risk-taking as means of "feeling alive."

Fails to realize the consequences of risk-taking; believes that social rules are unnecessarily confining of own sense of adventure.

Eschews normal desire for safety as evidence of cowardice.

Proves own mettle as a means of proving self-esteem and worthiness to self and others.

The Disingenuous Psychopath

Superficial sociability (or even seductiveness) hides an impulsive, moody, and resentful core.

Emotionally labile, prone to excitement-seeking, stimulus-dependent behavior, lacking in forethought, with a high potential for painful consequences.

Rationalizes and projects blame onto others when attempts to solicit attention go awry.

(continued)

Table 2.3 *Continued*

The Spineless Psychopath

Aggression not intrinsically rewarding; psychopathic acts intended to show others that the psychopath is not weak.

Has first-strike mentality; strikes whenever own fearfulness peaks (perhaps in episodes of panic), regardless of objective degree of threat.

Experiences fantasies of vulnerability; sees others as sadistic or exploiting.

The Abrasive Psychopath

Prefers to be overtly contentious, confrontational, antagonistic rather than indirectly manipulative.

Expects hostility from others, and preempts insults with own abrasiveness.

Prefers to escalate arguments; experiences pleasure by frustrating others, making them back down.

Inherently oppositional to any form of external control; seeks to break constraints simply because they exist.

The Tyrannical Psychopath

Realizes pleasure through total control of others.

Employs violence instrumentally, to force perceived opponents to cower or submit.

Projects image of power and brutality; supports self-image of power and superiority by inflicting pain and suffering, if not terror.

The Explosive Psychopath

Low frustration threshold, resulting in episodes of uncontrollable rage and violent attack.

Episodes may be instantaneous reaction to frustration or perceived insult, and thus may be perceived by others as random and unprovoked.

The Malevolent Psychopath

Hateful, destructive defiance of values of social life.

Inherently distrustful, ruthless, cold-blooded, revengeful, punitive.

The Malignant Psychopath

Often isolated, paranoid, with ruminative fantasies of power and revenge.

Sees others as inherently persecutory or treacherous.

Uses hostility as a means of armoring self, forcing adversaries to take pause and withdraw.

---

use with psychopathic subtypes constitutes a useful direction. For example, Craig, Bivens, and Olson (1997) administered the MCMI-III to a large sample of heroin and cocaine addicts. As with previous generations of the MCMI, the modal code type was Antisocial Personality Disorder. Craig (2000) found a base rate of 60% of Antisocial Personality Disorder in a similar sample. Logically, in populations where the base rate of a particular disorder is known to be extremely high, the second- and third-highest scales become a more intense focus of clinical attention. Why not bypass problems associated with inferences concerning the "correct code type" and instead measure the personality subtypes directly?

One of the fundamental principles in instrument construction is that validity should be built into an instrument from the beginning. Loevinger (1957), Jackson (1971), Millon (1981), and Skinner (1986) have each discussed test construction as a three-stage process. In the first, rational or theoretical stage, the content of each construct to be measured is defined as precisely as possible. Items may be written and refined by multiple so-called experts in the theory of the construct, sorted according to their discriminative characteristics, ranked in terms of difficulty level, and so on, all before being put to actual subjects. For our purposes, each of the 10 subtypes would be abstracted into short, descriptive or bulleted paragraphs that could more easily be compared against each of the personality items on the MCMI-III. Special attention would be given to the essential, discriminant characteristics of each subtype, the ultimate purpose being the development of a "psychopathic profile" against which any particular Antisocial personality or criminal would be assessed. To make the process more objective, some set of candidate judges could be employed to rate each item in terms of the degree to which it was believed to scale each subtype. Judges would be treated similarly to items, their ratings assessed for reliability and any individual whose judgments were found deviant would be eliminated from the judge pool.

In the second, internal-statistical stage, the items are presented to real individuals in order to gather response data. Various statistics, usually Cronbach's alpha, are then calculated to ensure that the items tap a single dimension. Items with strong relationships to scales for which they were not intended may be deleted or reassigned. In addition, a correlation matrix of the instrument's scales may be examined for anomalies to bring this pattern in line with theoretical expectations. Because the subtypes are intrinsically related, the pattern of intercorrelations among the scales would be examined for failures of discriminative validity. Items that are too general, though immensely valuable in assessing their major personality construct, would be identified and probably discarded or would have their item weights adjusted to better tease apart the scales. In addition, given a critical mass of empirical data, it is possible to refine one's theoretical postulates based on psychometric considerations. For example, it might be found that what were previously believed to be separate subtypes could not be teased apart during scale creation. This might well lead to reconsideration of the entire constellation of subtypes, with some being merged into others or deleted completely as too narrow to sustain further examination. Alternatively, other subtypes might be written and the whole process repeated.

In the third, external stage, the newly developed scales would be compared to instruments of established reputation as well as to clinical judgments. Rather than simply use diagnostic efficiency statistics, however, which are probably too methodologically coarse for scale creation within narrow domains of content, the clinical judges would be asked to provide their own personality subtype ratings for each individual in the development pool. Test items would then be selected or weighted to maximize similarity between instrument profiles and clinician judgments, thus capitalizing on the original intentions of the instrument construction: to encode validity directly into the inventory from the beginning. Items that pass through all three stages are said to have been validated theoretically, statistically, and empirically.

The Millon inventories have essentially been constructed according to this tripartite logic. Eventually, the item pool of such subtype instruments could be expanded and migrated completely away from their dependence on the MCMI. Other behavioral and clinical indices specific to an antisocial population could be added, so that the resulting multiaxial inventory would be optimized on both Axis I and Axis II.

Obviously, the same strategy could be pursued in developing scales for subtypes of any personality disorder, though the Antisocial and Borderline are the most obvious candidates simply because the high base rates of these disorders in clinical settings makes the additional specificity promised by a dedicated instrument highly attractive.

THEORETICAL REVISIONS

In the first section, we concentrated on developing an interpretive logic for the assessment of personality subtypes with the MCMI-III. In the second section, we asked how the subtypes might be assessed if we were free to tinker with the items to produce subtype scales, thus overcoming some of the inferential problems inherently associated with personality profiles by measuring the subtypes directly. In this final section, we ask how the theory itself might be rejiggered to ultimately optimize its utility with the MCMI-III in generating a taxonomy of personality constructs and in psychodiagnosis.

In *Toward a New Personology*, Millon (1990) wrote about the virtues of integration of various domains of clinical science. A historical perspective shows that he was absolutely correct: Clinical practice is not well served by a psychology that consists of disjointed perspectives, instruments, and therapies. Consider two of the most widely used tests in psychological assessment, the MMPI and the Rorschach. Any coordination between these instruments with the *DSM-IV-TR* would involve retrofitting existing test items and blots to *DSM* diagnoses, not generating new items on the basis of psychological theory. If new disorders are best assessed by blots or items not already in existence, then that's too bad. Although their norms are updated periodically, these dinosaurs of psychological assessment just keep hanging on, year after year after year, resisting extinction because they are entrenched in clinical practice.

Surely, Millon's paragraphs advocating integration are seminal in the literature of personality disorders. In particular, it is these paragraphs that crystallize the logic that distinguishes Millon from every other author writing in the area. Please take a moment now to revisit Figure 2.1, presented earlier in this chapter. Unlike other thinkers, who were content to construct theoretical models from various "part-functions" (Millon, 1990), Millon realized that because personality is integrative, a taxonomy of constructs consistent with the surplus meaning inherent in the term could not be derived from within any domain or perspective of psychology itself. To do so would simply be to commit the same error as previous thinkers: to argue that personality is primarily biological (e.g., Cloninger, 1986, 1987), or primarily cognitive (e.g., Beck & Freeman, 1990), or even primarily psychodynamic (e.g., Kernberg, 1984, 1996). Developments in each of these areas, though not actually irrelevant, were regarded simply as "horizontal refinements" (Millon, 1990). Rather than continue to wage wars of attribution against thinkers and model builders in other domains, it was necessarily to step outside psychology to seek other organizing principles—here, the principles of evolution.

Despite these auspicious foundations, the full promise of integration was never fully realized in Millon's work. This was not because the evolutionary polarities of the model lacked theoretical currency, but because the principle of integration was not pushed to its logical conclusions, resulting in certain theoretical inconsistencies. A full explication of these is beyond the scope of this chapter; we will discuss only two. First, if personality is an inherently integrative construct, then why are the personality disorders derived as combinations of the evolutionary polarities taken two at a time, rather than as combinations of all three polarities simultaneously? The former strategy leads to a complex matrix that appears nearly everywhere the theory is explained in detail. In addition, a close reading of the theory shows that additional ideas are required to actually derive the personalities, namely, imbalance of polarities, reversal of the pleasure-pain polarity, and conflict between self and other. Finally, a close reading shows that the structurally defective personalities are not actually derived from the polarities of the evolutionary theory at all; instead, it is posited that there are three ways that personality can be structurally defective, corresponding to the Borderline, Paranoid, and Schizotypal personalities. Collectively, these features substantially complicate the parsimony of the theory.

Second, Millon (1981; Millon & Davis, 1996) discusses the development of personality as a stage theory. Given the synthetic properties of personality as a construct, putting forward a model of personality development is obviously far different from simply tracing the antecedents of a particular personality trait. Disorders or styles are considered to be clusters of traits, so development becomes an exceedingly complex proposition. Nevertheless the theory does hold that at the highest level of generality, the themes of personality development are mainly concerned with the contents of the polarity model: Issues related to pain and pleasure constitute the first stage. Those related to active versus passive constitute the second stage, and those related to self and other constitute the third stage.

The problem lies with synthesizing the developmental model with the derivation of the personality constructs from the theory, namely, the fact that every personality construct derived by Millon (1981, 1990) reflects a combination of two and only two polarities. Consider the Sadistic and Masochistic personalities. According to Millon and Davis (1996), these reflect a passive versus active reversal of pleasure and pain. Likewise, the interpersonally imbalanced personalities reflect some combination of self versus other and active versus passive. The Narcissist, for example, is conceptualized by Millon as being passive and self-oriented. But how does a Masochist or a Narcissist or an Avoidant "know" that his or her development should be limited to extreme loadings on two of the polarities rather than three? How does development "know" that once personality is loaded on two polarities, it's effectively time for further development to stop? Or, how does development "know" to skip loading on pleasure-pain so that the individual can develop into some amalgam of the interpersonally imbalanced personalities, for example? The answer, of course, is that no developmental imperative exists that confines personality development to two polarities rather than three. Instead, it can be expected that the experiences of each person, in combination with biological variables, synergistically interacting across all domains of personality, result at the highest level of generality in attainments on each of the polarities that can be measured quantitatively by psychological assessment.

The way forward is to arrange the polarities so that they form the axes of a single, integrated, personologic space, that is, a geometric framework that breaks out its major personality constructs as a synthesis of all three polarities simultaneously. Note that such a framework is neither a contrivance nor a convenience; it is explicitly required by the philosophy that undergirds the model. Regardless of whether or not the reader agrees with the particular framework put forward in this chapter, some geometric framework will be required to put the evolutionary model on a logically consistent foundation. Indeed, it is our opinion that operationalizing personality constructs as a combination of two polarities rather than three may explain why comorbidity is so pervasive on Millon inventories, and in the personality disorders generally: Any client with loadings on all three polarities, which would include most normal individuals, must be diagnosed with at least two personality styles or disorders if his or her individuality is to be captured by the current constellation of constructs. As Millon (1990) himself noted, "The intrinsic cohesion of persons is not merely a rhetorical construction, but an authentic substantive unity. Personologic features may often be dissonant, and may be partitioned conceptually for pragmatic or scientific purposes, but they are segments of an inseparable biopsychosocial entity" (p. 12). If we believe that real personalities are complex composites, then we must also believe that comorbidity is built into system. How then, can the evolutionary model be revised such that the above problems are eliminated?

THE REVISED EVOLUTIONARY MODEL

The simplest way forward is to consider the three evolutionary polarities of the evolutionary model as axes of a three-dimensional space (see Figure 2.3). Personality constructs correspond to regions of this space that reflect combinations of the basic polarities. Because these constructs are all part of a single integrated model, the content of each becomes a

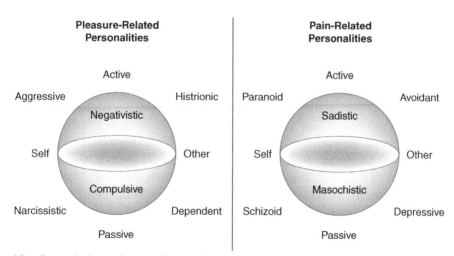

Visualize each circumplex as a dome or hemisphere. A horizontal slice has been taken out of the middle of each dome in order to illustrate Conflictedness as a third dimension rising up from the surface of each circumplex. The slice is horizontal because Conflict can only exist between the Self and the Other. Each slice is shaded in the center to create the impression of depth. Two hemispheres are presented because one dimension has been split along its extremes of Existentially-Engaged and Existentially-Breached.

Figure 2.3
The personologic space of the revised evolutionary
model, diagrammed as two circumplexes.

reference point for comparison and contrast when deriving and refining the content of the others. Each fixes the others against the possibility of construct drift that might occur were the constructs simply broken out as a list to be operationalized and memorized (as with the *DSM-IV*). The revised evolutionary model contains numerous comparisons that allow us to validate it against clinical intuition. For example, every personality construct has several "polarity opposites" and a "diametrical opposite." Within the pleasure circumplex, the Histrionic personality is the opposite of the Narcissist. Certainly they may look alike on the surface, but in terms of their deeper motivations, the attention seeking of the Histrionic personality is essentially other-oriented and thus opposite to the self-oriented admiration seeking of the Narcissistic personality. Constructs that are opposite in along every polarity are "diametrically opposite." The Dependent is pathologically attached, seeking loyal companions from whom to derive an endless supply of nurturant resources, whereas its diametrical opposite, the Paranoid, is too interpersonally suspicious to attach to anyone and may actually recoil from feelings of vulnerability that naturally accompany warm feelings in human relationships. The Narcissist exhibits inflated self-esteem, leading to fantasies of grandiose ability or success, whereas its diametrical opposite, the Avoidant, entertains fears of social humiliation and defeat. The Aggressive personality (self-active-pleasure) is self-confident and expansive, while its diametrical opposite, the Depressive, is self-doubting, submissive, resigned.

Personality constructs described on the pain circumplex can be seen as more dysfunctional variants of those on the pleasure circumplex. Because fantasy and fear are so closely aligned to pleasure and pain, we can speculate that the personality constructs on the pleasure circumplex secretly fear (whether consciously or not) that they will become the equivalent personality on the pain circumplex, and those on the pain circumplex fantasize about their successful personality style analogue on the pleasure circumplex. Thus, the Avoidant would like to be a successful Histrionic, socially smooth, the center of attention, with no self-consciousness in social situations that might sabotage interpersonal relationships. Likewise, the Depressive would like to be indissolubly attached to an infinite source of understanding and nurturance. The Schizoid would like to be completely absorbed in the real talents and capabilities of the self and would like to be admired for legitimate accomplishments. The Paranoid would like to expand the boundaries of self-influence without fear, rather than retreat behind walls raised to protect an insecure autonomy. As these descriptions show, a comparison and contrast of the personalities residing on the pain circumplex with those on the pleasure circumplex becomes a metric of the personality pathology severity that is built in to the revised evolutionary model but either is not present or is not fully re-alized in the original formulation.

The revised evolutionary model is interesting, but three dimensions generate only eight personality disorders; the Compulsive, Masochistic, Negativistic, and Compulsive personalities have no place in the three-dimensional version. To integrate these constructs into the model, conflict-edness is added as a dimension. Existing at the same level as the content dimensions, conflict is seen as a fundamental organizing principle for the whole personality. Conflict occurs only between self and other, and its in-clusion in the revised evolutionary model essentially recognizes the rich contributions of the psychodynamic perspective to the history of personal-ity theory, specifically that early attachment experiences with caretakers (Bowlby, 1969/1982) have long-lasting effects that are incorporated into cognitive-motivational-affective schemas for reward and punishment, evo-lutionary mechanisms that the psychodynamic perspective would refer to as "superego introjects." The revised evolutionary model is identical to Millon's original formulation in this respect, again differing only in terms of how the taxonomic constructs are derived. Once conflict has been added, the revised evolutionary model may be seen as possessing four of the di-mensions of the five-factor model. Indeed, if we consult the list of subtypes given in Millon and Davis (1996), we find the name "Conscientious Com-pulsive" given to the pure 7 subtype.

Looking again at Figure 2.3, with conflictedness added, a horizontal slice is removed from the middle of each hemisphere to illustrate conflict-edness as a dimension rising up from the surface of each circumplex. The slice is horizontal because conflict exists only between self and other. Of the four conflicted personalities, only the Compulsive appears in the main body of *DSM-IV-TR*. The Negativistic has been put forward as a provi-sional disorder requiring further study. The Masochistic and Sadistic per-sonalities, first seen in the revised third edition of the *DSM* (1987), have now been dropped from the official taxonomy. Nevertheless, in accor-dance with the generativity and falsifiability we expect from a good the-ory, the revised evolutionary model predicts that all four are valid personality constructs that can be meaningfully related both to each other and to the other personalities of the model. For example, the Masochist emerges as a kind of "failed Compulsive." Both possess hypertrophied superego introjects, but the Compulsive still believes that blame can be purged through the pursuit of perfection and that the introjects can be pleased, or at least appeased. In contrast, the Masochist owns the judg-ment of its introjects and deliberately arranges scenarios that have a high potential for painful consequences, many designed to humiliate the subject. Likewise, the Sadist may be considered the opposite of the Negativistic personality. With the Negativist, the idea of "conscientious protest" (the opposite of conscientious conformity) takes on pathological dimensions. Whereas the normal-range social activist believes that authority will ultimately respond conscientiously if rule breaking honestly seeks to make a larger moral point, with the Negativist, authority is no longer viewed as being responsive or even moral. Rather than act overtly, as a social activist does, the Negativist acts covertly to pervert the system behind the scenes. In contrast, by deliberately inflicting needless pain and disappointment, the Sadist stands on its head the idea of moral relations that honor the dignity of creatures. As these examples show, the idea that pleasure and pain are somehow reversed, as in the original evolutionary model, is only a surface characteristic. The theater in which the Masochistic and Sadistic personalities act out their pathology has a distinctive interpersonal aspect. In contrast, Millon describes these disorders as having an active versus passive orientation to pain, respectively. Self and other do not play a primary part in the derivation of these disorders. In contrast, the revised evolutionary model predicts that issues relating to self versus other are so fundamental to Sadistic and Masochistic personalities that these constructs could not otherwise be generated.

The resulting four-dimensional space directly generates 12 of the 14 personality disorders listed in the *DSM-III, III-R, IV,* and *IV-TR* and their appendixes and interrelates and differentiates all of its constructs in a single, integrated, personologic space. In contrast, Millon's model generates 11 of the 14, does so in a more complicated way (requiring the idea of reversal in addition to conflict), and leaves the relationship between many personalities obscure and free to drift relative to others.

Both models recognize the existence of structurally defective personalities, but the revised evolutionary model does not directly generate the Schizotypal or the Borderline from its polarities. In contrast, the original formulation does not directly generate the Schizotypal, Borderline, or Paranoid. The Paranoid, in particular, provides a notable contrast between the revised evolutionary model and Millon's original formulation, receiving its content from the three evolutionary polarities in the revised model. In general, the notion of a structurally defective personality has tremendous merit, recognizing that personality itself is a heuristic construct. Just as psychoanalysts view personality as having different levels of organization, there is no reason to suppose that real individuals should be equal in terms of their level of personality integration. Accordingly, the notion of structurally defective personalities allows us to explore parts of the psychopathologic landscape where the very idea of a personality disorder begins to break down, an area that exists, by definition, somewhere between Axis I and Axis II. In fact, because these constructs are concerned primarily with personality structure rather than content, the model predicts that they should have a long and problematic taxonomic history, which they certainly do.

ASSESSMENT OF PERSONALITY SUBTYPES WITH THE REVISED EVOLUTIONARY MODEL

Can the personality subtypes given in Millon and Davis (1996) be assessed using the revised evolutionary model and the MCMI-III? Because the derivation of the personality constructs in Millon's original formulation lacked an integrated personologic space, the content of the personality constructs could not be fixed relative to each other. Thus, it cannot be assumed that the MCMI-III is optimized as a measure of the revised model's personality constructs. In fact, the revised evolutionary model is not the only circumplical model of Millon's constructs to have been developed. In the manual for the MCMI-II (Millon, Millon, & Green, 1987), Millon himself suggested a circumplical structure, based on an Impassive-Expressive dimension and an Autonomous-Enmeshed dimension. Strack, Choca, and Gurtman (2001) examined Millon's (1987) circumplex of personality disorders in a sample of over 2,400 psychiatric patients who completed the MCMI-III. Their findings replicate Strack, Lorr, and Campbell (1990): Instead of an Autonomous-Enmeshed dimension, they found an Impulsivity-Compulsivity dimension, concluding that "changes are needed to rectify discrepancies between the theory and empirical findings" (quoted from abstract). To fully realize the potential of the revised evolutionary model, a new inventory would need to be constructed (and it probably would not correspond as directly to the *DSM-IV-TR* as the current MCMI-III because its goal would be internal theoretical consistency and power, not *DSM* compatibility; at the current time, clinicians can only map the MCMI-III elevations into the revised model space and assess for themselves whether the additional surplus meaning afforded by the revised model is clinically helpful).

Moreover, there are certain important differences in the interpretive principles. With the MCMI-III, the arrangement of the scales has limited meaning. The order of the scales on the personality profile could be changed without much affecting the interpretive process. In contrast, the revised evolutionary model encodes numerous principles related to the degree of personality pathology directly into its geometric space. Many of the interpretive principles appropriate to the Interpersonal Circle (e.g., Kiesler, 1983) also apply to the revised model. First, the ideas of flexibility versus rigidity can quickly be assessed by determining the extent to which the profile is circular versus lop-sided. A circular profile indicates a relatively rich and balanced behavioral repertoire consisting of a variety of strategies that might be matched against a particular situation. A lop-sided profile indicates a paucity of coping strategies, with only a limited response set from which behaviors appropriate to any given situation might be selected. Second, the intensity of the profile can be assessed as the distance from the center of the circle to the edge of the profile. The more extreme the profile is in a particular direction, the greater the degree of pathology. A combination of intensity and lack of flexibility is thus doubly pathological because the individual can express only a few kinds of responses to an extreme degree. In theory, such patients could be especially prone to the development of structural pathologies. The original formulation cannot make theoretical predictions that are as precise and testable.

Another defining characteristic of the revised evolutionary model is its view of normality. Whereas most theorists hold that the difference between normality and pathology is simply a matter of degree (see Benjamin, 1996, for a notable exception), the revised model argues that normality and pathology differ both quantitatively and qualitatively. The revised model holds that the balance of normality resides primarily on the pleasure circumplex. These styles believe that their characteristic strategies will ultimately bring happiness and success, and in moderate amount, they do. In contrast, the pain circumplex reflects themes of withdrawal, resignation, detachment, and defeat. While a modicum of painful experiences is necessary for successful adaptation, normality intrinsically requires that pleasure outweigh pain. For example, if we draw a line through personologic space from the Dependent to the Paranoid and view the resulting continuum as running, in the interpersonal domain, from the pathological fusion of the Dependent, to normal trust, to mistrust, and finally to the alienation of the Paranoid, it is mostly trust combined with some mistrust that constitutes the greatest potential for psychological health. Finally, the revised evolutionary model holds that a moderate amount of conflictedness is adaptive, simply because this allows the objectives of the self to be balanced with the needs and desires of others, to be profitably expressed in the normal range as either conscientiousness or constructive protest, normal-range traits of the Compulsive and Negativistic personalities, respectively. More severely compromised are personalities that exist on the pain circumplex, particularly those that are conflicted, the Sadistic and Masochistic. Most severe are personalities experiencing symptoms of structural decompensation.

Millon may well have had certain similar ideas. The personality scales of the MCMI-III are loosely arranged from left to right in terms of their degree of pathology. The Schizoid (scale 1) reflects the near absence of personality, and the Avoidant (scale 2A) likewise appears withdrawn or turned inward. The Depressive (scale 2B), the Dependent (scale 3), and the Narcissist (scale 5) are all passive styles; the Histrionic is at least other-oriented (scale 4). We might argue that the Compulsive (scale 7) should be moved before the Antisocial (scale 6A) and Sadistic (scale 6B), but from the perspective of the revised model, the conflicted personalities should indeed be grouped together. The Negativistic (scale 8A) and Masochistic (scale 8B) finish up this set, with the structurally defective personalities following (scales S, C, and P).

Where does this leave the assessment of the personality subtypes? The profile pattern is literally intended to function as a theoretically based schematic of the person, on which rests the validity of the whole assessment. The theory provides a promissory note that these dimensions are not randomly selected, but are instead sufficient to both exhaust each individual nature and organize the resulting information in a manner optimal for understanding and treating psychopathology. From this perspective, the personality subtypes are, in their original formulation, an attempt to adapt a set of personality constructs formulated in the absence of an integrated personologic space to the complexity of real patients, by converting the co-morbidity of an unintegrated taxonomic schema into what are genuinely useful clinical reference points. And to a great extent, the narratives given in Millon and Davis (1996) are both interesting and helpful, and they do help us capture a degree of interpretive specificity that the major constructs cannot. But in another sense, the subtypes are simply a list, the way the personality disorders are presented in the *DSM-IV-TR* as a list.

At the beginning of this chapter, we noted that the subtypes and the major constructs exist on a different ontological footing. We said that the subtypes may be seen as a bridge from the abstract and eternal realm of theoretical necessary, which is the evolutionary model, to the particular, transient, and temporal realm of historical accident and contingency, which constitutes the individual human life. The revised evolutionary model is an attempt to put the subtypes on the same firm theoretical footing as the major constructs. Its ambition is to press the surplus meaning inherent in the term *personality* to its logical conclusion, maximize the generativity of the theory, and put the subtypes on the same ontological foundation as the major constructs by showing how both are part and parcel of the same integrated personologic space, interrelated and differentiated through the same domains as the major types. Whereas the original formulation simply operationalizes the major constructs by selecting attributes from the domains of personality that seem consonant with our intuition (e.g., the Paranoid is interpersonally suspicious, the Histrionic cognitively scattered), the argument being made is that both the major types and subtypes can be expressed as part and parcel of a single integrated

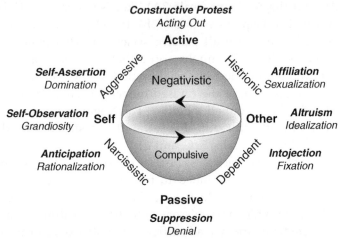

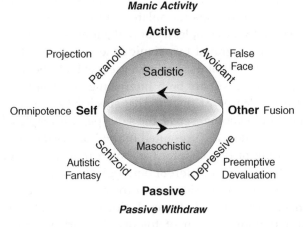

Figure 2.4
Defense mechanisms and personality.

space that organizes attributes from the personality domains and does so precisely. Perhaps nowhere is such order needed more than in psychodynamic psychology, where the definitions of various defense mechanisms tend to be overlapping, incomplete, or obscure. Drawing strongly on Millon (1990), Figure 2.4 uses the revised evolutionary model to impose theoretical cohesiveness on this otherwise unruly arena. Doubling the precision of the original formulation, defense mechanisms are given for every 45 degrees of every circumplex within the revised model, with healthy variants of personality represented on the pleasure circumplex. As with the major constructs, it is necessary that any structural models erected within the personality domains obey the geometric rules intrinsic to the revised model itself. Thus, we would assert that omnipotence is a pathological opposite of self-observation, as are pathological fantasies of fusion. Likewise, the rationalization of the Narcissist, which excuses self-oriented behavior, stands in opposition to the autistic fantasy of the Schizoid, as well as to preemptive devaluation of the Depressive. Similar circumplical models could be constructed for every clinical domain identified by Millon (1990).

In addition, because personality styles that are closer together in personologic space can be expected to co-occur more frequently than those further apart, the geometrical representation afforded by the revised evolutionary model actively suggests personality subtypes. The analogue of the MCMI-III Antisocial personality is the revised model's Aggressive (a full discussion of the relationship between the revised model and psychopathy is beyond the scope of this chapter, but psychopaths are, quite obviously, likely to cluster on the self-oriented circumplex). Here, the model actively suggests, in addition to the subtypes outlined by Millon and Davis (1996), the possibility of a Compulsive Psychopath which should be at least as common as the Spineless Psychopath, an amalgam of the Antisocial and Avoidant personalities. Such individuals would be highly systematic in their exploitation of others. Wearing the "mask of sanity" (Cleckley, 1950), they could exhibit extensive knowledge of the system, working its codes and power structures instrumentally with great effectiveness to enlarge their domain of power. Some would seek to control the system from within, to put the stamp of their own personality on its operation. They would respond ferociously and rigorously to competition or opposition of any kind, would actively recruit the loyalties of others in doing so, and would use the rules and formal powers of their station ruthlessly for their own purposes. As the elevation of Aggressive traits increases, they would, more and more, subvert the spirit of the rules for their own pathological purposes, arguing all the while that the end justifies the means. Indecisiveness would not be a characteristic of these individuals, as that trait belongs to the more Dependent half of the Compulsive construct.

FROM PERSON TO PATHOLOGY: AXIS I HYPOTHESES

The idea that personality forms the immune system of the psychological matrix is an important axiom of Millon's (1981) work. Axis I diagnoses are seen to result from the interaction of Axis II and the psychosocial stressors of Axis IV. When the immunological matrix is no longer adequate to external demands, that is, when the mismatch between person and environment is too great, the result is symptom production. Figures 2.5 and 2.6 examine

AGGRESSIVE: Depression occurs when sense of strength, power, or ability to control flow of objective events so central to self-image are somehow falsified. Being defeated by others may induce feelings of weakness or submission. Random misfortune may induce feelings of helplessness. Feelings of boredom and inefficacy may set in when forced to work in highly structured or conventional settings that do not allow for competitive individuality.

NEGATIVISTIC: Depression ensues when world seems even more inherently amoral and unjust and self as misunderstood and cosmically jinxed, if not actively persecuted, than usually viewed by the subject. This may occur after abandonment by frustrated lovers, demotion at work, or other serious shortfall, usually provoked by the negativist, or when the negativist is prevented from complaining about or sabotaging the ruling regime, their favorite coping mechanism, or forced into highly structured surroundings, where they feel helpless to vent rebellious feelings.

HISTRIONIC: Sees attractiveness of self as guaranteeing steady stream of instrumental surrogates. Depression occurs when entertaining, charming, vivacious self-image is punctured, resulting in feelings of emptiness that disappear once attentiveness can be resolicited. Boredom and depression may be readily confused, with dramatic somatic complaints providing relief from respites of inattentiveness from omnipotent and omniscient surrogates.

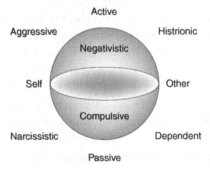

NARCISSISTIC: Sees self as superior and talented, and thus, automatically worthwhile. Self-esteem is assumed, not earned. Depression occurs when sense of specialness is repeatedly invalidated by objective events, public humiliations, or social comparison with persons even more "special," or through frustrated sense of entitlement, as when subjects are unable to obtain relief from tedium they so thoroughly deplore.

COMPULSIVE: Depression ensues when the criticism of superego introjects cannot be assuaged, either because of objectively imperfection in performances, leading to actual or feared harsh criticism by authority figures in real world, and thus a realistic foundation for repressed guilt. Depression may also occur when compulsive is forced to work in settings where objective standards of success, approval, or performance feedback are ambiguous due to insufficient structure, leading to feelings of loss of control. Somatic symptoms provide objective excuse for poor performances.

DEPENDENT: Sees self as weak and inadequate; bonds with strong surrogates immunize against depressive feelings; depression most likely when relationship with primary instrumental surrogate is threatened, either through abandonment or death, when feelings of aloneness and helplessness become overwhelming; somatic complaints function to defeat demands for greater responsibility and instrumental competency; subjects may blame self when relationships fail, increasing their own sense of guilt and negative self-worth.

Figure 2.5
Depressive inputs: Pleasure-related personalities.

PARANOID: Uses paranoid feelings to defend against depression; disavows feelings of resignation and inadequacy through projection, thus saving self-image of potency and confidence; depression is a sign of weakness that others are trying to inflict upon the subject; hopelessness and helplessness run counter to autonomous self-ideal and must be fought against as imposed from without.

SCHIZOID: Depression results from seeing self as having failed in all important aspirations, as being a disappointment to self and others and voided own potentialities; refusal to relate through isolation inside the self represents fallback position, an unwillingness to put objective inadequacies of self on public display; lack of motivation becomes logical way to prevent objective evaluation and feedback about feared inadequacies; attempts to solve problem by evolving autistic criteria for self-esteem, thereby providing foundation for a personalized creativity that frees self from total depressive collapse.

MASOCHISTIC: Depression constitutes a pervasive affect, but is characterized by excessive self-criticism, rather than resignation, as in depressive personality. Unlike the compulsive, the masochist has concluded that sadistic introjects cannot be placated, and has joined forces with them as a kind of self-sadism. Depressive feelings worsen when guilt cannot be expiated through overwork and self-sabotage, or when the subject feels overbenefited in relationships in some way. Somatic symptoms may provide a needed albatross when things are going too well.

AVOIDANT: Sees self as so shamed and unattractive that scorn and contempt are provoked from others, thereby foreclosing all hope of relatedness and intimacy; faults are imagined and magnified, leading to self-hatred; longs for creative expression, but evaluates own productions so harshly that motivation becomes impossible to sustain.

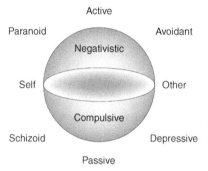

SADISTIC: Depression ensues when victims seem to have finally escaped punishment or become immune to its effects, leaving the sadist unable to work out their hostile enmeshment on the world. Such individuals feel extremely frustrated, alone, and impotent when unable to create pain in others and savor their suffering. Others inflict pain as a means of reacting against the shame they believe the world should heap upon themselves. Lack of a victim only legitimizes sense of shame, creating a desperation that can turn to resignation when search for a sufferer looks dim.

DEPRESSIVE: Sees self as so needy and pathetic that no helper will champion its causes, as abandoned and despised, and helpless before a myriad of life challenges; paralyzed by the complexity of life; and resigned to a state of being alone and misunderstood, seeing self with a capacity for empathy and feeling to which no one apparently can relate; somatic complaints may be used to provide objective evidence of disability, excusing shortcomings, propping up need for instrumental surrogates, and coercing nurturance from others.

Figure 2.6

Depressive inputs: Pain-related personalities.

65

the relationship between depression and personality, organized in terms of the revised evolutionary model, for each of the personality disorders. Thus, we find that, for the Negativist, depression ensues when the world seems even more inherently amoral and unjust and the self more misunderstood and cosmically persecuted than is usual. This may occur after abandonment by frustrated lovers, demotion at work, or other serious shortfall, may be in part provoked by the Negativist, or may occur when the Negativist has been prevented from complaining about or sabotaging the ruling regime or forced into highly structured surroundings that essentially coerce behavior, leaving him or her helpless to vent rebellious feelings. The Histrionic grooms the self-presentation to attract a steady stream of instrumental surrogates. Depression occurs when that entertaining, charming, vivacious self-image is punctured, resulting in feelings of emptiness that disappear once attentiveness can be resolicited. Boredom and depression may be readily confused, with dramatic somatic complaints providing relief from respites of inattentiveness from ideally omnipotent and omniscient surrogates. Subtypes of personality simply offer diverse sets of hypotheses for clinicians to entertain. As with domains of personality, the revised evolutionary model suggests that vulnerabilities to depression, and to most Axis I conditions, can be interrelated and differentiated in a single space. In theory, a personality subtype would possess the greatest vulnerability to depression (or any other Axis I disorder) when the mismatch between person and environment was greatest for its primary pattern. Like personality traits, situations vary in terms of their generality. Accordingly, subtypes formed by adjacent personality constructs (e.g., a Compulsive-Dependent) could be more vulnerable to symptom production than subtypes whose major elevations occur at a distance, as such individuals could encounter situations broad enough to frustrate the full range of their coping mechanisms.

CONCLUSION

In this chapter, we looked at the diagnosis of personality subtypes in Millon's theory and on the MCMI-III. We examined the psychometric structure of the MCMI-III and suggested certain clinical pearls that might assist in the interpretive process, particularly the use of diagnostic efficiency statistics, as well as strategies for disambiguating code types where 3, 4, or 5 scales are approximately equally elevated. We argued that the items of the MCMI-III could be used to derive scales designed to assess specific types, using 10 subtypes of psychopathy as an example. Finally, we argued that the theoretical basis on which the subtypes of personality are generated and assessed could be revised so that comorbidity is no longer an artifact of the diagnostic system, but instead emerges as a complement to the natural relationships that exist in an integrated personologic space termed the revised evolutionary theory. Principles of normality and pathology were contrasted with typical dimensional views of personality and with those of Millon's original formulation. It was suggested that the revised evolutionary model could guide the operationalization of personality subtypes in a much more precise manner than the original theory, and a structural model of the defense mechanisms was put forward. Finally, vulnerabilities to the Axis I conditions were also structurally strategized, these constituting causal hypotheses that might be applicable to any given personality subtype.

REFERENCES

Albeniz, A., & Holmes, J. (1996). Psychotherapy integration: Its implications for psychiatry. *British Journal of Psychiatry, 169*(5), 563–570.

Allport, G. W., & Odbert, H. S. (1936). Trait names: A psycholexical study. *Psychological Monographs, 47*(whole issue).

American Psychiatric Association. (1980). *Diagnostic and statistical manual of mental disorders* (3rd ed.). Washington, DC: Author.

American Psychiatric Association. (1987). *Diagnostic and statistical manual of mental disorders* (3rd ed., rev.). Washington, DC: Author.

American Psychiatric Association. (1994). *Diagnostic and statistical manual of mental disorders* (4th ed.). Washington, DC: Author.

Beck, A. T., & Freeman, A. F. (1990). *Cognitive therapy of personality disorders.* New York: Guilford Press.

Benjamin, L. S. (1974). Structured analysis of social behavior. *Psychological Review, 81,* 392–425.

Benjamin, L. S. (1986). Adding social and intrapsychic descriptors to Axis I of *DSM-III.* In T. Millon & G. L. Klerman (Eds.), *Contemporary directions in psychopathology: Toward the* DSM-IV (pp. 599–638). New York: Guilford Press.

Benjamin, L. S. (1993). *Interpersonal diagnosis and treatment of personality disorders.* New York: Guilford Press.

Benjamin, L. S. (1996). *Interpersonal diagnosis and treatment of personality disorders.* New York: Guilford Press.

Blackburn, R., Donnelly, J. P., Logan, C., & Renwick, S. J. (2004). Convergent and discriminative validity of interview and questionnaire measures of personality disorder in mentally disordered offenders: A multitrait-multimethod analysis using confirmatory factor analysis. *Journal of Personality Disorders, 18*(2), 129–150.

Blount, C., Evans, C., Birch, S., Warren, F., & Norton, K. (2002). The properties of self-report research measures: Beyond psychometrics. *Psychological Psychotherapy, 75*(Pt 2), 151–164.

Bowlby, J. (1982). *Attachment and loss: Vol 1. Attachment.* New York: Basic Books. (Original work published 1969)

Campbell, D. T., & Fiske, D. W. (1959). Convergent and discriminant validation by the multitrait-multimethod matrix. *Psychological Bulletin, 56,* 81–105.

Charter, R. A., & Lopez, M. N. (2002). Millon Clinical Multiaxial Inventory (MCMI-III): The inability of the validity conditions to detect random responders. *Journal of Clinical Psychology, 58*(12), 1615–1617.

Clark, L. A. (1990). Toward a consensual set of symptom clusters for assessment of personality disorder. In J. N. Butcher & C. D. Spielberger (Eds.), *Advances in personality assessment* (Vol. 8, pp. 243–266). Hillsdale, NJ: Erlbaum.

Clark, L. A. (1993). *Manual for the Schedule for Nonadaptive and Adaptive Personality (SNAP).* Minneapolis, MN: University of Minnesota Press.

Clark, L. A., & Watson, D. W. (1990). *General Temperament Survey (GTS).* Unpublished manuscript, Southern Methodist University.

Cleckley, H. (1950). *The mask of sanity.* St Louis: C. V. Mosby.

Cloninger, R. C. (1986). A unified biosocial theory of personality and its role in the development of anxiety states. *Psychiatric Developments, 3,* 167–226.

Cloninger, R. C. (1987). A systematic method for clinical description and classification of personality variants. *Archives of General Psychiatry, 44,* 573–588.

Costa, P. T., & McCrae, R. R. (1992). The five-factor model of personality and its relevance to personality disorders. *Journal of Personality Disorders, 6,* 343–359.

Craig, R. J. (1999). Testimony based on the Millon Clinical Multiaxial Inventory: Review, commentary, and guidelines. *Journal of Personality Assessment, 73*(2), 290–304.

Craig, R. J. (2000). Prevalence of Personality Disorders among Cocaine and Heroin Addicts. *Substance Abuse, 21*(2), 87–94.

Craig, R. J., Bivens, A., & Olson, R. (1997). MCMI-III-derived typological analysis of cocaine and heroin addicts. *Journal of Personality Assessment, 69*(3), 583–595.

Cronbach, L. J., & Gleser, G. C. (1965). *Psychological tests and personnel decisions.* Urbana: University of Illinois Press.

Davis, R. D. (1996). *Foundational studies in the creation of MCMI-III abbreviated forms.* Unpublished dissertation, University of Miami.

Davis, R. D., & Millon, T. (1999). Models of personality and its disorders. In T. Millon, P. Blaney, & R. D. Davis (Eds.), *The Oxford textbook of psychopathology.* New York: Oxford University Press.

Davis, R. D., & Wenger, A. (1997). Validation of the MCMI-III. In T. Millon (Ed.), *The Millon Inventories: Clinical and personality assessment.* New York: Guilford Press.

Dreessen, L., Arntz, A., Hendriks, T., Keune, N., & van den Hout, M. (1999). Avoidant personality disorder and implicit schema-congruent information processing bias: A pilot study with a pragmatic inference task. *Behavioral Research and Therapy, 37*(7), 619–632.

Fromm, E. (1973). *The anatomy of human destructiveness.* New York: Holt, Rinehart and Winston.

Hempel, C. G. (1965). *Aspects of scientific explanation.* New York: Free Press.

Hsu, L. M. (2002). Diagnostic validity statistics and the MCMI-III. *Psychological Assessment, 14*(4), 410–422.

Jackson, D. N. (1971). The dynamics of structured tests. *Psychological Review, 78,* 229–248.

Kass, F., Spitzer, R. L., Williams, J. B., & Widiger, T. (1989). Self-defeating personality disorder and *DSM-III-R:* Development of the diagnostic criteria. *American Journal of Psychiatry, 146*(8), 1022–1026.

Kennedy, S. H., Katz, R., Rockert, W., Mendlowitz, S., Ralevski, E., & Clewes, J. (1995). Assessment of personality disorders in anorexia nervosa and bulimia nervosa. A comparison of self-report and structured interview methods. *Journal of Nervous and Mental Diseases, 183*(6), 358–364.

Kernberg, O. F. (1984). *Severe personality disorders.* New Haven, CT: Yale University Press.

Kernberg, O. F. (1996). A psychoanalytic theory of personality disorders. In J. F. Clarkin & M. F. Lenzenweger (Eds.), *Major theories of personality disorder* (pp. 106–140). New York: Guilford Press.

Kiesler, D. J. (1983). The 1982 Interpersonal Circle: A taxonomy for complementarity in human transactions. *Psychological Review, 90,* 185–214.

Kuhn, T. S. (1970). *The structure of scientific revolutions* (2nd ed.). Chicago: University of Chicago Press.

Lenzenweger, M. F., Clarkin, J. F., Kernberg, O. F., & Foelsch, P. A. (2001). The Inventory of Personality Organization: Psychometric properties, factorial composition, and criterion relations with affect, aggressive dyscontrol, psychosis proneness, and self-domains in a nonclinical sample. *Psychological Assessment, 13*(4), 577–591.

Livesley, W. J., Jackson, D. N., & Schroeder, M. L. (1989). A study of the factorial structure of personality pathology. *Journal of Personality Disorders, 3,* 292–306.

Livesley, W. J., & Jang, K. L. (2000). Toward an empirically based classification of personality disorder. *Journal of Personal Disorders, 14*(2), 137–151.

Livesley, W. J., Schroeder, M. L., Jackson, D. N., & Jang, K. L. (1994). Categorical distinctions in the study of personality disorder: Implications for classification. *Journal of Abnormal Psychology, 103*(1), 6–17.

Loevinger, J. (1957). Objective tests as instruments of psychological theory. *Psychological Reports, 3,* 635–694.

Marks, I. M. (2002). The maturing of therapy: Some brief psychotherapies help anxiety/depressive disorders but mechanisms of action are unclear. *British Journal of Psychiatry, 180,* 200–204.

McCann, J. T., & Dyer, F. J. (1996). *Forensic assessment with the Millon Inventories.* New York: Guilford Press.

McCrae, R. R., Yang, J., Costa, P. T., Jr, Dai, X., Yao, S., Cai, T., et al. (2001). Personality profiles and the prediction of categorical personality disorders. *Journal of Personality, 69*(2), 155–174.

McDermut, W., Zimmerman, M., & Chelminski, I. (2003). The construct validity of depressive personality disorder. *Journal of Abnormal Psychology, 112*(1), 49–60.

Meehl, P. E. (1978). Theoretical risks and tabular asterisks: Sir Karl, Sir Ronald, and the slow progress of soft psychology. *Journal of Consulting and Clinical Psychology, 46,* 806–834.

Millon, T. (1969). *Modern psychopathology: A Biosocial Approach to maladaptive learning and functioning.* Philadelphia: Saunders.

Millon, T. (1981). *Disorders of personality:* DSM-III, *Axis II.* New York: Wiley.

Millon, T. (1990). *Toward a new personology: An evolutionary model.* New York: Wiley.

Millon, T., Everly, G., & Davis, R. D. (1993). How can knowledge of psychopathology facilitate psychotherapy integration? A view from the personality disorders. *Journal of Psychotherapy Integration, 3,* 331–352.

Millon, T., & Davis, R. D. (1996). Disorders of Personality: *DSM-IV* and Beyond. New York: Wiley.

Millon, T., Millon, C., & Green, C. (1987). Millon Clinical Multiaxial Inventory – II. Minneapolis: National Computer Systems.

Pepper, S. C. (1942). *World hypotheses.* Berkeley: University of California Press.

Pincus, A. L. (1994). The interpersonal circumplex and the interpersonal theory: Perspectives on personality and its pathology. In S. Strack & M. Lorr (Eds.), *Differentiating normal and abnormal personality* (pp. 114–136). New York: Springer.

Retzlaff, P., Stoner, J., & Kleinsasser, D. (2002). The use of the MCMI-III in the screening and triage of offenders [International]. *Journal Offender Therapy and Comprehensive Criminology, 46*(3), 319–332.

Reynolds, S. K., & Clark, L. A. (2001). Predicting dimensions of personality disorder from domains and facets of the Five-Factor Model. *Journal of Personality, 69*(2), 199–222.

Rossi, G., Van den Brande, I., Tobac, A., Sloore, H., & Hauben, C. (2003). Convergent validity of the MCMI-III personality disorder scales and the MMPI-2 scales. *Journal of Personality Disorders, 17*(4), 330–340.

Schoenberg, M. R., Dorr, D., & Morgan, C. D. (2003). The ability of the Millon Clinical Multiaxial Inventory—third edition to detect malingering. *Psychological Assessment, 15*(2), 198–204.

Shapiro, D. A., Barkham, M., Stiles, W. B., Hardy, G. E., Rees, A., Reynolds, S., et al. (2003). Time is of the essence: A selective review of the fall and rise of brief therapy research. *Psychological Psychotherapy, 76*(Pt 3), 211–235.

Sinha, B. K., & Watson, D. C. (2001). Personality disorder in university students: A multitrait-multimethod matrix study. *Journal of Personality Disorders, 15*(3), 235–244.

Skinner, H. (1986). Construct validation approach to psychiatric classification. In T. Millon & G. L. Klerman (Eds.), *Contemporary directions in psychopathology: Towards the* DSM-IV (pp. 307–329). New York: Guilford Press.

Spitzer, R. L., Feister, S., Gay, M., & Pfohl, B. (1991). Results of a survey of forensic psychiatrists on the validity of the sadistic personality disorder diagnosis. *American Journal of Psychiatry, 148*(7), 875–879.

Strack, S., Choca, J. P., & Gurtman, M. B. (2001). Circular structure of the MCMI-III personality disorder scales. *Journal of Personality Disorders, 15*(3), 263–274.

Strack, S., Lorr, M., & Campbell, L. (1990). An evaluation of Millon's circular model of personality disorders. *Journal of Personality Disorders, 4,* 353–361.

Waldeck, T. L., & Miller, L. S. (2000). Social skills deficits in schizotypal personality disorder. *Psychiatry Research, 93*(3), 237–246.

Westen, D., & Muderrisoglu, S. (2003). Assessing personality disorders using a systematic clinical interview: Evaluation of an alternative to structured interviews. *Journal of Personality Disorders, 17*(4), 351–369.

Widiger, T. A., & Costa, P. T., Jr. (2002). FFM personality disorder research. In P. T. Costa, Jr. & T. A. Widiger (Eds.), *Personality disorders and the five-factor model of personality.* Washington, DC: American Psychological Association.

CHAPTER 3

Alternative Interpretations for the Histrionic, Narcissistic, and Compulsive Personality Disorder Scales of the MCMI-III™

ROBERT J. CRAIG

THE RESEARCH evidence suggests that elevated scores on the MCMI Histrionic and Compulsive scales are most often obtained by nonclinical, healthy-functioning groups and may suggest normal traits associated with a histrionic and compulsive style. When they appear in clinical groups, which is atypical, they tend to be associated with less severity of the disorder and better treatment outcomes. However, elevated scores on the Narcissistic scale may suggest either a healthy confidant personality style or traits associated with the Narcissistic Personality Disorder. Caution is warranted when interpreting these scales.

The Millon Clinical Multiaxial Inventory (MCMI), as revised (Millon, 1983, 1987, 1994a), is a popular instrument for the assessment of personality disorders and major clinical syndromes (Piotrowski, 1997; Watkins, Campbell, Nieberding, & Hallmark, 1995). Along with a solid literature and research base (Butcher & Rouse, 1996; Craig, 1993a, 1997), there are published interpretive manuals (Choca, 2004; Craig, 1993b), two commercially available computer interpretive services (Craig, 1994; Millon, 1994b), and several specialty books to aid in the clinical interpretation of this test (McCann & Dyer, 1996; Millon, 1997; Retzlaff, 1995). However, unless one is aware of the research evidence on the test's scales, there may be a tendency to misinterpret MCMI scales and thereby arrive at faulty conclusions or recommendations. This is especially true for the Histrionic, Narcissistic, and Compulsive Personality Disorder scales because research evidence suggests that these scales may not be measuring the disorders implied by their scale designations. This will be elaborated on shortly.

The MCMI-III currently consists of four validity measures (called "modifying indices"; i.e., a Validity Index and Disclosure, Desirability, and Debasement scales), 11 "clinical personality patterns" (i.e., personality disorder scales; Schizoid, Avoidant, Depressive, Dependent, Histrionic, Narcissistic, Antisocial, Aggressive [Sadistic], Compulsive, Passive-Aggressive [Negativistic], and Self-Defeating), and three scales assessing severe personality pathology (i.e., Schizotypal, Borderline, and Paranoid). Finally, the test provides scales that assess major clinical syndromes (Anxiety, Somatoform, Bipolar: Manic, Dysthymia, Alcohol, Drug, and Posttraumatic Stress Disorders) and three severe syndromes (Thought Disorder, Major Depression, and Delusional Disorder).

It is critical for any test to have a body of research that supports the basic dimensions purportedly measured by its scales. It is also critical for the clinician to be aware of this research to avoid interpretive errors. For example, the Major Depression scale of the MCMI-I and II was meant to measure psychotic depression (Millon, 1983, 1987). However, the research evidence demonstrated poor convergent validity with similar measures for this scale. This was because there were no vegetative items in the scale that reflected the more severe form of the depression spectrum disorders. The presence of the vegetative signs was the hallmark of the diagnostic criteria for Major Depression, yet they were absent from the item pool of the scale. Thus, there was low agreement between the MCMI Major Depression scale(s) and other measures of Major Depression. This has been rectified in the MCMI-III scale for Major Depression, which brings the item content more in line with the official diagnostic criteria for the disorder.

This was one of the more egregious findings in MCMI-based research, but there are others. The most contentious ones may be the meaning of elevated scores on the Histrionic, Narcissistic, and Compulsive disorders of the MCMI. The research evidence to date seems to suggest that these scales may not be measuring the disorders implied by their names. The evidence includes (1) convergent validity studies correlating these scales with similar measures, (2) research findings correlating these scales with measures of mental health and measures of maladjustment, and (3) code types associated with clinical and nonclinical populations. It is the purpose of this chapter to present this evidence and then to offer other interpretations for elevations on these scales.[1]

CONVERGENT VALIDITY

Table 3.1 presents research data on the convergent validity of the Histrionic, Narcissistic, and Compulsive Personality Disorder scales. As there is no gold standard with which to demonstrate the validity of a given personality disorder scale, researchers have had to correlate these scales with similar measures. Although this strategy sounds acceptable, it may result in comparing a solidly developed and standardized instrument or scale with one that is less than adequate scientifically.

The clearest evidence for a lack of convergent validity is that seen for the Compulsive Personality Disorder scale. This scale almost uniformly correlates *negatively* with other measures of Compulsive Personality Disorder, particularly with the MMPI, ranging from .00 to −.50, with a median of −.27. The scale shows low and mostly negative correlations with other measures of Compulsive Personality Disorder as well.

The convergent validity of the MCMI Histrionic scale (all versions) appears quite satisfactory. Its correlation ranged from .57 to .85, with a median correlation of .68 with the MMPI Histrionic. Similarly, MCMI Narcissism correlated with MMPI Narcissistic, ranging from .49 to .78, with a median of .65, suggesting good correspondence to similar measures.

When data were aggregated for all self-report measures of PDs (MMPI PD), Personality Disorder Questionnaire (PDQ), Wisconsin PD, and Coolidge Axis II Inventory, the MCMI Histrionic correlated ranging from −.05 to .85, with a median of .68, based on 18 data sets; MCMI Narcissistic correlated ranging from −.05 to .78, with a median of .61; MCMI Compulsive correlated ranging from .00 to −.50, with a median of −.26.

Another consistent finding across the data is that these three scales tend to have higher correlations, generally in the moderate range, with their scale counterparts when both are derived from self-report measures. Their convergent validity is low when they are compared to structured clinical interviews measuring these same disorders.

MCMI Histrionic correlations with the Structured Clinical Interview for *DSM* Personality Disorders (SCID I/II) ranged from −.03 to .32, with a median of .11; MCMI Narcissistic correlations ranged from −.02 to .31, with a median of .13; MCMI Compulsive correlations ranged from .00 to

---

[1] The stimulus for this review was several psychologists calling me to inquire about the interpretation of these scales, especially in custody evaluations and in civil damage suits.

Table 3.1

Correspondence of MCMI Histrionic, Narcissistic, and Compulsive
Scales with Similar Measures from Other Personality Disorder Measures

Authors	Instrument	MCMI	Hist r′	Narc r′	Comp r′
Morey & Levine (1988)	MMPI PD	I	.85	.68	.00
Dubro & Wetzler (1989)	MMPI PD	I	.66	.55	−.42
McCann (1989)	MMPI PDI	I	.68	.78	−.30
Zarella, Schuerger, & Ritz (1990)	MMPI PD	I	.71	.70	−.50
		I	.44	.49	−.49
Chatham, Tibbals, & Harrington (1993)	MMPI PD	I	X	.66	X
Schuller, Bagby, Levitt, & Joffe (1993)	MMPI PD	I.	69	.73	−.27
Wise (1994)	MMPI PD	I	.63	.66	−.13
McCann (1991)	MMPI PD	II	.74	.65	−.04
Hicklin & Widiger (2000)	MMPI PD	III	.73	.65	−.26
Wise (1996)	MMPI-2 PD	II	.57	.68	−.10
Wise (2001)	MMPI-2 PD	II	.61	.54	−.02
Lindsay ,Sankis, & Widiger (2000)	MMPI-2 PD	III	.73	.55	X
	PDQ-4	III	−.05	.27	X
Hogg, Jackson, Rudd, & Edwards (1990)	SIDP	I.50	.32	.43	
Torgersen & Alnaes (1990)	SIDP	I.20	.18	-.05	
Turley, Bates, Edwards, & Jackson (1992)	SIDPII	.07	.02	X	
Klein et al. (1993)	WISCPD	I	.36	.16	−.32
Coolidge & Merwin (1992)	Coolidge	II	.73	−.05	.56
Renneberg, Chambliss, Dowdall, Fauerbach, & Gracely (1992)	SCID	II	.14	.16	.38
Kennedy et al. (1995)	SCID-II	II	−.03	−.02	.09
Hills (1995)	SCID-II	II	.09	.11	.00
Marlowe, Husband, Bonieskie, Kirby, & Platt (1997)	SCID-II	II	.32	.31	.03
Soldz, Budman, Demby, & Merry (1993)	PDE	II	.56	.41	−.05

Authors	Instrument	MCMI	Hist r'	Narc r'	Comp r'
Hart, Dutton, & Newlove (1993)	PDE	II	.36	.22	−.01
Wierzbicki & Gorman (1995)	PDQ-R	II	.61	.47	.14
Lindsay et al. (2000)	PDQ-R	III		.27	
	MMPI-PD	III	.73	.27	X
Silberman, Roth, Segal, & Burns (1997)	Coolidge	II	.10	.40	−.11

Coolidge = Coolidge Axis II Inventory (now called the Coolidge Assessment Battery); MMPI PD = Personality Disorder scale from the Minnesota Multiphasic Personality Inventory; PDE = Personality Disorder Evaluation; PDQ-R = Personality Disorder Questionnaire-Revised; r' = Correlation coefficient; SCID = Structured Clinical Interview for DSM Disorders-Personality Disorder Module; SIDP = Structured Inventory for DSM Personality Disorders; WISCPD = Wisconsin Personality Disorders: Narcissism.

.38, with a median of .06 (all based on four studies). MCMI Histrionic correlations with the Structured Inventory for *DSM* Personality Disorders (SIDP) ranged from .07 to .50, with a median of .20; for MCMI Narcissistic, correlations ranged from .02 to .32, with a median of .18. These data were based on only three studies. Correlations of MCMI Compulsive were based on two studies, with data showing correlations of .43 and −.05, respectively. If we compute MCMI correlations by combining all structured clinical interviews (i.e., SCID, SIDP, Personality Disorder Evaluation), we find that the Histrionic scale showed correlations ranging from −.03 to .56, with a median of .14; Narcissism correlated from −.02 to .41, with a median of .18; and Compulsive correlated from −.05 to .43, with a median of .02. These correlations were based on nine data sets. This finding is not specific to the MCMI but is a general finding in the research literature when different methodologies are compared to assess personality disorders (Craig, 2002; Farmer, 2000).

Another strategy is to correlate the scales with measures with which they should show a positive correlation given the underlying construct assessed by the scale. The data from this strategy appear in Table 3.2. The data are largely within these expectations for MCMI Histrionic and Narcissism scales but inconsistent for the Compulsive scale.

Convergent validity data with other tests of personality disorders do not tell the whole story. For these measures to demonstrate ecological validity, they should not appear in code types in nonclinical groups and should appear in the code types of patients with the underlying disorder

Table 3.2

Correspondence of MCMI Histrionic, Narcissistic, and
Compulsive Scales with Similar Measures

Authors	Instrument	MCMI	Hist r′	Narc r′	Comp r′
Broday (1988)	Perfectionism	I	X	X	−.37
Prifitera & Ryan (1984)	NPI	I	X	.66	X
Auerback (1984)	NPI	I	X	.55	X
Emmons (1987)	NPI	I	X	.27	X
Chatham et al. (1993)	NPI	I	X	.75	X
Morey (1985)	ICL Narc	I	X	.51	X
McAllister, Baker, Mannes, Stewart, & Sutherland (2002)	Self-Esteem	II	X	.43	X
Chick, Martin, Nevels, & Cotton (1994)	*DSM-III-R*	I	.00	.09	.05
Frost, Krause, & Steketee (1996)	Hoarding Scale II	X	X	.13	
Costa & McCrae (1990)	NEO				
	Neuroticism	I	X	X	−.39
		II	X	X	−.09
	Extroversion	I	.60	.47	−.09
		II	.57	.42	−.03
	Agreeableness	I	X	X	.09
		II	X	X	.15
	Conscientiousness	I	X	X	.38
		II	X	X	.52
Lehne (1994)	NEO	I			
	Neuroticism		X	X	−.63
	Extroversion		.63	.57	.21
	Agreeableness		X	X	.58
	Conscientiousness		X	X	.36
Strack (1991)	PACL Sociable	.59	X	X	
	Confidant	X	.46	X	
	Respectful	X	X	.59	
Wise (1994)	MBHI	I			
	Sociable		.51	X	X
	Confidant		X	.53	X
	Respectful		X	X	.15
Millon (1994a)	SCL-90-R O/C III	X	X	−.37	
	MMPI Pt	III	X	X	−.47
	MMPI Hy	III	−.11	X	X

Authors	Instrument	MCMI	Hist r′	Narc r′	Comp r′
Gough & Bradley (1996)	CPI Social	I			
	Presence–men	.60	X	X	
	Women	.69	X	X	
	CPI Self-				
	Acceptance Men		X	.64	X
	Women		X	.60	X
Bayon, Hill,	TCI Novelty	II	.38	X	X
Svrakic, Przybeck,					
& Cloninger (1996)	Seeking				

CPI = California Psychological Inventory; ICI Narc = Interpersonal Adjective Checklist: Narcissism; MBHI Conf = Millon Behavioral Health Index Confidence; NEO Ext = Extroversion Factor from the Neuroticism Extroversion Openness to Experience Personality test; NPI = Narcissistic Personality Inventory; O/C = Obsessive/Compulsive scale from the Symptom Checklist-90-Revised; Pt = Psychasthenia; r′ = Correlation coefficient; SCL-90-R Hy = Hysteria; SM-III-R Cklt = A checklist from *DSM-III-R* personality disorders; TCI = Temperament and Character Inventory.

measured by the scale. They should correlate positively with measures of psychopathology and personality pathology and negatively with measures of mental health. We inspect these data next.

HISTRIONIC SCALE

There are four lines of evidence that suggest that this scale is measuring a histrionic style but not a histrionic disorder.

1. *This scale correlates positively with measures of mental health and negatively with measures of maladjustment.* The Histrionic scale correlated positively and moderately with the California Psychological Inventory (CPI) scales of Social Poise (.63), Sociability (.62), and Self-Acceptance (.55; Holliman & Guthrie, 1989); in the CPI's most recent revision (CPI-R), Histrionic correlated with Social Poise .60 for men and .69 for women; Self-Acceptance correlated .55 for men and .68 for women (Gough & Bradley, 1996); MCMI Histrionic correlated moderately and positively with the 16 Personality Factor (16PF) primary factors of Dominant (E), Enthusiastic (F), and Venturesome (H), and with the second-order factors of Extroversion (.64) and Independent (Craig & Olson, 1993; Hyer, Woods, Boudewyns, Harrison, & Tamkin, 1990) and had negative correlations with Conscientiousness on scales measuring the five-factor model of personality (Costa & McCrae, 1990;

Soldz, Budman, Demby, & Merry, 1993) and with the Sociable scale (.50) of the Personality Adjective Check List (Strack, 1991). It positively correlated with the MMPI-derived Ego Strength (Es) scale and negatively (−.72) with Wiggins Social Maladjustment (Millon, 1983). Elevated scores on Histrionic were associated with higher scores on the Eysenck Personality Inventory factor of Extroversion (Gabrys et al., 1988). The Histrionic scale shows generally low and negative correlations with many scales from the Profile of Mood States (POMS; McMahon & Davidson, 1985) and with the Symptom Check List-90-Revised (SCL-90-R) scales for both the MCMI-I and III (Millon, 1983, 1994a). Higher scores on MCMI-III Histrionic scale were associated with lower scores on the Emotional Neglect subscale of the Childhood Trauma Questionnaire among 147 females with PTSD. Higher scores on the Adult Attachment scale (e.g., secure attachment) were associated with higher scores on the Histrionic scale (Allen, Coyne, & Huntoon, 1998).

Finally, factor studies for all three versions of the MCMI clearly demonstrate that the Histrionic scale correlates positively with items dealing with extroverted traits and ego-inflated self-evaluations and behaviors and negatively with items pertaining to general maladjustment and with isolation and withdrawal (Choca, 2004; Craig & Bivens, 1998).

2. *Nonclinical, healthy-functioning populations tend to obtain elevated scores on the Histrionic scale.* Researchers have reported that the following healthy groups had elevated scores on the Histrionic scale as their highest score: Air Force pilots in training (mean BR score 71) who actually had low scores on need for Exhibition—a histrionic trait—based on scores from the Personality Research Form (Retzlaff & Gibertini, 1987, 1988), undergraduates (Barrett & Etheridge, 1994; Boyle & Le Dean, 2000; Jay, Grove, & Grove, 1987; Richman & Nelson-Gray, 1994; Sinha & Watson, 1999; Terpylak & Schuerger, 1994), graduate students in psychology (mean BR score of 76; Jay et al., 1987), normal females (mean BR score of 74; Tisdale, Pendleton, & Marler, 1990), and normal community members (Hastings & Hamberger, 1994; Sugihara & Warner, 1999; Wall, Schuckit, Mungas, & Ehlers, 1990).[2]

3. *Similarly, this scale is relatively absent in the code types of clinical populations (Craig, 1995; see also Chapter 5).* When it does appear, it seems to be a favorable prognostic sign.[3] Only one study (Stark & Campbell, 1988) has

---

[2] Although the test manual states that BR scores > 84 reflect traits associated with the disorder at the diagnostic level and BR scores of 74 to 84 reflect traits associated with the disorder but not at the diagnostic level, researchers have generally used BR > 74 as an operational measure of the diagnosis. This is particularly true when computing diagnostic power statistics (not presented here).

[3] The finding of an isolated group with this code type does not establish the scale's validity with this group as a clinical entity. In most cases, other researchers found that these groups have had code types that were not associated with this scale. For example, male batterers tend to score highest on Antisocial, Aggressive, or Passive-Aggressive (Negativistic). Substance abusers tend to score highest on Antisocial (Craig, 1995).

found clinical patients (drug abusers) with a modal code type reflecting elevated base rate scores on Histrionic at the diagnostic (i.e., BR > 84) level. A few others have found clinical populations with their highest scores on Histrionic elevated at the subclinical (BR 74 to 84) levels. These include bulimics (Garner, Olmsted, Davis, & Rocket, 1990), females in outpatient psychotherapy (Tisdale et al., 1990), male and female alcoholics (Matano, Locke, & Schwartz, 1994), male batterers (Hastings & Hamberger, 1994), patients with Late Luteal Phase Dysphoria (i.e., PMS; Parry, Ehlers, Mostofi, & Phillips, 1996), patients with attention-deficit disorders (May & Bos, 2000), and female child custody litigants (Lampel, 1999; McCann et al., 2001). (Note that most of these populations are primarily women, though there are a few exceptions.)

4. *Patients (N = 54) treated for at least 15 sessions with rational-emotive psychotherapy and who also had higher Histrionic scale scores had better outcomes, including better mental health and higher self-esteem* (Leaf, Ellis, DiGiuseppe, & Mass, 1991; Leaf et al., 1990). Elevated scores were also associated with less distress and more positive life events and fewer social problems and were negatively correlated with measures of irrationality and positively correlated with measures of rationality (Leaf, Alington, Ellis, DiGiuseppe, & Mass, 1992; Leaf, Alington, Mass, DiGiuseppe, & Ellis, 1991). Other populations whose elevated Histrionic scores predicted good outcomes include bulimics (Garner et al., 1990) and male batters with a good premorbid history (Hastings & Hamberger, 1994).

COMPULSIVE SCALE

Four lines of evidence suggest that this scale is measuring generally healthy-functioning people. The data come from many of the same research studies cited for the Histrionic scale.

1. *As with the Histrionic scale, the Compulsive scale correlates positively with measures of mental health and negatively with measures of maladjustment.* For example, this scale moderately correlated with MMPI measures of Ego Strength (Langevin et al., 1988; Millon, 1983; Smith, Carroll, & Fuller, 1988). It moderately correlated with CPI scales of Well-Being, Self-Control, Achievement via Conformance, and Intellectual Efficiency (Holliman & Guthrie, 1989). Patients with higher Compulsive scores had better outcomes, including better mental health and higher self-esteem (Leaf et al., 1990; Leaf, Ellis, et al., 1991). Elevated Compulsive scores were also associated with less distress and more positive life events and fewer social problems and were negatively correlated with measures of irrationality and positively correlated with measures of rationality (Leaf

et al., 1992; Leaf, Alington, et al., 1991). The scale shows consistent negative relationships with the symptoms scales of the POMS (McMahon & Davidson, 1985) and with the SCL-90 (Millon, 1983). The Compulsive scale correlated .59 with the Respectful personal style of the Personality Adjective Checklist (PACL; Strack, 1991). In factor studies, high scores on the Compulsive scale, across all three versions of the scale, are positively associated with items dealing with controlled behaviors and emotions and negatively with items pertaining to maladjustment. Items on the Compulsive scale load negatively on Factor I (General Maladjustment) and negatively on Factor III (Antisocial Acting-Out; Choca, 2004; Craig & Bivens, 1998).

2. *Elevations on this scale tend to appear in psychologically healthy-functioning groups.* For example, the following groups attained their highest elevations on the Compulsive scale: first-year seminary students ($N = 52$; mean BR 75; Piersma, 1987), family practice residents ($N = 67$; mean BR 69; Lemkau, Purdy, Rafferty, & Rudisill, 1988), aviators ($N = 82$; mean BR 69; King, 1994), Air Force student pilots ($N = 73$; Retzlaff & Gibertini, 1987), nonabused males (Beasley & Stoltenberg, 1992), laminectomy patients (Herron, Turner, & Weiner, 1986), patients with eye disease (Mannis, Morrison, Holland, & Krachmer, 1987), chronically obese patients (Chandarana, Conlon, Holliday, Deslippe, & Field, 1990), low alpha-wave normals (Wall et al., 1990), and normal women (Tisdale et al., 1990).

3. *Scale elevations on Compulsive are absent in most clinical groups (Craig, 1995; see also Chapter 5). When it is present, it tends to occur as a positive predictive sign and reflect less severity in a given disorder.* Elevated scores on this scale predicted less severe depression and alcoholism and predicted a positive response to treatment (Joffe & Regan, 1991; McMahon, Flynn, & Davidson, 1985). Some groups of alcoholics, mostly in cluster analytic studies, have found a type with subclinical elevations on the Compulsive scale (Donat, 1988; Donat, Walters, & Hume, 1991, 1992; Matano et al., 1994; Mayer & Scott, 1988), but these scores were associated with higher functioning in male alcoholics (McMahon, Davidson, & Flynn, 1986), with transient depression (i.e., depression that abated after 1 month of treatment) among female alcoholics (McMahon & Tyson, 1990), with patients in remission from depression (Joffe & Regan, 1991), and in patients successfully treated for panic disorders (Reich, 1991).

4. *Patients with an Obsessive-Compulsive Disorder did not obtain elevated scores on the Compulsive scale.* In the only published study featuring patients with a primary Obsessive-Compulsive Disorder, the mean base rate score on the Compulsive Personality Disorder scale was 56 (i.e., in the normal range; Joffe, Swinson, & Regan, 1988).

NARCISSISTIC SCALE

Research on the Narcissistic scale shows a somewhat inconsistent pattern, suggesting that this scale may be measuring either a healthy personality style or a Narcissistic Personality Disorder.

1. *The scale correlates both positively and negatively with measures of mental health and maladjustment, depending on the measure.* The MCMI Narcissistic scale correlates moderately and positively with the CPI scales of Sociability, Dominance, Social Poise, and Self-Acceptance (Holliman & Guthrie, 1989); with the 16PF primary factors of Dominant, and with the second-order factors of Extroversion and Independent (Craig & Olson, 1992; Hyer et al., 1990); and with Extroversion of the five-factor model of personality (Costa & McCrae, 1990; Soldz et al., 1993). It correlated .40 with MMPI-derived Ego Strength scale, and −.71 with Wiggins Social Maladjustment (Millon, 1983) and .31 with Sociable, .46 with Confident, and .50 with Forceful relational styles of the PACL (Strack, 1991). Higher scores on MCMI-III Narcissism were associated with lower scores on the Emotional Neglect subscale of the Childhood Trauma Questionnaire among 147 females with PTSD. Higher scores on the Adult Attachment Scale (e.g., secure attachment) were associated with higher scores on Narcissism (Allen et al., 1998). MCMI-III Narcissism elevations predicted the need for less mental health service among 10,000 Colorado inmates (Retzlaff, Stoner, & Kleinsasser, 2002). However, it significantly and positively correlates with scores on the Narcissistic Personality Disorder (see Table 2.1).

As with the Histrionic scale, the Narcissistic scale generally shows low and negative correlations with many POMS scales (McMahon & Davidson, 1985) and with many symptom scales from the SCL-90-R (MCMI-III; Millon, 1994a). Factor studies with all versions of the MCMI clearly demonstrate that the Narcissism scale correlated positively with items dealing with extroverted traits and behaviors and negatively with items pertaining to general maladjustment and with isolation and withdrawal (Choca, 2004; Craig & Bivens, 1998).

2. *Elevations on this scale appear in nonclinical populations.* These include college students (Barrett & Etheridge, 1994; Holliman & Guthrie, 1989; Retzlaff, Sheehan, & Fiel, 1991), happily married men (Murphy, Meyer, & O'Leary, 1993), and Air Force pilot trainees (Butters, Retzlaff, & Gibertini, 1986; Retzlaff & Gibertini, 1987).

3. *Elevations on this scale also appear in clinical populations.* Only four studies have found clinical populations whose modal MCMI profiles were at the subclinical level on Narcissism yet were highest in the code type. These populations were patients with Schizophrenia (Jackson, Greenblatt,

Davis, Murphy, & Trimakas, 1991) and felons (Chantry & Craig, 1994; Hastings & Hamberger, 1994). Retzlaff and Bromley (1991) reported that alcoholic patients had elevated scores (mean BR 78; highest in the code type on the Narcissistic scale) but were labeled a "Healthy Subtype," based on their scores on the Basic Personality Inventory.

Patients ($N = 54$) treated for at least 15 sessions with rational-emotive psychotherapy and who also had higher scores on the Narcissistic scale had better outcomes, including better mental health and higher self-esteem, had less distress and more positive life events with fewer social problems, and had scores that correlated with measures of rationality rather than irrationality (Leaf, Ellis, et al., 1991; Leaf et al., 1992). The patients with Schizophrenia who scored at the subclinical level were those who were able to suppress their symptoms (Jackson et al., 1991), and the felons (batterers) were in a group with a good premorbid history (Hastings & Hamberger, 1994).

DISCUSSION

Evidence has been presented suggesting that the MCMI scales of Histrionic and Compulsive Personality Disorders may not be measuring a personality disorder at all. Rather, they seem to measure normal, non-clinical traits associated with those styles. Correlations with a variety of self-report measures and scales show that they consistently correlate positively with measures of mental health and life satisfaction and correlate negatively with measures of psychopathology. The Narcissistic scale appears to measure either a healthy ego functioning state or a Narcissistic Personality Disorder, as the scale correlates moderately with other measures of narcissism but also with measures of mental health and positive adjustment. This general conclusion has appeared across a variety of sample populations and in a variety of (treatment) settings (Leaf et al., 1990).

How should these scales be interpreted when they are elevated? When, in the clinician's judgment, the patient does have a personality disorder associated with elevations on either the Histrionic, Narcissistic, or Compulsive Personality Disorder scales, then the clinician's description of that personality should be congruent with the domains, traits, and behaviors associated with that disorder. If, however, clinical judgment determines that the patient does not meet the diagnostic criteria for that disorder, despite clinical elevations on the parent scale, then it is recommended that the clinical description of that personality be descriptive of personality traits associated with that style.

S. Strack (personal communication, April 2003) has suggested that, in such cases, the clinician interpret scale elevations as if they were elevations on the PACL (Strack, 1987; see also Chapter 4) and not on the MCMI. The logic behind this recommendation is that the PACL was developed to assess Millon personality styles in a nonclinical (i.e., nonpathological) population. There is evidence (Strack, 1991) that PACL scales are significantly related to MCMI counterpart scales and share common variance. Whether one uses the interpretive principles associated with PACL elevations or uses attenuated traits associated with the disorder at the diagnostic level, the clinician needs to seriously consider alternative interpretations when these scales are clinically elevated.

PERSONALITY DISORDERS VERSUS PERSONALITY STYLES

In this section we present for consideration common descriptions for these scale elevations based on whether or not the patient has the personality disorder or the personality style.

HISTRIONIC DISORDER

Clinical elevations describe a person who is likely to be excessively dramatic, theatrical, and attention getting to receive attention and approval. Such personalities profess undying adoration and approval of valued others. Others view these behaviors as phony and superficial, but Histrionics' unconscious use of denial prevents them from this self-observation. Often seductive in style, dress, or speech, they seek frequent stimulation and excitement and behave in an exhibitionistic manner to get praise and attention. They are impulsive and changeable, even fickle. Because they are emotionally labile, they are easily excited and prone to emotional outbursts, particularly when things do not go their way. They have strong needs for social acceptance and approval and hence are very gregarious, assertive, and socially outgoing. Due to their enchanting and seductively engaging manner, others are initially drawn to them, but relationships are usually shallow and strained due to their emotional outbursts and self-centeredness. They place their own needs above those of others, and this insensitivity irritates others. Beneath this aura of self-assurance and confidence may be a fear of autonomy and independence that compels the individual to constantly seek acceptance and approval. They may use denial and repression as their main defenses. When stressed, they are at risk for somatoform disorders and marital problems.

Histrionic Style

This personality style is characterized by traits of extroversion, attention seeking, sociability, gregariousness, and spontaneity. These individuals are outgoing, lively, animated, talkative, and often colorful and dramatic. They appear enthusiastic but also emotional and changeable and are easily bored. They enjoy novelty and excitement and like being in public but have a tendency to become angry and disgusted when things do not go their way. They may appear somewhat superficial and fickle. As long as they get their need for attention met, they are quite enjoyable and entertaining.

Narcissistic Disorder

Narcissistic patients are extremely self-centered, expect others to recognize them for their special qualities, and require constant praise and admiration. They have excessive expectations of entitlement and demand special favors simply on the basis of who they are. They appear arrogant, haughty, conceited, boastful, snobbish, pretentious, and supercilious. They can be momentarily charming but show a social imperturbability and exploit social relationships. Sometimes they behave in an autocratic manner because they feel they are superior to others. Although their basic personality style tends to alienate people, they seem rather indifferent and treat others with contempt. They may use rationalization as their main defense. Beneath this façade may be feelings of inadequacy and insecurity; hence, they may become overly sensitive to feelings of rejection. When they experience a narcissistic injury, they are prone to develop an Affective Disorder and perhaps Paranoia.

Narcissistic Style

These personality types are charming, self-centered, self-assured, self-reliant, confidant, and vain and have an attention-seeking personality style with feelings of entitlement and even uniqueness. They think well of themselves and may even demonstrate facts that back up their grandiose statements. They may act with an air of superiority, expecting others to quickly accede to their wishes, and behave selfishly. They generally are socially adept and can be witty. They enjoy status and recognition and act confidently. They are generally self-sufficient and tend to blame others for any failures.

COMPULSIVE DISORDER

These patients may be behaviorally rigid, constricted, meticulous, respectful, polite, conscientious, overconforming, organized, respectful, perhaps perfectionistic, formal, cooperative, moralistic, judgmental, efficient, and inflexible and may suppress their strong resentments and anger toward those, usually authority figures, whose approval they seek. They generally have a repetitive lifestyle of patterned behaviors. They impress people with their conscientiousness, but unconsciously they fear making mistakes and receiving disapproval. Unconsciously they feel inadequate and fear failure, so they behave in a polite, organized, meticulous, respectful, and overly serious manner. They are extremely respectful and deferential with superiors but may treat subordinates autocratically. They have a strong sense of duty and are models of propriety and restraint. With an anxious conformity, they try to avoid criticism. Their behavior stems from a conflict over felt hostility toward authority, which they wish to express, and a fear of social disapproval and rebuke should they expose this oppositional resentment. This forces them to become overly conforming and highly controlled, placing excessive demands on themselves to win favor, as they are plagued by self-doubts. They constantly worry over meeting external standards, and obsessive fear of social disapproval results in their being a model of proper behavior. They tend to have a strong sense of duty and strive to avoid criticism. They rely on achievement and accomplishment of personal goals to feel worthwhile. Obsessional thinking may or may not be present. They are at risk for developing an obsessive-compulsive clinical syndrome and psychophysiological disorders.

COMPULSIVE STYLE

These people are highly organized, efficient, duty-bound, obliging, respectful, reliable, self-reliant, conscientious, cooperative, productive, emotionally restrained, methodical, persistent, goal-directed, and socially conforming. They are rigid and not easily distracted from their high achievement needs. They strive to conform to conventional standards and to their own high standards of personal conduct. They are not necessarily competitive, prefer jobs that are highly structured with clear goals and standards, and may rely on superiors to provide them with a sense of direction. In fact, they possess many of the same traits as seen in the Compulsive personality but without the functional impairment. Their qualities are often valued in business, industry, and military venues.

COMMENT

It should be pointed out that these conclusions are primarily based on research evidence derived from the MCMI-I and II. Limited research data are available from the MCMI-III scales. The extent to which these conclusions apply to other measures of these disorders is also a matter of conjecture and future research. Because the MCMI has a substantial research base, we are able to generate conclusions and hypotheses that we cannot garner from most other measures of personality disorders that lack this firm research base.

Furthermore, the findings reported here may not be specific to the MCMI scales, but rather may be a result of the constructs assessed by the scales. In other words, it may be that there are definitional and criteria-set problems associated with the diagnosis, rather than problems with the scales that measure them. This is also a matter for future research. However, until further data become available, the clinician is cautioned against possible overinterpretation of the Histrionic, Narcissistic, and Compulsive scales of the MCMI-III.

REFERENCES

Allen, J. G., Coyne, L., & Huntoon, J. (1998). Complex posttraumatic stress disorder in women from a psychometric perspective. *Journal of Personality Assessment, 62,* 277–298.

Auerback, J. S. (1984). Validation of two scales for narcissistic personality disorder. *Journal of Personality Assessment, 48,* 649–653.

Barrett, T., & Etheridge, J. R. (1994). Verbal hallucinations in normals: III. Dysfunctional personality correlates. *Personality and Individual Differences, 16,* 57–62.

Bayon, C., Hill, K., Svrakic, D. M., Przybeck, T. R., & Cloninger, C. R. (1996). Dimensional assessment of personality in an outpatient sample: Relations of the systems of Millon and Cloninger. *Journal of Psychiatric Research, 30,* 341–352.

Beasley, R., & Stoltenberg, C. D. (1992). Personality characteristics of male spouse abusers. *Professional Psychology: Research and Practice, 23,* 310–317.

Boyle, G. J., & Le Dean, L. (2000). Discriminant validity of the illness behavior questionnaire and Millon Clinical Multiaxial Inventory-III in a heterogeneous sample of psychiatric outpatients. *Journal of Clinical Psychology, 56,* 779–791.

Broday, S. E. (1988). Perfectionism and the Millon basic personality patterns. *Psychological Reports, 63,* 791–794.

Butcher, J. N., & Rouse, S. V. (1996). Personality: Individual differences and clinical assessment. *Annual Review of Psychology, 47,* 87–111.

Butters, M., Retzlaff, P., & Gibertini, M. (1986). Non-adaptability to basic training and the Millon Clinical Multiaxial Inventory. *Military Medicine, 151,* 574–576.

Chandarana, P. C., Conlon, P., Holliday, M. D., Deslippe, T., & Field, V. A. (1990). A prospective study of psychosocial aspects of gastric stapling surgery. *Psychiatric Journal of the University of Ottawa, 15,* 32–35.

Chantry, K., & Craig, R. J. (1994). MCMI typologies of criminal sexual offenders. *Sexual Addiction and Compulsivity, 1,* 215–226.

Chatham, P. M., Tibbals, C. J., & Harrington, M. E. (1993). The MMPI and the MCMI in the evaluation of narcissism in a clinical sample. *Journal of Personality Assessment, 60,* 239–251.

Chick, D., Martin, S. K., Nevels, R., & Cotton, C. R. (1994). Relationship between personality disorders and clinical symptoms in psychiatric inpatients as measured by the Millon Clinical Multiaxial Inventory. *Psychological Reports, 74,* 331–336.

Choca, J. P. (2004). *Interpretive guide to the Millon Clinical Multiaxial Inventory* (3rd ed.). Washington, DC: American Psychological Association.

Coolidge, F. L., & Merwin, M. M. (1992). Reliability and validity of the Coolidge Axis II Inventory: A new inventory for the assessment of personality disorders. *Journal of Personality Assessment, 59,* 233–238.

Costa, P. T., & McCrae, R. R. (1990). Personality disorders and the five-factor model of personality. *Journal of Personality Disorders, 4,* 362–371.

Craig, R. J. (Ed.). (1993a). *The Millon Clinical Multiaxial Inventory: A clinical research information synthesis.* Hillsdale, NJ: Erlbaum.

Craig, R. J. (1993b). *Psychological assessment with the Millon Clinical Multiaxial Inventory (II): An interpretive guide.* Odessa, FL: Psychological Assessment Resources.

Craig, R. J. (1994). *MCMI-II/III interpretive system.* Odessa, FL: Psychological Assessment Resources.

Craig, R. J. (1995). Clinical diagnoses and MCMI code types. *Journal of Clinical Psychology, 51,* 352–360.

Craig, R. J. (1997). A selected review of the MCMI empirical literature. In T. Millon (Ed.), *The Millon inventories* (pp. 303–326). New York: Guilford Press.

Craig, R. J. (2002). Assessing personality and psychopathology with interviews. In J. R. Graham & J. A. Neglieri (Eds.), *Assessment psychology* (Vol. 10, pp. 487–508). New York: Wiley.

Craig, R. J., & Bivens, A. (1998). Factor structure of the MCMI-III. *Journal of Personality Assessment, 70,* 190–196.

Craig, R. J., & Olson, R. E. (1992). Relationship between MCMI-II scales and normal personality traits. *Psychological Reports, 71,* 699–705.

Donat, D. C. (1988). Millon Clinical Multiaxial Inventory (MCMI) clusters for alcohol abusers: Further evidence of validity and implications for medical psychotherapy. *Medical Psychotherapy, 1,* 41–50.

Donat, D. C., Walters, J., & Hume, A. (1991). Personality characteristics of alcohol dependent inpatients: Relationship of MCMI subtypes to self-reported drinking behavior. *Journal of Personality Assessment, 57,* 335–344.

Donat, D. C., Walters, J., & Hume, A. (1992). MCMI differences between alcoholics and cocaine abusers: Effects of age, sex, and race. *Journal of Personality Assessment, 58,* 96–104.

Dubro, A. F., & Wetzler, S. (1989). An external validity study of the MMPI personality disorder scales. *Journal of Clinical Psychology, 45*, 570–575.

Emmons, R. A. (1987). Narcissism: Theory and measurement. *Journal of Personality and Social Psychology, 52*, 11–17.

Farmer, R. F. (2000). Issues in the assessment and conceptualization of personality disorders. *Clinical Psychology Review, 7*, 823–851.

Frost, R. O., Krause, M. S., & Steketee, G. (1996). Hoarding and obsessive-compulsive symptoms. *Behavior Modification, 20*, 116–132.

Gabrys, J. B., Utendale, K. A., Schumph, D., Phillips, N., Peters, K., Robertson, G., et al. (1988). Two inventories for the measurement of psychopathology: Dimensions and common factorial space on Millon's Clinical and Eysenck's General Personality Scales. *Psychological Reports, 62*, 591–601.

Garner, D. M., Olmsted, M. R., Davis, R., & Rocket, W. (1990). The association between bulimic symptoms and reported psychopathology. *International Journal of Eating Disorders, 9*, 1–15.

Gough, H. G., & Bradley, P. (1996). *CPI manual* (3rd ed.). Los Angeles: Consulting Psychologists Press.

Hart, S. D., Dutton, D. G., & Newlove, T. (1993). The prevalence of personality disorder among wife assaulters. *Journal of Personality Disorders, 7*, 329–341.

Hastings, J. E., & Hamberger, L. K. (1994). Psychosocial modifiers of psychopathology for domestically violent and nonviolent men. *Psychological Reports, 74*, 112–114.

Herron, L., Turner, J., & Weiner, P. (1986). A comparison of the Millon Clinical Multiaxial Inventory and the Minnesota Multiphasic Personality Inventory as predictors of successful treatment by lumbar laminectomy. *Clinical Orthopaedics and Related Research, 203*, 232–238.

Hicklin, J., & Widiger, T. A. (2000). Convergent validity of alternative MMPI-2 personality disorder scale. *Journal of Personality Assessment, 75*, 502–518.

Hills, H. A. (1995). Diagnosing personality disorders: An examination of the MMPI-2 and MCMI-II. *Journal of Personality Assessment, 65*, 21–34.

Hogg, B., Jackson, H. J., Rudd, R. P., & Edwards, J. (1990). Diagnosing personality disorders in recent-onset schizophrenia. *Journal of Nervous and Mental Diseases, 179*, 194–199.

Holliman, N., & Guthrie, P. (1989). A comparison of the MCMI and the CPI in assessment of a nonclinical population. *Journal of Clinical Psychology, 45*, 373–382.

Hyer, L., Woods, M. G., Boudewyns, P. A., Harrison, W. R., & Tamkin, A. S. (1990). MCMI and 16PF with Vietnam veterans: Profiles and concurrent validation of MCMI. *Journal of Personality Disorders, 4*, 391–401.

Jackson, J. L., Greenblatt, R. L., Davis, W. E., Murphy, T. T., & Trimakas, K. (1991). Assessment of schizophrenic inpatients with the MCMI. *Journal of Personality Assessment, 51*, 243–253.

Jay, G. W., Grove, R. N., & Grove, K. S. (1987). Differentiation of chronic headache from non-headache pain patients using the Millon Clinical Multiaxial Inventory (MCMI). *Headache, 27*, 124–129.

Joffe, R. T., & Regan, J. J. (1991). Personality and family history of depression in patients with affective illness. *Journal of Psychiatric Research, 25,* 67–71.

Joffe, R. T., Swinson, R. P., & Regan, J. J. (1988). Personality features of obsessive-compulsive disorder. *American Journal of Psychiatry, 145,* 1127–1129.

Kennedy, S. H., Katz, R., Rockert, W., Mendlowitz, S., Ralevski, E., & Clewes, C. J. (1995). Assessment of personality disorders in anorexia nervosa and bulimia nervosa: A comparison of self-report and structured interview methods. *Journal of Nervous and Mental Diseases, 183,* 358–364.

King, R. E. (1994, March). Assessing aviators for personality pathology with the Millon Clinical Multiaxial Inventory (MCMI). *Aviation, Space, and Environmental Medicine.* 227–231.

Klein, M. H., Benjamin, L. S., Rosenfeld, R., Treece, C., Husted, J., & Greist, J. H. (1993). The Wisconsin Personality Disorders Inventory: Development, reliability, and validity. *Journal of Personality Disorders, 7,* 285–303.

Lampel, A. K. (1999). Use of the Millon Clinical Multiaxial Inventory-III in evaluating child custody litigants. *American Journal of Forensic Psychology, 17,* 19–31.

Langevin, R., Lang, R., Reynolds, R., Wright, P., Garrels, D., Marchese, V., et al. (1988). Personality and sexual anomalies: An examination of the Millon Clinical Multiaxial Inventory. *Annals of Sex Research, 1,* 13–32.

Leaf, R. C., Alington, D. E., Ellis, A., DiGiuseppe, R., & Mass, R. (1992). Personality disorders, underlying traits, social problems, and clinical syndromes. *Journal of Personality Disorders, 6,* 134–152.

Leaf, R. C., Alington, D. E., Mass, R., DiGiuseppe, R., & Ellis, A. (1991). Personality disorders, life events, and clinical syndromes. *Journal of Personality Disorders, 5,* 264–280.

Leaf, R. C., DiGiuseppe, R., Ellis, A., Mass, R., BackX, W., Wolf, J., et al. (1990). "Healthy" correlates of MCMI scales 4, 5, 6, and 7. *Journal of Personality Disorders, 4,* 312–328.

Leaf, R. C., Ellis, A., DiGiuseppe, R., & Mass, R. (1991). Rationality, self-regard and the "healthiness" of personality disorders. *Journal of Rational and Cognitive Behavior Therapy, 9,* 3–37.

Lehne, G. K. (1994). The NEO-PI and the MCMI in the forensic evaluation of sex offenders. In P. T. Costa & T. A. Widiger (Eds.), *Personality disorders and the five-factor model of personality.* (pp. 175–188). Washington, DC: American Psychological Association.

Lemkau, J. P., Purdy, R. R., Rafferty, J. P., & Rudisill, J. R. (1988). Correlates of burnout among family practice residents. *Journal of Medical Education, 63,* 682–691.

Lindsay, K. A., Sankis, L. M., & Widiger, T. A. (2000). Gender bias in self-report personality disorder inventories. *Journal of Personality Disorders, 14,* 218–232.

Lindsay, K. A., & Widiger, T. A. (1995). Sex and gender bias in self-report personality disorder inventories: Item analysis of the MCMI-II, MMPI, and PDQ-R. *Journal of Personality Assessment, 65,* 1–20.

Mannis, M. J., Morrison, T. L., Holland, E. J., & Krachmer, J. H. (1987). Personality trends in keratoconus: An analysis. *Archives of Ophthalmology, 105,* 798–800.

Marlowe, D. B., Husband, S. D., Bonieskie, L. M., Kirby, K. C., & Platt, J. J. (1997). Structured interview versus self-report test vantages for the assessment of personality pathology in cocaine dependence. *Journal of Personality Disorders, 11*, 177–190.

Matano, R. A., Locke, K. D., & Schwartz, K. (1994). MCMI personality subtypes for male and female alcoholics. *Journal of Personality Assessment, 63*, 250–264.

May, B., & Bos, J. (2000). Personality characteristics of ADHD adults assessed with the Millon Clinical Personality Inventory-II: Evidence of four distinct subtypes. *Journal of Personality Assessment, 75*, 237–246.

Mayer, G. S., & Scott, K. J. (1988). An exploration of heterogeneity in an inpatient male alcoholic population. *Journal of Personality Disorders, 2*, 243–255.

McAllister, H. A., Baker, J. D., Mannes, C., Stewart, H., & Sutherland, A. (2002). The optimal margin of illusion hypothesis: Evidence from the self-serving bias and personality disorders. *Journal of Social and Clinical Psychology, 21*, 414–426.

McCann, J. T. (1989). MMPI personality disorder scales and the MCMI: Concurrent validity. *Journal of Clinical Psychology, 45*, 365–369.

McCann, J. T. (1991). Convergent and discriminant validity of the MCMI-II and MMPI personality disorder scales. *Psychological Assessment: A Journal of Consulting and Clinical Psychology, 3*, 9–18.

McCann, J. T., & Dyer, F. J. (1996). *Forensic assessment with the Millon inventories.* New York: Guilford Press.

McCann, J. T., Flens, J. R., Campagna, V., Collman, P., Lazzaro, T., & Connor, E. (2001). The MCMI-III in child custody evaluations: A normative study. *Journal of Forensic Psychology Practice, 1*, 27–44.

McMahon, R. C., & Davidson, R. S. (1985). An examination of the relationship between personality patterns and symptom/mood patterns. *Journal of Personality Assessment, 49*, 552–556.

McMahon, R. C., Davidson, R. S., & Flynn, P. M. (1986). Psychological correlates and treatment outcomes for high and low social functioning alcoholics. *International Journal of the Addictions, 21*, 819–835.

McMahon, R. C., Flynn, P. M., & Davidson, R. S. (1985). The personality and symptom scales of the Millon Clinical Multiaxial Inventory: Sensitivity to posttreatment outcomes. *Journal of Clinical Psychology, 41*, 862–866.

McMahon, R. C., & Tyson, D. (1990). Personality factors in transient versus enduring depression among inpatient alcoholic women: A preliminary analysis. *Journal of Personality Disorders, 4*, 150–160.

Millon, T. (1983). *Millon Clinical Multiaxial Inventory manual.* New York: Holt, Rinehart and Winston.

Millon, T. (1987). *Millon Clinical Multiaxial Inventory-II: Manual for the MCMI-II.* Minneapolis, MN: National Computer Systems.

Millon, T. (1994a). *Millon Clinical Multiaxial Inventory-III.* Minneapolis, MN: National Computer Systems.

Millon, T. (1994b). *Millon Clinical Multiaxial Inventory-III interpretive service.* Minneapolis, MN: National Computer Systems.

Millon, T. (1997). *Millon Clinical Multiaxial Inventory-III: Manual* (2nd ed.). Minneapolis: MN: Pearson Assessments.

Morey, L. C. (1985). An empirical approach of interpersonal and *DSM-III* approaches to classification of personality disorders. *Psychiatry, 48,* 358–364.

Morey, L. C., & Levine, D. J. (1988). A multitrait-multimethod examination of Minnesota Multiphasic Personality Inventory (MMPI) and Millon Clinical Multiaxial Inventory (MCMI). *Journal of Psychopathology and Behavioral Assessment, 10,* 333–344.

Murphy, C. M., Meyer, S. L., & O'Leary, K. D. (1993). Family of origin violence and MCMI-II psychopathology among partner assaultive men. *Violence and Victims, 8,* 165–176.

Parry, B. L., Ehlers, C. L., Mostofi, N., & Phillips, E. (1996). Personality traits in LLPDD and normal controls during follicular and luteal menstrual-cycle phases. *Psychological Medicine, 26,* 197–202.

Piersma, H. L. (1987). The use of the Millon Clinical Multiaxial Inventory in the evaluation of seminary students. *Journal of Psychology and Theology, 15,* 227–233.

Piotrowski, C. (1997). Use of the Millon Clinical Multiaxial Inventory in clinical practice. *Perceptual and Motor Skills, 84,* 1185–1186.

Prifitera, A., & Ryan, J. J. (1984). Validity of the Narcissistic Personality Inventory (NPI) in a psychiatric sample. *Journal of Clinical Psychology, 40,* 140–142.

Reich, J. (1991). The effect of personality on placebo response in panic patients. *Journal of Nervous and Mental Diseases, 178,* 699–702.

Renneberg, B., Chambless, D. L., Dowdall, D. J., Fauerbach, J. A., & Gracely, E. J. (1992). The Structured Clinical Interview for *DSM-III-R,* AXIS-II and the Millon Clinical Multiaxial Inventory: A concurrent validity study of personality disorders among anxious patients. *Journal of Personality Disorders, 6,* 117–124.

Retzlaff, P. (1995). *Tactical psychotherapy for the personality disorders: An MCMI-III-based approach.* Boston: Allyn & Bacon.

Retzlaff, P., & Bromley, S. (1991). A multi-test alcoholic taxonomy: Canonical co-efficient clusters. *Journal of Clinical Psychology, 47,* 299–309.

Retzlaff, P., & Gibertini, M. (1987). Air Force pilot personality: Hard data on "The Right Stuff." *Multivariate Behavioral Research, 22,* 383–399.

Retzlaff, P., & Gibertini, M. (1988, July). Objective psychological testing of U.S. Air Force officers in pilot training. *Aviation, Space, and Environmental Medicine,* 661–663.

Retzlaff, P., Sheehan, E. P., & Fiel, A. (1991). MCMI-II report style and bias: Profile and validity scales analyses. *Journal of Personality Assessment, 56,* 466–477.

Retzlaff, P., Stoner, J., & Kleinsasser, D. (2002). The use of the MCMI-III in the screening and triage of offenders. *International Journal of Offender Therapy and Comparative Criminology, 46,* 319–332.

Richman, H., & Nelson-Gray, R. (1994). Nonclinical panicker personality: Profile and discriminative ability. *Journal of Anxiety Disorders, 8,* 33–47.

Schuller, D. R., Bagby, R. M., Levitt, A. J., & Joffe, R. T. (1993). A comparison of personality characteristics of seasonal and nonseasonal major depression. *Comprehensive Psychiatry, 34,* 360–362.

Silberman, C. S., Roth, L., Segal, D. L., & Burns, W. J. (1997). Relationship between the Millon Clinical Multiaxial Inventory-II and Coolidge Axis II Inventory in chronically mentally ill older adults: A pilot study. *Journal of Clinical Psychology, 53,* 559–566.

Sinha, B. K., & Watson, D. C. (1999). Predicting personality disorder traits with the Defense Style Questionnaire in a normal sample. *Journal of Personality Disorders, 13,* 281–286.

Smith, D., Carroll, J. L., & Fuller, G. (1988). The relationship between the Millon Clinical Multiaxial Inventory and the MMPI in a private outpatient mental health clinic population. *Journal of Clinical Psychology, 44,* 165–174.

Soldz, S., Budman, S., Demby, A., & Merry, J. (1993). Representation of personality disorders in circumplex and five-factor space: Explorations with a clinical sample. *Psychological Assessment, 5,* 41–52.

Stark, M. J., & Campbell, B. K. (1988). Personality, drug use, and early attrition from substance abuse treatment. *American Journal of Drug and Alcohol Abuse, 14,* 475–485.

Strack, S. (1987). Development and validation of an adjective checklist to assess the Millon personality types in a normal population. *Journal of Personality Assessment, 51,* 572–587.

Strack, S. (1991). Factor analysis of MCMI-II and PACL basic personality scales in a college sample. *Journal of Personality Assessment, 57,* 345–355.

Sugihara, Y., & Warner, J. A. (1999). Mexican-American male batterers on the MCMI-III. *Psychological Reports, 85,* 163–169.

Terpylak, O., & Schuerger, J. M. (1994). Broad factor scales of the 16PF fifth edition and Millon personality disorder scales: A replication. *Psychological Reports, 74,* 124–126.

Tisdale, M. J., Pendleton, L., & Marler, M. (1990). MCMI characteristics of *DSM-III-R* bulimics. *Journal of Personality Assessment, 55,* 477–483.

Torgersen, S., & Alnaes, R. (1990). The relationship between the MCMI personality scales and *DSM-III,* Axis II. *Journal of Personality Assessment, 55,* 698–707.

Turley, B., Bates, G. W., Edwards, J., & Jackson, H. J. (1992). MCMI-II personality disorders in recent-onset bipolar disorders. *Journal of Clinical Psychology, 48,* 320–329.

Wall, T. L., Schuckit, M., A., Mungas, D., & Ehlers, C. L. (1990). EEG alpha activity and personality traits. *Alcohol, 7,* 461–464.

Watkins, C. E., Campbell, V. L., Nieberding, R., & Hallmark, R. (1995). Contemporary practice of psychological assessment by clinical psychologists. *Professional Psychology: Research and Practice, 26,* 54–60.

Wierzbicki, M., & Gorman, J. L. (1995). Correspondence between students' scores on the Millon Clinical Multiaxial Inventory-II and Personality Diagnostic Questionnaire-Revised. *Psychological Reports, 77,* 1079–1082.

Wise, E. A. (1994). Personality style code type concordance between the MCMI and MBHI. *Journal of Clinical Psychology, 50,* 367–380.

Wise, E. A. (1996). Comparative validity of MMPI-2 and MCMI-II personality disorder classifications. *Journal of Personality Assessment, 66,* 569–582.

Wise, E. A. (2001). The comparative validity of MCMI-II and MMPI-2 personality disorder scales with forensic examinees. *Journal of Personality Disorders, 15,* 275–279.

Zarrella, K. L., Schuerger, J. M., & Ritz, G. H. (1990). Estimation of MCMI *DSM-III* Axis II constructs from MMPI scales and subscales. *Journal of Personality Assessment, 55,* 195–201.

CHAPTER 4

Combined Use of the PACL and MCMI-III™ to Assess Normal Range Personality Styles

STEPHEN STRACK

SINCE THE introduction of the MCMI in 1977, it has become one of the most frequently used assessment instruments for the examination of personality disorders and major clinical syndromes. Only the Rorschach and MMPI-2 have produced more research within the past 10 years. There are now over 400 empirical studies based on this measure and six books (Craig, 2002).

There have been numerous changes in the MCMI as it has evolved through three editions (Millon, 1983a, 1987, 1997; Strack, 1999), but some things have not changed. For example, all versions were based on Millon's (1996, 1997) comprehensive model of personality and psychopathology, all contain scales aligned with the *Diagnostic and Statistical Manual of Mental Disorders* (*DSM;* e.g., American Psychiatric Association [APA], 2000), all were developed and normed on psychiatric patients rather than normals, and all of the personality and clinical syndrome scales were standardized using base rate (BR) scores rather than T-scores. T-scores were considered inappropriate by Millon (1997) because they assume an underlying normal population distribution, and the MCMI-III normative sample consists of psychiatric patients. BR scores reflect the diagnoses of the individuals Millon used to develop the test. For the MCMI-III (Millon, 1997), he had expe-

Preparation of this manuscript was supported by the U.S. Department of Veterans Affairs.

rienced clinicians providing *DSM-III-R* (APA, 1987) multiaxial diagnoses for all of the patients in the normative group. By knowing the scores of these patients on the MCMI-III, and their clinical diagnoses, Millon was able to create anchor points for his scales that would reflect the prevalence, or BR, of each psychiatric condition. BR scores of 60 were set as the median raw score obtained by all patients. BR scores of 75 were assigned to the minimum raw score obtained by patients who met criteria for the particular disorder or condition. BR scores of 85 were given to the minimum raw score of patients who were judged to have a particular disorder or condition as their primary problem.

From a clinician's point of view, perhaps the greatest strength of this instrument is its ability to assign probabilities for diagnosis of a variety of *DSM* Axis I and Axis II disorders in persons presenting for mental health treatment. Millon (1983a, 1987, 1997) developed the test for this purpose, and his narrative reports were written with the assumption that the test taker is in the initial phases of mental health evaluation or treatment.

Over the years, the MCMI (Millon, 1983a, 1987, 1997) has been employed for many purposes beyond that of establishing diagnoses among psychiatric patients entering treatment. It is currently used to evaluate college counseling students, persons referred to employee assistance programs, worker's compensation claimants, child custody examinees, and individuals being screened for employment in high-risk jobs such as law enforcement. Potential problems of the test when used in relatively normal populations, and when the examinee does not wish to have psychiatric treatment, are that (1) it does not assess a broad range of healthy personality features, including strengths, and (2) the psychiatric norms create a situation where most normal persons obtain elevated scores on a small set of the personality scales (i.e., Histrionic, Narcissistic, and Compulsive; Choca & Van Denburg, 1997; Craig, 2002; Millon, 1997).

In circumstances where the MCMI-III is used with relatively high-functioning clients or persons who do not wish to have psychiatric treatment, it is advisable to seek additional information about these persons from tests that don't depend on psychiatric norms or focus strongly on psychopathology. One relevant source is the Personality Adjective Checklist (PACL; Strack, 1987, 1991c, 2002), a 153-item self-report and rating measure of Millon's (1969/1983b) eight basic personality patterns that was developed for use with normal adults. It features a Problem Indicator scale that taps aspects of Millon's three severe Schizoid, Cycloid, and Paranoid styles and may be used as a gauge of possible personality disorder. PACL personality scales measure theoretically derived, *normal* versions of the character types most frequently seen in clinical settings. Test results yield rich descriptions of respondents in a language that closely resembles that found in the *DSM* (APA, 2000). The measure is often used by therapists and personnel psychologists who work with relatively high-functioning individuals and who want to understand the *strengths* of their clients as well as their weaknesses. The PACL has been used in numerous research studies that tested various propositions of Millon's theory and addressed the interface between normal and abnormal personality (e.g., Strack, 1991c, 1997; Strack & Guevara, 1999).

In this chapter, I present the provenance and development of the PACL and its empirical base and relationship to the MCMI and demonstrate ways that the measure can be fruitfully used in conjunction with the MCMI-III to assess client strengths and obtain personality ratings in a variety of evaluative settings.

NORMAL AND ABNORMAL PERSONALITY ON A CONTINUUM

An attractive feature of Millon's (1969/1983b, 1981, 1986a, 1986b, 1990, 1994, 1996, 1997, 1999) model is its assumption that normal and abnormal personalities of the same type lie along a continuum, with disordered character representing an exaggeration or distortion of normal traits. Normal and abnormal persons are viewed as sharing the same basic styles. Disordered individuals are depicted as a small subset of the pool of all persons who, for various biological, psychological, environmental, and social reasons, have developed traits that are rigid and maladaptive.

In deriving his personalities, Millon (1981, 1986a, 1986b, 1990, 1994, 1996, 1997) distinguished four points along the normal-abnormal continuum: normal character and styles exhibiting mild, moderate, and severe pathology. Eight personality types are considered to exist in normal form and in mild or moderate pathological form: Asocial, Avoidant, Submissive (Dependent), Gregarious (Histrionic), Narcissistic, Aggressive, Conforming (Compulsive), and Negativistic. Three severe styles—Schizoid (Schizotypal), Cycloid (Borderline), and Paranoid—are thought to be variants of the mildly and moderately pathological personalities and not to have direct counterparts in the normal domain.

Two sets of concepts were outlined by Millon to distinguish his personalities at the various continuum points. One set of concepts defines the relative position of normal and pathological individuals on three of his evolutionary polarities: active-passive, pleasure-pain, and self-other (Millon, 1990). Normal individuals are thought to be balanced in each of these areas, for example, possessing both moderate self-esteem and empathic regard for others. Mild or moderate pathology is apparent among persons showing excesses or deficits in self- or other-regard, active or passive coping, and/or pleasure-pain orientation. Severe pathology is marked by extremes or distortions on these polarities.

A second set of ideas used by Millon (1969/1983b, 1986a) to distinguish normal and abnormal personalities focuses on interpersonal functioning, namely, an individual's level of flexibility, stability, and tendency to foster vicious cycles. Healthy persons are viewed as interpersonally flexible, adaptive in coping, ego-resilient, and able to avoid, escape from, or move beyond pathogenic attitudes, behaviors, or situations. In contrast, mildly and moderately pathological persons exhibit rigidity in interpersonal relations, nonadaptive coping, low ego strength, and a tendency to become mired in dysfunctional schemas or transactions with others and the environment. More severely disturbed individuals are viewed as strongly rigid and inflexible, lacking in adaptive coping skills, possessing extreme ego deficits, and unable to avoid, escape, or move through pathological thought processes and relationships.

In a recent expansion of his theory, Millon (1994, 2004; Millon & Davis, 1994, 2000) explicated a number of new dimensions that he believes underlie the manifest forms of normal personality. His pathological personality styles, and their normal variants measured by the PACL, were conceived on the basis of three *motivating* aims: active-passive, pleasure-pain, and self-other. To encompass a wider array of normal personality forms, Millon introduced four new axes differentiating various *cognitive* styles and five axes delineating *interpersonal* styles.

DEVELOPMENT OF THE PACL

The checklist was developed using a method outlined by Loevinger (1957), which was used by Millon and his colleagues for creating his clinical measures. In this method, test construction is theory-driven and follows a step-by-step process, with development and validation occurring together.

In the first stage of development and validation, 405 theory-derived adjectives were selected to measure normal versions of Millon's (1969/1983b) eight basic and three severe personality styles. Items were drawn from numerous sources, including *Modern Psychopathology* (Millon, 1969/1983b), and were selected based on rater judgments that each item had a clear best fit for one style (for details, see Strack, 1987, 1991c).

The second, structural validity phase of test construction involves creating scales that match the underlying theory. Toward this end, the 405-item experimental check list was given to 207 men and 252 women from colleges in Ohio and Florida. Preliminary scales were created from items that were endorsed by at least 5% and no more than 80% of subjects and had minimum item-scale correlations of .25 and maximum within-scale item-item correlations of .49 (to prevent redundancy; Strack, 1987, p. 577). Using these criteria, measures were created for each of Millon's eight basic styles that had satisfactory internal consistency and temporal reliability. Alpha coefficients ranged from .76 to .89 (new sample median = .83; p. 578), and test-retest correlations over a 3-month period ranged from .60 to .85 (median = .72 across sexes; p. 578). Additional data showed the scales to be relatively free from social desirability bias (p. 581).

Unfortunately, measures could not be developed for the three severe Schizoid, Cycloid, and Paranoid personalities because of extremely low endorsement rates (<5%) for most keyed items. Rather than throw away the handful of good items that remained for these measures, they were combined into an experimental Problem Indicator scale, PI, which we thought might be useful in identifying persons with personality disorders.

In addition to the personality and experimental scales, I developed three response bias indices to aid in the detection of faked protocols (Strack, 1991c), namely, Random (R), Favorable (F), and Unfavorable (UF). Separate groups of college students were asked to complete the PACL randomly or with intent to give an overly favorable or overly unfavorable self-report. Discriminant function analyses were used to distinguish the faked tests from PACLs completed under the normal instructional set. Equations were derived from these analyses (separately for men and women) and were cross-validated with independent samples. The equations were able to correctly identify a large majority of faked (75% to 91%) and normal tests (60% to 94%).

In accordance with the third stage of test development, extensive external validity data have been reported for the PACL in the form of correlations with tests of personality, mood, and dispositional variables, and reports from subjects about current and past behavior (Horton & Retzlaff, 1991; Pincus & Wiggins, 1990; Strack, 1987, 1991b, 1991c, 1994; Strack & Guevara, 1999; Strack & Lorr, 1990; Strack, Lorr, & Campbell, 1989; Wiggins & Pincus, 1989, 1994). My own research demonstrated that each PACL scale is in line with theoretical expectations and measures milder versions of Millon's (1969/1983b) pathological styles. For example, the scale measuring the Avoidant personality (Inhibited) was positively associated with measures of shyness, submissiveness, and social anxiety, and negatively associated with measures of sociability, dominance, and emotional well-being (Strack, 1991c). The scale measuring Aggressive traits (Forceful) was positively linked to measures of arrogance, dominance, assertiveness, and autonomy, and negatively linked to measures of deference, submissiveness, and conscientiousness (Strack, 1991c). In a study comparing the PI scores of psychiatric patients ($n = 124$) and normal adults ($n = 140$) who completed the PACL using standard instructions, I (Strack, 1991a) found that 84% of the PI scores T > 60 were obtained by patients (only 16% of the normals had T-scores over 59).

Other investigators have reported expected relationships between PACL scales and a variety of measures. For example, Horton and Retzlaff (1991) correlated the PACL with Moos's Family Environment Scale in a sample of 65 undergraduates. They found that family cohesion and expressiveness were strongly associated with cooperative and sociable personality styles, and conflict was most prevalent in the families of sensitive and forceful persons. High scores on the Respectful scale were linked to family environments in which cohesion, organization, and religiosity were salient features.

Wiggins and Pincus (1989; Pincus & Wiggins, 1990) examined the PACL in the context of MMPI personality disorder scales, big five Interpersonal Adjective Scales (IAS-B5), the NEO Personality Inventory (NEO-PI), and a circumplex version of Horowitz's (Horowitz, Alden, Wiggins, & Pincus, 2000), Inventory of Interpersonal Problems. PACL scales exhibited anticipated relationships with each of the tests in correlational, canonical, and factor analyses. For example, PACL Introversive and Sociable were loaded (in opposite directions) on a factor that included the MMPI Schizoid and Histrionic scales, NEO-PI Extraversion, and IAS-B5 Dominance. PACL Forceful was correlated .59 with interpersonal problems associated with dominance behavior, and PACL Cooperative was correlated .48 with problems involving exploitation by others.

The PACL was recently correlated and factor-analyzed with MMPI-2 scales in independent samples of psychiatric patients ($n = 196$) and normal adults ($n = 124$; Strack & Guevara, 1999). Consistent with previous research, PACL scales measuring Millon's neurotic, introverted styles (Introversive, Inhibited, Sensitive, PI) were positively associated with MMPI-2 scales measuring introversion (Si), affective states (D, Pt), and disturbed thinking (Sc); PACL scales measuring extroverted, socially dominant Millon styles (Sociable, Confident, Forceful) were negatively associated with the same MMPI-2 scales. PACL and MMPI-2 scales were reliably associated along two bipolar dimensions measuring Neuroticism/Introversion versus Extroversion and Emotional Distress versus Emotional Stability that accounted for 45% of the variance. A third General Distress factor loaded only MMPI-2 scales. Congruency coefficients indicated that the factors for patients and normals were very similar. Results highlighted the consistency of the links between MMPI-2 basic scales, the PACL, and other Millon instruments, as well as the utility of the PACL as a measure of Millon's personality styles in a mental health population.

In keeping with the emphasis on normality, PACL scales were normed as T-scores rather than BR scores. Normative data (Strack, 1991c) were obtained from 2,507 normal adults between the ages of 16 and 72. Men composed 47.4% of the sample and women 52.6%. Ethnic makeup was 65.2% non-Hispanic White, 17.3% Hispanic, 9.1% Black, 7.6% Asian, and 0.8% Native American Indian or Eskimo.

The PACL is available as a paper-and-pencil measure that can be hand-scored or entered into a computer file via optical scanner. Full-color, computerized versions of the checklist for Windows (WinPACL; Robbins, 1998) are available that permit computer administration of the test, scoring, and printing of profile plots of scores as well as narrative interpretations. The narrative interpretations were written for use in counseling and personnel settings and were based on Millon's writings, empirical information obtained during test construction and validation, and clinical experience with the test. These programs allow for unlimited use on a single computer and, as an aid to researchers, can produce exportable files containing test data for multiple subjects.

Now that clinicians, researchers, and their clients have access to the World Wide Web, the PACL can also be securely administered and scored via the Internet using PACLOnline and IPACL. Go to the Internet site http://www.21stcenturyassessment.com for information about these services.

COMPARISON WITH THE MCMI

The PACL was designed exclusively on the basis of Millon's (1969/1983b) original model of personality and measures normal trait characteristics. This is in contrast to the three editions of the MCMI, which were designed to match *DSM* Axis II criteria for personality disorders. Additionally, Millon's original model differs somewhat from that found in his more recent writings (Millon, 1986a, 1986b, 1990, 1994, 1996, 1997).

In accordance with Millon's (1969/1983b, 1987, 1994, 1997) model and akin to the MCMI, PACL personality scales contain varying numbers of overlapping items, ranging from one for the Respectful scale to nine for the Sensitive scale. The percentage of overlapping items on PACL scales is substantially lower than that for MCMI scales, and ranges from 5% to 35%. As a result, scale intercorrelations for the PACL are somewhat lower than those for the MCMI (median $r = |.35|$ across sexes; Strack, 1987, p. 579). Also as a result, PACL scales containing only nonoverlapping

Table 4.1

Corresponding Scales for the PACL, MCMI-I, MCMI-II, and MCMI-III

PACL	MCMI-I	MCMI-II	MCMI-III
1. Introversive	1. Schizoid	1. Schizoid	1. Schizoid
2. Inhibited	2. Avoidant	2. Avoidant	2A. Avoidant
			2B. Depressive
3. Cooperative	3. Dependent	3. Dependent	3. Dependent
4. Sociable	4. Histrionic	4. Histrionic	4. Histrionic
5. Confident	5. Narcissistic	5. Narcissistic	5. Narcissistic
6. Forceful	6. Antisocial	6A. Antisocial	6A. Antisocial
		6B. Aggressive	6B. Sadistic
7. Respectful	7. Compulsive	7. Compulsive	7. Compulsive
8. Sensitive	8. Passive-	8A. Passive-	8A. Negativistic
	Aggressive	Aggressive	
		8B. Self-Defeating	8B. Masochistic
PI. Problem	S. Schizotypal	S. Schizotypal	S. Schizotypal
Indicator	C. Borderline	C. Borderline	C. Borderline
	P. Paranoid	P. Paranoid	P. Paranoid

The PACL PI scale measures aspects of the Schizotypal, Borderline, and Paranoid styles but does not directly assess these personalities.

items have been found to be quite reliable on their own and to yield essentially the same factors as the overlapping scales (Pincus & Wiggins, 1990; Strack, 1991c; Wiggins & Pincus, 1989).

Table 4.1 lists corresponding personality measures for the PACL, MCMI-I, MCMI-II, and MCMI-III. Two MCMI scales are listed for PACL Inhibited, Forceful, and Sensitive. This is because Millon (1986a, 1986b, 1994, 2004) divided his original Avoidant (Inhibited) personality into Avoidant and Depressive types, his original Aggressive (Forceful) style into Antisocial and Aggressive/Sadistic, and his original Negativistic (Sensitive) style into Passive-Aggressive/Negativistic and Self-Defeating/Masochistic. An examination of items for these scales suggests that MCMI Avoidant, Aggressive, and Passive-Aggressive may be closer to the PACL Inhibited, Forceful, and Sensitive scales, respectively, than MCMI Depressive, Antisocial, and Self-Defeating, although research is needed to verify this impression.

In practice, correspondence between the PACL and various versions of the MCMI is reduced by the dissimilar test formats (adjectives versus statements), models used, and focus on normality versus pathology. In spite of these differences, I (Strack, 1991b) found the 8 PACL and 10 MCMI-II basic personality scales to be correlated between .39 and .67 (median = .52, using MCMI-II weighted raw scores) in a sample of 65 male and 75 female college students. The lowest values were found for PACL Sensitive/MCMI-II Self-Defeating (.39) and PACL Forceful/MCMI-II Antisocial (.41), suggesting that these MCMI-II scales are not strongly aligned with Millon's original (1969/1983b) model. By comparison, the MCMI-II Aggressive scale was correlated .53 with PACL Forceful, and the MCMI-II Passive-Aggressive scale was correlated .51 with PACL Sensitive.

Factor analyses of PACL, MCMI-I, and MCMI-II personality scales have revealed very similar results. The three higher-order dimensions found in the PACL (Strack, 1987), that is, Neuroticism, Assertiveness-Aggressiveness, and Social Extroversion-Introversion, correspond to the three factors found by Retzlaff and Gibertini (1987) for the 8 MCMI-I basic scales among psychiatric patients and normal adults, and by Strack, Lorr, Campbell, and Lamnin (1992) for the 13 MCMI-II personality scales with patients. A joint factor analysis of PACL and MCMI-II basic personality scales among college students also yielded three factors (using residual scores), with corresponding PACL and MCMI-II scales loading on the same dimensions (Strack, 1991b).

Strack, Lorr, and Campbell (1990) examined the circular ordering of MCMI-II personality disorder scales in a mixed group of psychiatric patients and compared results with those from the PACL among normal adults. Plotted against the orthogonally rotated first two principal components, they found a reasonably good circle for MCMI-II scales (using residual scores) that, for the most part, followed Millon's (1987, p. 20) predictions. Ordering for the PACL scales was similar, although a less complete circle was noted: Sociable, Confident, and Forceful were loaded opposite Introversive, Inhibited, and Sensitive on one dimension, and Cooperative and Respectful defined one end of a second dimension but had no opposing scales.

MILLON'S PERSONALITIES AS MEASURED BY THE PACL

Correlational evidence demonstrates that normal versions of Millon's basic styles are milder variants of the personalities as disorders. Unfortunately, behavioral studies and side-by-side comparisons of matched groups of normals and patients on the PACL and MCMI have not yet been carried out. As a result, important data are still needed to address the precise nature of similarities and differences between normal and disordered forms of Millon's personalities.

With regard to the appearance of Millon's personalities in normal form, what can be offered at this point is a portrait of each style based on Millon's theory, empirical findings from studies associating PACL scales with other measures, and clinical experience with the test. Summaries of empirical findings can be found in Strack (1991c, 1993, 2002, in press). The following descriptions present normal prototypes of persons who obtain high scores on individual scales.[1] In practice, people are seldom prototypical, instead exhibiting a mixture of traits from multiple styles. Nevertheless, the descriptions flesh out various aspects of normal personality not readily grasped by extrapolations from Millon's writings on pathological character. Especially noteworthy among the normal styles are their positive dispositional features and interpersonal attitudes. Even less desirable traits are placed within a normal frame of reference.

SCALE 1: INTROVERSIVE

Aloof, introverted, and solitary, these persons usually prefer distant or limited involvement with others and have little interest in social activities, which they find unrewarding. Appearing to others as nonchalant and untroubled, they are often judged to be easygoing, mild-mannered, quiet, and retiring. They frequently remain in the background of social life and work quietly and unobtrusively at a job. At school or in the workplace, these people do well on their own, are typically dependable and reliable, are nondemanding, and are seldom bothered by noise or commotion around them. They are often viewed as level-headed and calm. However, these individuals may appear unaware of or insensitive to the feelings and thoughts of others. These characteristics are sometimes interpreted by others as signs of indifference or rejection but reveal a sincere difficulty in being able to sense others' moods and needs. Introversive persons can be slow and methodical in demeanor, lack spontaneity and resonance, and be awkward or timid in social or group situations. They frequently view themselves as being simple and unsophisticated and are usually modest in appraising their own skills and abilities. At the same time, their placid demeanor and ability to weather ups and downs without being ruffled are traits frequently prized by friends, family members, and coworkers.

Individuals with this personality style are frequently attracted to intellectual or mechanical occupations that allow them to be on their own. They often pursue goals that permit them to regulate the amount of information and stimulation they receive. Given a choice, they seek a stable work environment with few people and little commotion. Nevertheless,

[1] Personality characteristics of individuals obtaining low scores (T < 40) on PACL Cooperative, Sociable, Confident, Forceful, and Respectful scales can also be interpreted (see Strack, 2002, pp. 199–201). For example, low Cooperative scores indicate a minimal need for approval, communality, and dependency, and low Respectful scores suggest that the respondent is not rule-bound and may lack organizational skills.

most of these individuals perform well in noisy, stimulating environ-ments, if they are allowed to work independently at a pace they set for themselves. These individuals are usually reliable and dependable em-ployees who are not bothered by repetitive tasks. They are quiet, slow-paced, pleasant, and nondemanding and usually maintain a calm demeanor. They do not respond well if asked to assume leadership posi-tions or participate actively in groups. At times, coworkers may find these individuals frustrating to be with because they often tune out those around them and may seem insensitive to their needs.

SCALE 2: INHIBITED

As with the introversive style, the inhibited personality is marked by a tendency toward social withdrawal. However, for inhibited individuals, this pattern is motivated not by disinterest, but by a fear of negative con-sequences. Inhibited persons tend to be sensitive to their own feelings and to those of others. They often anticipate that others will be critical or rejecting of them, and because of this, they frequently seem shy or skit-tish in unfamiliar surroundings. In this regard, family members and ac-quaintances may see them as being unnecessarily nervous, wary, and fearful. Although inhibited persons tend to get along reasonably well with others, they are often difficult to get to know on a personal level. These individuals usually wish that they could be at ease with others and tend to desire closeness, but they often are just too uncertain of the con-sequences of closeness and intimacy to let their guard down. As a result, they may experience feelings of loneliness but be unable or unwilling to do anything about them. Because of their sensitivity to others, inhibited persons are often described as kind, considerate, and empathic by close acquaintances. Inhibited persons often prefer to work alone or in a small group with people they can come to know well. They do best in a stable work environment where stimulation and commotion are kept at low to moderate levels. Persons working with inhibited types need to appreciate their sensitivity to both positive and negative feedback, as well as their need to build trust over a long period of time.

Individuals with this personality style frequently seek intellectual, conventional, and artistic occupations that permit them to regulate the amount of stimulation and information they receive from their environ-ment. They prefer stable work settings where they can operate alone or with a few close associates. They do not thrive in busy, social environ-ments, which they frequently find too taxing of their personal resources. In a stable, safe environment, these personalities are known for being kind, considerate, and loyal. They are often perceptive and tuned in to the feelings and thoughts of others. However, they are typically slow in adjusting to change and find it difficult to be assertive or active in group situations. Supervisors will do well to appreciate their sensitivity and need for interpersonal space. Because these individuals are usually not forthcoming with their feelings, it is important to request regular feedback from them about their work experiences.

SCALE 3: COOPERATIVE

Cooperative persons can be identified by a need for approval and affection and by a willingness to live in accord with the desires of others. They usually adapt their behavior to the standards of others but in the process may deny their own needs. Interpersonally, these individuals are often cooperative, reliable, considerate of others, and deferential. They may appear even-tempered, docile, obliging, self-effacing, ingratiating, or naive. Cooperative individuals often see themselves as being modestly endowed in terms of skills and abilities. They are often pleased when they can rely on others and may feel insecure when left on their own. Especially when faced with difficult or stressful situations, cooperative persons seek others to provide authority, leadership, and direction. They often prefer group work environments and will typically excel in them if given support and guidance. They are usually willing to follow directions and co-operate with coworkers in team efforts.

Known as team players who thrive in large, social work environments, these individuals perform best in supportive work roles under the guidance of strong leaders. They are cordial, agreeable, and reliable and strive to get along well with colleagues. They enjoy many conventional, social, and intellectual occupations. Their cheerful optimism helps them weather workplace stress and change relatively well. They are thoughtful of others, willing to please, and good at smoothing over conflicts and disagreements. When things are gloomy and the going gets tough, they can often find the silver lining. These individuals are usually uncomfortable being assertive and often avoid problems rather than face them head-on. They are followers rather than leaders and struggle when asked to act independently or be on their own.

SCALE 4: SOCIABLE

Like cooperative personalities, sociable individuals have a need for attention and approval. However, unlike cooperative persons, sociable types take the initiative in assuring their reinforcements by being center-stage. They are characterized by an outgoing, talkative, and extroverted style of behavior and tend to be lively, dramatic, and colorful. These people are typically viewed by others as spontaneous, clever, enthusiastic, and vigorous. They can be quite sensitive to the needs and wants of others, at least to those aspects that will help them get the attention they seek. Sociable individuals may also be seen as fickle in their attachments. They may have quickly shifting moods and emotions and may come across as shallow and ungenuine. These persons tend to prefer novelty and excitement and are bored by ordinary or mundane activities. Like cooperative personalities, sociable individuals seem uncomfortable or deflated when left on their own. Not surprisingly, sociable types often excel in group work environments where they can exercise their showy style. They often do well interacting with the public, may be skilled and adept at rallying or motivating others, and will usually put their best side forward even in difficult circumstances.

Individuals with this personality style often seek social, enterprising, and artistic occupations where they can exercise their need for stimulation and attention. Easily bored with repetition, they enjoy unusual duties and tasks that change frequently. They do well in large groups and seem to thrive in boisterous environments with little structure. They are extroverted, lively, and energetic. They often enjoy working with the public and make good salespersons. They are attentive to their appearance and keep a cheerful optimism, even in difficult circumstances. However, these individuals can be exasperating to some colleagues because of their quickly shifting interests and emotions. They find it difficult to stick with something once they have lost interest and seldom hesitate to change loyalties if an alternative gives them more of what they want. Attitudes and feelings can likewise vacillate from intense enthusiasm to disgruntled negativism in a short span of time. However, angry outbursts are just as short-lived as intense reactions in the other direction. When the air has cleared, these individuals return to their upbeat disposition as if nothing had happened.

Scale 5: Confident

Aloof, calm, and confident, these personalities tend to be egocentric and self-reliant. They may have a keen sense of their own importance, uniqueness, or entitlement. Confident individuals enjoy others' attention and may be quite bold socially, although they are seldom garish. They can be self-centered to a fault and may become so preoccupied with themselves that they lack concern and empathy for others. These persons have a tendency to believe that others share, or should share, their sense of worth. As a result, they may expect others to submit to their wishes and desires and to cater to them. Ironically, the confident individual's secure appearance may cover feelings of personal inadequacy and sensitivity to criticism and rejection. Unfortunately, they usually do not permit others to see their vulnerable side. When feeling exposed or undermined, these individuals are frequently disdainful, obstructive, or vindictive. In the workplace, confident persons like to take charge in an emphatic manner, often doing so in a way that instills confidence in others. Their self-assurance, wit, and charm often win them supervisory and leadership positions.

Confident individuals are frequently attracted to enterprising occupations that give them the status and power they seek. They are self-driven and work hard to attain their goals. They are competitive and shrewd. They do equally well on their own and in social settings, but in groups they have a need to be one up and will often resist roles that place them in an equal or deferential position. The self-assured, bold style of these individuals often wins them leadership positions. Colleagues frequently feel secure that these individuals will work hard to succeed and will accomplish their objectives in spite of obstacles. On the negative side, these individuals are usually more concerned with themselves than with others and can be insensitive and uncaring about the effects of their behavior on coworkers. Their need for success and tribute may, at times, take precedence over company rules, ethics, and social propriety.

Scale 6: Forceful

Like confident persons, forceful individuals can be identified by an inclination to turn toward the self as the primary source of gratification. However, instead of the confident personality's internalized sense of self-importance, forceful people seem driven to prove their worthiness. They are characterized by an assertive, dominant, and tough-minded personal style. They tend to be strong-willed, ambitious, competitive, and self-determined. Feeling that the world is a harsh place where exploitiveness is needed to assure success, forceful individuals are frequently gruff and insensitive in dealing with others. In contrast to their preferred, outwardly powerful appearance, these individuals may feel inwardly insecure and be afraid of letting down their guard. In work settings, these personalities are often driven to excel. They work hard to achieve their goals, are competitive, and do well where they can take control or work independently. In supervisory or leadership positions, these persons usually take charge and see to it that a job gets done. However, they often need to temper an inclination to demand as much of others as they do of themselves.

Forceful persons often aspire to mechanical and enterprising occupations that give them independence and a sense of being in control. Their strong competitive spirit gives them an edge in jobs that require a steadfast pursuit of goals in difficult circumstances. These persons are known for their hard work, toughness, and determination. They can tolerate group settings, but they prefer to be outside the bounds of community rules and regulations. They are self-oriented and do not readily consider the needs of others. They can be gruff and insensitive to colleagues and seldom hesitate to step on toes if doing so helps them achieve their ends. Their assertive, forthright style and desire to win typically earns them confidence and respect from colleagues. In many job situations, their lack of sensitivity and warmth may be overlooked because of their perseverance and ability to succeed in spite of opposition.

SCALE 7: RESPECTFUL

Responsible, industrious, and respectful of authority, these individuals tend to be conforming and work hard to uphold rules and regulations. They have a need for order and are typically conventional in their interests. These individuals can be rule-abiding to a fault, however, and may be perfectionistic, inflexible, and judgmental. A formal interpersonal style and notable constriction of affect can make some respectful persons seem cold, aloof, and withholding. Underneath their social propriety there is often a fear of disapproval and rejection or a sense of guilt over perceived shortcomings. Indecisiveness and an inability to take charge may be evident in some of these persons due to a fear of being wrong. However, among coworkers and friends, respectful personalities are best known for being well-organized, reliable, and diligent. They have a strong sense of duty and loyalty, are cooperative in group efforts, show persistence even in difficult circumstances, and work well under supervision.

Individuals with this personality style are frequently attracted to conventional, mechanical, and intellectual occupations that offer a structured work environment and clear guidelines for performance. Given a job to accomplish, they use their organizational skills and strong work ethic to see that it gets done accurately and on time. In the workplace, they are often prized for their loyalty, conscientiousness, and willingness to persist at difficult, even repetitive tasks. They take their responsibilities seriously and are motivated to please supervisors and respected colleagues. These individuals do well on their own, but they are also good team players and thrive in group settings. They are willing to cooperate and follow the lead of others. They are astute at recognizing the implicit rules of the workplace and will internalize these quickly. It is difficult for these individuals to operate successfully if tasks and goals are not well defined and when a freewheeling, unstructured approach is required. They are uncomfortable making decisions on their own and asserting a point of view that is not shared by others. Coworkers often value their ability to keep their nose to the grindstone and their emotions under wrap, but some individuals may come across as so task-oriented and constricted that they are viewed as impersonal, insensitive, and uncaring. They can be tough on subordinates, whom they hold to the same perfectionist standards they have for themselves.

SCALE 8: SENSITIVE

Sensitive personalities tend to be unconventional and individualistic in their response to the world. They march to the beat of a different drummer and are frequently unhappy with the status quo. They may be quick to challenge rules or authority deemed arbitrary and unjust. They may also harbor resentment without expressing it directly and may revert to passive-aggressive behavior to make their feelings known. Many sensitive people feel as if they don't fit in and view themselves as lacking in interpersonal skills. In fact, to others they often appear awkward, nervous, or distracted and seem angry or dissatisfied with themselves and others. They can be indecisive and have fluctuating moods and interests. An air of uncertainty and general dissatisfaction may reflect an underlying dependency and sense of personal inadequacy. With their best side forward, sensitive persons can be spontaneous, creative, and willing to speak out for what they believe in. These qualities make them especially suited to jobs that are not rule-bound, that give them a certain independence from supervision, and that require unusual duties or creative expression.

Artistic and intellectual occupations are frequently favored by people with this personality style. They seek loosely structured work environments that allow them freedom and autonomy in interpreting task requirements. They do not respond well to strict rules and regulations. They like to determine the pace at which they work and to choose the goals they strive for. Although they appreciate stable group settings and can operate successfully within them, these persons tend to be freethinking and not inclined to follow group norms. Their sensitive, temperamental nature requires a measure of tolerance and support from supervisors and colleagues. Because they often react quite negatively to criticism and heavy-handed authority, these should be avoided or downplayed. The talents of these persons are most likely to be realized in a workplace that is nurturing and supportive of their individuality.

SCALE PI: PROBLEM INDICATOR

Items for this scale were compiled from adjectives measuring the Schizoid, Cycloid, and Paranoid personalities, for example, "chaotic," "fragmented," "depressed," and "suspicious." Although the scale does not define a personality style, high scores are indicative of personality problems and the potential for disorder. High scorers possess personality disorder traits and symptoms such as low ego strength and affective instability. They are likely to appear anxious, dysphoric, and fearful, exhibit strong self-doubt, and express dissatisfaction with themselves and others. They may have long-standing adjustment problems in major areas of life such as work, school, and relationships. Those who score high on this scale are not likely to fit the same picture of normality as are low scorers (e.g., by exhibiting interpersonal rigidity and maladaptiveness), but further assessment is advised before drawing conclusions regarding the presence of a disorder.

USING THE PACL WITH THE MCMI-III

The PACL (Strack, 1991c, 2002) is appropriate for use with persons 16 years and older who read at minimally the 8th-grade level. It has been successfully employed in conjunction with the MCMI-III by therapists working in college counseling centers and employee assistance programs; by vocational counselors, personnel psychologists, marriage and family counselors; by therapists doing custody and worker's compensation evaluations; and by general practitioners who work with relatively high-functioning clients. Because the PACL is quick (10 mins.) and easy to administer, it is often given during initial screening visits to assess personality style and identify persons who may have serious problems. Clinicians have found it to be useful with people who can't or won't complete questionnaire measures, for example, some medical patients, adolescents, and the elderly. A number of clinicians use the PACL to rate their clients' personality styles and to have couples and family members assess each other, employing the norms in the PACL Manual (Strack, 1991c) for scoring. Although the norms are based on self-reports, they have worked remarkably well with a variety of ratings.

PSYCHIATRIC POPULATIONS

When using the PACL in psychiatric settings it is important to keep in mind that the test measures *normal* trait characteristics, not personality disorder (PD) features. High scores on the PACL indicate that an individual possesses *more* of the traits of a particular normal personality style than other adults in the general population. For example, the higher an individual's score is above T = 50 on any particular scale, the more likely it is that he or she will fit the prototype descriptions given earlier. The test doesn't assess PD features beyond those measured by the PI scale and, as indicated previously, this scale should not be interpreted as suggesting the presence of personality problems unless elevated at T > 60.

Nevertheless, there are circumstances where clinicians find the PACL to be helpful with psychiatric patients who demonstrate clinically significant scores on the MCMI-III: (1) assessing strengths of the client, including vocational and school interests; (2) giving feedback to clients about their personality style; and (3) obtaining personality ratings. Each of these areas is discussed in turn.

Because the MCMI-III (Millon, 1997) was designed as a diagnostic instrument and was normed on patients, BR score elevations are associated with increased probability of psychiatric diagnosis and higher degrees of psychopathology. Furthermore, studies have not been done on the characteristics of those who obtain low BR scores on the clinical scales. Except for research studies showing that normal functioning is frequently associated with moderate scores on the Histrionic, Narcissistic, and Compulsive PD scales (Choca & Van Denburg, 1997; Craig, 2002; McCann et al., 2001; Millon, 1997; Strack, 1993), positive personality correlates are not available for MCMI-III clinical scales. When therapists are seeking to understand the positive personality features of their clients, including goals for school and work, results of the PACL can provide valuable information, as the prototype descriptions given previously demonstrate.

The MCMI-III narrative test printouts provided by Pearson Assessments clearly indicate that they should not be disclosed to the patient and his or her family. Although trained clinicians are usually adept at communicating clinical findings to patients and families in a language they can understand, there are circumstances where the client wants to see for himself or herself what the results actually say. The interpersonal behavior and work/school sections of the PACL narrative reports were written with counseling clients in mind; because of this, these sections can be read to, or given to, the client as feedback.[2] The decision about whether or not to read or give the client sections of his or her narrative PACL results must be determined by the clinician doing the assessment. When I provide testing feedback to my clients, I preface my remarks by explaining the strengths and limitations of self-report testing in general, along with the strengths and limitations of the PACL (Strack, 1991c). I indicate that the narrative test results are blind to the respondent's unique circumstances, but, as a result of the norming process, the PACL can give

---

[2] I do not recommend giving clients the entire PACL narrative report because it contains far more technical information than they can readily interpret, and the section focusing on treatment issues may give information that is detrimental to the client.

clients a generally accurate portrait of their feelings, attitudes, behaviors, and interests vis-à-vis others in the general population. I tell clients that we can discuss their feelings and reactions after they have listened to or read their test results, and they can let me know what fits and what doesn't fit. In my experience over many years, this feedback process is almost universally beneficial. It affords an opportunity for a transparent and collaborative interaction between the mental health provider and the client that can build trust, provides the client with limited (digestible) knowledge about psychological assessment, sets the stage for treatment planning, and helps build an expectation that self-knowledge is an important part of the assessment and treatment experience.

I mentioned that clinicians use the PACL to rate their clients' personality styles and to have couples and family members assess each other. In this context, self-report data can be readily contrasted with ratings to reveal similarities and differences between self-other viewpoints. If more than one person rates an individual, scores can be combined or weighted to produce composite profiles. Of course, self-report doesn't have to be limited to one's *current* personality. Clients can be asked to describe their ideal self, how they were as a child or before a major life event, and how they imagine themselves in a variety of roles and personas (for an example, see Strack, 1997).

CASE EXAMPLE: TOM AND SUSAN

To illustrate how one can use the PACL and MCMI-III in a psychiatric setting, I offer a case involving a married couple, Tom and Susan. Tom is a 45-year-old Mexican American army veteran with a high school diploma. He has a long-standing diagnosis of Schizoaffective Disorder and has been under psychiatric care continuously for 10 years. His psychiatrist referred him to me when Tom asked for psychotherapy to improve his marriage. Tom grew up in a working-class neighborhood in East Los Angeles. He is a third-generation American whose family spoke both English and Spanish in the household. Because he has no trace of an accent when speaking English and looks Anglo (non-Hispanic White), many people assume that he is not Mexican American. As is common among U.S. military veterans of all ethnic backgrounds, Tom identifies strongly with mainstream American culture and values.

Tom has been married to Susan for 20 years. This is his second marriage and her first. They have no children, but Tom has a grown son by his first wife, who lives in a nearby community. Susan is 43 years old and also has a high school education. She is Anglo and grew up as the only, but adopted, child of a middle-class couple in Southern California.

Tom and Susan met when he was "making good money" as a management-level employee at a large technology firm. Susan had turned her childhood love of horses into a career and was working as a local representative for a saddlery firm based in Europe. Both look back on the first 10 years of their marriage—before Tom got seriously ill—as "wonderful." They were "good friends" who shared interests in the outdoors, music, and traveling. They had "lots of money" and "no responsibilities" and so were able to indulge their hobbies and interests. They bought a home together in a middle-class neighborhood and were "very happy" there.

Always energetic (even hyperactive) and ready for a good time, Tom recalled using recreational drugs, including cocaine, fairly often at parties with his military buddies before he suffered his first psychotic breakdown at the age of 35. He was hospitalized and released after 3 weeks with "a cocktail" of antipsychotic medications. In spite of heavy doses of a variety of medications, Tom reported that his mental condition was never stable for more than a few weeks after his first breakdown, even though he was compliant with his treatment plan and became completely sober from illicit drug and alcohol use. He eventually had to quit his job and was placed on social security disability after about 2 years of unemployment.

Susan was exasperated by the failure of doctors to cure her husband. Every time he would become stable for a short time, she hoped that "the old Tom" would return, but this was not to be. When doctors told her that Tom would probably never fully recover from his illness and might never work again, she became "depressed" and walled herself off from him. She poured herself into her job and began taking on more and more of their previously mutual responsibilities, but she never sought psychological treatment and felt that no one in their immediate families provided more than moral support.

When Tom stopped working, their lifestyle changed drastically. They could no longer travel or buy the things they used to take for granted. They eventually lost their home, had to declare bankruptcy, and ended up in a mobile home park, something Susan feels is "degrading."

In spite of her anger and frustration at their change of fate, Susan reported that divorce was never a serious option. "I love Tom," she said during a phone interview. However, after 10 years of living with a mentally ill husband, she still feels "cheated" by life, and she is angry with Tom for not performing his previously strong roles in their marriage. She and Tom stopped socializing, and they stopped doing the things that they used to enjoy doing together. Although they currently spend a lot of their free time at home, they live separate lives. Tom absorbs himself in a ham radio club (something he can do at home) and enjoys building electronics that he purchases via the Internet. Susan enjoys her small garden and caring for her two cats.

Tom was referred to me when he demonstrated 6 months of stability, with only minor psychotic symptoms, after being placed on an atypical antipsychotic medication in combination with an antidepressant and mood stabilizer. During my initial interviews, he reported having hypomanic and depressive mood swings 4 to 5 days each month, which were the days preceding and immediately following the first of the month, when his disability check would arrive. He reported having occasional psychotic symptoms in the form of visual hallucinations associated with nightmares, but these could be easily overcome by getting out of bed and refocusing his attention by watching television or listening to music.

Fairly satisfied with his current psychiatric treatment and manageable symptoms, Tom said he wanted to "start talking again" to his wife and see if they could resume a more normal marriage. He said that he felt Susan "is always angry at me and shuts me off when I start to say something." He felt that he had lost a lot of self-esteem due to his mental illness and inability to work. He was self-isolating, fearful of new experiences, and, most of all, fearful of his wife. "If she comes home looking angry I go to my room and shut the door," he said. He reported that, in the rare times when the two of them would try to communicate, he would "do the listening" and then try to say positive things that would not upset her. He said that he believed his mood swings around the first of the month were caused by the fact that Susan managed their money, and he would have to ask for permission to buy anything. He realized that he was unhappy about the financial arrangement but too afraid to do anything about it.

With Tom's permission, I called Susan and she verified much of his account of their marital situation. She said that she was "forced" to manage their money because Tom was "too sick" to do so. She felt that Tom was "irresponsible" about a lot of things and she would have to "nag him" to do simple tasks like take out the trash and vacuum the rug. She didn't believe that she was openly hostile toward him, but she acknowledged that she often came home from work tired and didn't feel like talking to him.

As Tom had earlier predicted, Susan declined my offer to come in for couple's counseling. She said that it would be too difficult to take time off from work, and she intimated that it wouldn't be helpful: "Tom's been sick a long time and I don't think he's going to change much at this point." Nevertheless, she said she was supportive of Tom's interest in seeking help and that she would consider participating in assignments I might give as part of his treatment.

Prior to developing a treatment plan, I conducted a series of interviews to gauge Tom's stability, maturity, verbal skills, potential for insight, and ability to carry out instructions. These meetings revealed Tom to be alert, oriented, and cooperative, energetic, bright, insightful, and talkative. His thoughts were cogent and clear, and there were no signs of psychosis. He had obviously taken time over the years to learn quite a bit about his mental illness and medications. He was able to tell me about every medication he had been prescribed since he became mentally ill, including their benefits and side effects. I was also able to observe the hypomanic-depressive period that occurred just prior to and after the first of the month, when his disability check would arrive. During this 4- to 5-day period, Tom had to isolate himself. He felt angry and emotionally out of control. He had racing thoughts about his money and having to ask his wife for permission to buy little things. He did not sleep for 48 to 72 hours and then would become deflated and depressed for another 24 to 48 hours, during which time he would take extra medication to catch up on his sleep.

As part of the initial evaluation, I gave Tom a battery of tests, including the MCMI-III and PACL. He was very interested in the testing process, asked lots of questions, and completed each measure with minimal assistance. All of his results were valid. With regard to the MCMI-III, the modifier indices showed a pattern of moderate self-disclosure (X BR = 77), low desirability (Y BR = 59), and moderate debasement (Z BR = 70). His exhibited clinical elevations on four Axis II PD scales, Avoidant (BR = 83), Depressive (BR = 78), Negativistic (BR = 78), and Masochistic (BR = 76), as well as two Axis I scales, Bipolar: Manic (BR = 83) and Dysthymic Disorder (BR = 80). None of the severe PD or Axis I scales was clinically elevated.

Tom's PACL personality scale results are presented in Figure 4.1. His response style scales (not displayed) were all well below the cut-offs for random, favorable, and unfavorable responding (< −10; Strack, 1991c, pp. 21–24). He endorsed a wide variety of adjectives ($n = 86$) and obtained a PI scale in the clinical range (T = 70). His personality profile showed a strong mixture of Inhibited (Avoidant; T = 74) and Cooperative (Dependent; T = 69) traits, with average scores on the next two highest scales, Sensitive (Negativistic; T = 55) and Introversive (Schizoid; T = 54). His lowest scale elevations were on Forceful (Antisocial/Aggressive; T = 27) and Confident (Narcissistic; T = 31).

When compared with psychiatric norms (MCMI-III), Tom's personality style suggests conflict between a desire for dependency, fear of independence, and a belief that others will reject and ridicule him if he reaches out to them. He probably has low self-esteem and high expectations for personal failure. He believes that others do, and will, criticize

Results for Tom

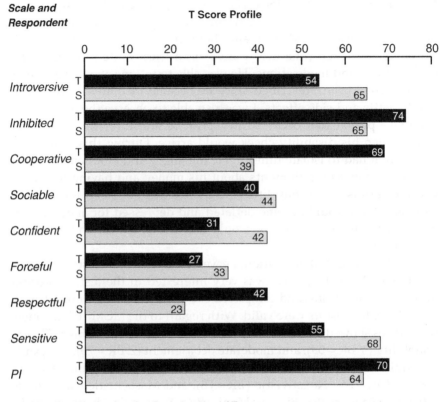

Note: T = Tom's self-rating; S = Susan's rating of Tom

Figure 4.1
PACL personality profiles for a married couple: Self-report and spouse rating.

and disapprove of any efforts he makes to build autonomy and self-sufficiency. He probably harbors anger and resentment toward those close to him and, when not displaying a "sad sack" demeanor, he may occasionally lash out with petulant and passive-aggressive behaviors aimed at communicating his dissatisfaction with a perceived lack of support.

In reference to normals (PACL), Tom comes across as a timid, deferential man who seeks harmonious relations with others and a safe, quiet environment populated with a few close friends and family members. He tends to be sensitive, worrisome, and lacking in self-esteem. He often feels vulnerable in social situations and limits his involvements to those people and circumstances where he can be assured of positive outcomes.

Results for Susan

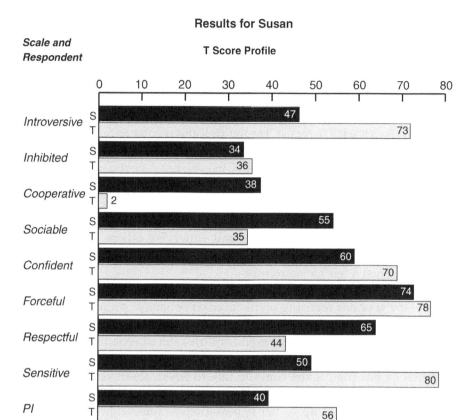

Note: S = Susan's self-rating; T = Tom's rating of Susan

Figure 4.1 *Continued*

He is typically pleasant, easygoing, and nondemanding. He is attentive to others' needs and will go out of his way to please those who are important to him. On the other hand, he tends to downplay his own skills and abilities and often seeks support and reassurance from people he views as stronger and more capable than he. A sense of being fragile or delicate can be detected in his efforts to keep his inner self hidden from almost everyone, as well as his avoidance of novelty, excitement, and conflict. These tendencies can make him seem self-preoccupied and anxious. Those close to him may feel exasperated by his self-limiting attitudes and lack of assertiveness, but they also value his gentle nature, kindness, concern, loyalty, and empathic responding.

The personality profiles from the two tests yielded similar findings. The major difference was that Tom's need for approval and communality was gauged as average among psychiatric patients (MCMI-III Dependent

BR = 62) and significantly above average in the normal population (PACL Cooperative T = 69). This is not a conflicting finding: It means that Tom is likely to appear average in dependency among psychiatric patients (i.e., this trait does not stand out), but among the general population, he will come across as obliging, helpful, and needy.

For feedback, I let Tom read his PACL interpersonal behavior narrative segment. I supplemented this with a verbal report of information contained in his MCMI-III report. He felt that the results of both tests were accurate. He told me that they show how much he has changed since his illness. He went on to describe his experiences in the military as a sergeant, where he had to give orders and be responsible for several men. He took the leadership skills he learned in the army with him into the civilian world and was promoted into a management position because of his ability to make good decisions and supervise others. At the same time, he admitted that he has always been emotionally sensitive and has always kept just a few close friends.

Following the initial assessment, Tom and I began individual psychotherapy sessions focusing on his marital behavior. According to Tom and Susan, he is too passive and unassertive in the relationship. Both feel that he has given up too many responsibilities since becoming ill. Tom reported that "Susan does just about everything; it's like I'm a boarder." He said that he has tried many times to talk to Susan about assuming more responsibilities, but she has been unreceptive. "She likes things done her way and I never meet up to her expectations," Tom said. Tom realized that without Susan's presence in therapy, his success would depend on whatever he could change in himself.

He was willing to operate under these circumstances, so we began our work with Tom identifying specific things he wanted to change in the marriage. His first priority was to become a partner with Susan in managing their money, because being dependent on her in this arena caused him a great deal of distress. His first homework assignment was to discuss the matter with Susan, which he did after two sessions of role-playing. Susan's response, according to Tom, was "How can you help me with the finances when you can't seem to help with cooking, cleaning, and shopping?" Tom admitted that he had become "lazy" and had let Susan take over the household chores. He agreed to assume more responsibility and started to do some of the shopping, cooking, and cleaning. After 3 weeks of this, Tom reported that he was exasperated by Susan's constant critical remarks. He said that she didn't like much of anything he did, and he felt hurt by her lack of support.

I reminded Tom that change would take considerable time because Susan had developed a negative attitude toward him due to his past instability. She had gotten used to a pattern where he would start positive behaviors and then relapse within a few weeks. I said that it was essential for him to keep up his efforts for change in spite of her criticism. With this encouragement, Tom continued his efforts, but he kept reporting that Susan was "never satisfied." After a few more weeks, Tom was ready to quit therapy.

At this point, I recommended to Tom that, before throwing in the towel, we should do some information gathering, or "recon" (reconnaissance), as he put it, to determine where the communication problems were occurring between him and Susan. We would do this using the PACL. Tom would complete the checklist by rating Susan's personality, and Susan would complete the PACL twice, first giving a report on herself and then one on Tom. Tom was skeptical about whether Susan would participate, but a phone call from me explaining the procedure to Susan resulted in no detectable resistance.

The results of these assessments are given in Figure 4.1. They were scored as self-reports, so Tom's rating of Susan was entered as if a woman were the respondent, and Susan's rating of Tom was measured against the norms for men.

As can be seen in the figure, there was appreciable agreement in the self-report and spouse ratings, but also areas where Tom and Susan did not see eye to eye. Focusing on the high-point scale scores, Susan sees Tom as having a problematic combination of Introverted (Schizoid), Inhibited (Avoidant), and Sensitive (Negativistic) traits, which is fairly consistent with Tom's view of himself. Susan did not agree with Tom's self-assessment of being Cooperative (Dependent), which includes seeking harmonious relations with others. Susan rated Tom lowest on traits of Conscientiousness (Respectful; MCMI-III Compulsive), indicating that she feels Tom does not follow directions well and is not orderly or timely in completing tasks.

Susan's self-report results were valid and revealed no unusual test-taking biases (i.e., the validity indices were within normal range). She endorsed a large number of adjectives (75) as self-descriptive and portrayed herself as having a normal (PI T = 40) but distinctly Forceful (Antisocial/Aggressive; T = 74) and Respectful (Compulsive; T = 65) personal style, with slightly above-average levels of Self-confidence (Narcissistic; T = 60) and Sociability (Histrionic; T = 55).

Her results suggest that she sees herself as a hard-nosed, self-disciplined, and unsentimental woman who adheres to rules and regulations as a way of maintaining an edge over competitors. She tends to view the world as a harsh place where toughness and efficiency are needed to excel. For her, survival of the fittest means being sharp, self-controlled, hard-working, and competent. She channels her competitive energies toward attaining personal goals and socially esteemed forms of success. In this regard, she can be something of a perfectionist. She can be insensitive to the needs of others and be overly stern, moralistic, and self-righteous. She may be noted for being somewhat hard-boiled and lacking in tender emotions, yet those close to her notice the tense, worrisome look in her eyes. In spite of the successes she enjoys in life, Susan is always on guard against potential problems and seldom feels confident enough to relax and let down her guard.

Tom rated Susan as having a normal personality style (PI T = 56). While he is impressed by her Forceful and Self-confident nature, he perceives her to be much more Sensitive and Introverted than she does, and he does not find her to be particularly Respectful (Compulsive) or Sociable (Histrionic). He rated her lowest on Cooperative traits, revealing that, in his mind, she does not desire communality or tenderness. Thus, while Tom views his wife (as she does) in terms of being tough-minded and self-confident, he sees her as being unpredictable, moody, irritable, and disinclined to build a relationship with him that is based on mutuality and love.

In our next session, I pointed out to Tom the areas of agreement and disagreement between himself and his wife. He was intrigued by the findings and reported that Susan was "impressed" by the information I was able to give her in a written summary (although not enough to coax her into joining the therapy). The results allowed us to map a strategy for changing Tom's attitudes and behaviors in relation to the marriage. First, Tom needed to change his expectations. I was able to convince him that although Susan is aware of his emotional sensitivity, it is not in her makeup to be emotionally sensitive toward him. She is a no-nonsense kind of person who has specific standards for performance. She admires fortitude and people who can adhere to goals in spite of obstacles. She is not inclined to display her feelings, even when asked to do so. She tends to ration praise and encouragement but not criticism. Although she probably wouldn't be helpful in guiding him back into his pre-illness roles and status in the relationship, she would surely welcome the outcome, and he would be aware of her pleasure as he moved toward success.

With these new expectations, I helped Tom identify some of the pre-illness behaviors and duties that Susan liked him to perform that he no longer did, as well as some of the current tasks and roles that Susan performs by herself that he knew she would like help with. For example, before his illness, Tom and Susan would negotiate cooking and cleaning chores based on who had more free time, energy, and available resources. Because Tom had essentially stopped doing all household tasks after becoming sick, it was easy for him to see that he needed to start doing more. He began with things that he knew he could do that would meet her standards, such as straightening up the living room and being clean, shaved, and dressed when she came home from work. At first, Susan rarely acknowledged his new behaviors, but Tom noted that she was less critical and irritable toward him at dinner time. Tom moved ahead by learning about Susan's work schedule and making dinner on days when she had long hours. As was his custom years ago when he worked, Tom found ways to surprise Susan with small gifts from time to time.

Over a period of several months, Tom's persistence paid off. Susan's mood toward him improved greatly, they began doing more things together during her off hours, and the two now meet at the beginning of each month to budget their income. Tom's self-esteem has increased, he no longer has hypomanic-depressive mood swings around the first of the month, and he has become more active in church activities.

Among the noteworthy features of this case example, let me point out that the MCMI-III was very useful in alerting me to the significant diagnostic features that had to be considered in assessing Tom's ability to engage in treatment. All of my therapeutic work was informed by the MCMI-III findings. With a fairly bright and stable client like Tom, whose spouse was at least somewhat cooperative, the PACL allowed me to provide direct feedback to Tom about his strengths and weaknesses, show him areas where he and Susan agreed and disagreed in their perceptions of one another, and create an intervention strategy based on real data that helped build Tom's confidence so that he could persist in his efforts to change the relationship during the early phases, when he felt discouraged by Susan's response.

EMPLOYMENT SCREENING, FITNESS FOR DUTY, AND CHILD CUSTODY EXAMINEES

Unlike persons who voluntarily seek mental health treatment, individuals referred for evaluation to determine their fitness to perform general or specific tasks are usually motivated to present themselves in a positive light. Clients who fall into this group include military personnel, individuals seeking (or seeking to keep) jobs in a variety of areas, including law enforcement, and persons referred for child custody evaluations. To be successful, the task for these individuals is not to reveal problems but to appear healthy and well-adjusted. Although the vast majority of these clients do not know specifically how to manipulate psychological tests in order to get or keep a particular job, obtain custody of their children, or avoid referral for mental health treatment, they typically know not to reveal too much negative material and to show

Table 4.2

MCMI-III Modifier Indices for Individuals Motivated to Present
Themselves Favorably or Instructed to Do So Deliberately

MCMI-III Scale	Law Enforcement Job Candidates		Child Custody Examinees		Psychiatric Fake Good	
	Mean	SD	Mean	SD	Mean	SD
X. Disclosure	29.6	15.9	31.6	16.1	55.9	19.9
Y. Desirability	78.1	16.4	75.6	13.1	73.5	22.8
Z. Debasement	19.5	18.7	23.1	21.9	40.5	29.7

The Law Enforcement Job Candidates (n = 54) were tested by the author and his colleagues for the VA and were undergoing actual job interviews. The Child Custody Examinees were 259 men and women from McCann et al.'s (2001) total sample who were
undergoing court-ordered assessment. The Psychiatric Fake Good sample consisted of
80 men and women psychiatric outpatients who were instructed by Daubert and Metzler
(2000) to "fake good in a credible manner" (p. 419).

that they possess the positive characteristics they believe are necessary
for obtaining their desired outcome. Evaluators can expect these clients
to present in a socially desirable way on self-report measures and to
downplay negative qualities.

Like the MMPI-2 (Butcher, 2001; Butcher et al., 2001), the majority of
MCMI-III (Millon, 1997) test items were written to detect specific problems. Most of these are face-valid and can be readily identified by respondents (Choca & Van Denburg, 1997; Millon, 1997). On the MMPI-2
(Butcher, 2001), job applicants usually obtain validity and standard clinical scale scores that are all within normal range. The most highly elevated
among these are the Superlative (S), Correction (K), and Lie (L) scales,
which are usually in the T = 60 to 70 range.

Large-scale job applicant studies have not been conducted with the
MCMI-III. However, assessments conducted by my colleagues and me on
54 men applying for jobs as armed police officers with the U.S. Department of Veterans Affairs (VA) yielded results that were consistent with
previous studies on normal samples and those focusing on persons who
presented themselves positively, either due to the circumstances of the
screening (e.g., child custody evaluations; McCann et al., 2001), or because they were instructed to do so (e.g., Craig, Kuncel, & Olson, 1994;
Daubert & Metzler, 2000; Millon, 1997). With regard to the modifier indices (see Table 4.2), the Disclosure (X) and Debasement (Z) scales were
very low among the VA job applicants and child custody examinees (BR <
35), whereas the Desirability (Y) scale was elevated, on average, above BR
75. It is significant that the X and Z scale scores of the psychiatric patients

asked to fake good (Daubert & Metzler, 2000) were more moderate than those of actual examinees who were motivated to present favorably.

The PD and clinical scale scores of the VA job applicants and child custody examinees (McCann et al., 2001) were universally low (BR M < 60), except for notable, and sometimes clinically significant, elevations on the Histrionic, Narcissistic, and Compulsive scales. The VA job applicants were most likely to have their highest elevation on the Compulsive scale (BR M = 72.1), followed by the Narcissistic scale (BR M = 65.3). Child custody examinees showed their highest elevations on the Histrionic (M = 69.8), Compulsive (M = 68.4), and Narcissistic (M = 65.2) scales (McCann et al., 2001, total sample). Research with non-help-seeking adults who completed the MCMI using normal instructions typically showed elevations on the same three PD scales (Choca & Van Denburg, 1997; Craig, 2002; Millon, 1997; Strack, 1993). Thus, VA job applicants and child custody examinees were frequently able to appear normal on the MCMI-III.

In situations where clients are motivated to present positively on the MCMI-III, the PACL can be useful because the test provides a normal frame of reference for assessing a range of *DSM* (APA, 2000; Sperry, 2003) personality traits. Recall that the PACL was normed on normal adults, uses T-scores rather than BR scores, and includes a PI scale. Because of these features, the PACL can be used to help rule out a PD when an examinee obtains one or more BR score elevations above 75 on the MCMI-III. It can also be useful in fleshing out the personality profiles of persons who, on the MCMI-III, show the restricted range of scale elevations associated with fake good and normal responding (i.e., elevations on Histrionic, Narcissistic, and Compulsive).

CASE EXAMPLE: PREEMPLOYMENT SCREENING

Let me use as an illustration the case of a 35-year-old African American married male military veteran, with 13 years of education. He was evaluated during the preemployment screening process that is used for hiring armed police officers at the VA. As is common practice in law enforcement hiring at state and local levels, the VA psychological evaluation is one of the last hurdles that a candidate must clear. Prior to reaching me, this candidate had to pass a thorough background check and at least three interviews. He was cleared by everyone in the law enforcement administration and now had to pass the medical checkup, which involved a physical and psychological examination.

The psychological evaluation was conducted on two consecutive days and involved a face-to-face structured interview and three self-report instruments, the MMPI-2, MCMI-III, and PACL. The candidate's relevant

MCMI-III modifier and PD scale elevations are given in Table 4.3 along with the results of the PACL. As is common with our applicant pool, this man had BR scores < 60 on all other MCMI-III PD and clinical scales.

On the MCMI-III validity indices, this man exhibited a typical *fake good* profile consistent with other VA law enforcement candidates and child custody examinees (see Table 4.2). He revealed very little about himself (X), and what he did reveal was of a socially desirable nature (Y). Except for scale 5 (Narcissistic), his item response pattern did not match that of a psychiatric diagnostic group. There is no indication of Axis I disturbance or severe Axis II personality pathology. Although a BR score of 79 on the Narcissistic scale would not be considered unusual for a normal adult in a research study, in an evaluative context like this there is a question of whether this man may be too egotistical for this particular job (e.g., defensive, haughty, contemptuous) or, worse yet, show the pattern of rigidity and inflexibility in interpersonal situations that is characteristic of someone with a PD.[3]

The PACL validity indices provide reassurance that the candidate's responses were neither too defensive (number of items checked = 22) nor too favorable to be usefully interpreted, although he was clearly presenting himself in a positive light. Compared with a normal population, there is no indication that this man has personality problems (PI = 44) or an unusual number of narcissistic traits (Confident = 50). The PACL personality profile suggests a strongly defined Cooperative and Respectful interpersonal style. He is likely to be agreeable, deferential, and devoted to hard work, as well as maintaining congenial relations with others. He is probably amiable, easygoing, and attentive to others' needs and wishes. He should be flexible and adaptable and willing to please those in authority and have a strong sense of propriety and morality. He is likely to be even-keeled emotionally (not impulsive) and to be a good team player, but he may be somewhat conventional and lacking in spontaneity. He may see himself as being modestly talented and socially awkward when outside his usual sphere of family, friends, and coworkers. He will probably do well working with the public in group settings but may have trouble if asked to assume a leadership position.

Readers unaccustomed to using the MCMI-III and PACL together may question the differences in test results noted by this example, but they are

---

[3] Recall that the MCMI-III (Millon, 1987, pp. 113–114) employs several methods to correct for positive and negative self-report biases. In this particular case, the candidate's low X score caused 5 BR points to be added to all of his Axis I and II scale scores, and an additional 8 BR points were added to his Narcissistic scale score as a result of a Denial/Complaint Adjustment (pp. 177–180). Thus, prior to these corrections, the candidate's Narcissistic BR score was 66, which is average and not in the clinically significant range.

Table 4.3
Test Scores for Law Enforcement Job Candidate

MCMI-III		PACL	
Scale	BR Score	Scale	Score
X. Disclosure	26	Number of items	
Y. Desirability	78	endorsed	22
Z. Debasement	10	R. Random	−17
4. Histrionic	59	F. Favorable	8
5. Narcissistic	79	UF. Unfavorable	−13
7. Compulsive	67	1. Introversive	41
		2. Inhibited	45
		3. Cooperative	70
		4. Sociable	46
		5. Confident	50
		6. Forceful	47
		7. Respectful	72
		8. Sensitive	41
		PI. Problem Indicator	44

Note. PACL scale scores 1 through PI are T scores.

not in conflict with one another. When this candidate's test responses are compared to those of a psychiatric population (i.e., people seeking help for emotional problems), he comes across as being overly defensive, overly positive, and possessing strong narcissistic traits (MCMI-III). He did not exhibit an Axis I disorder and, overall, did not fit very well with a patient population, which is good. When his responses are compared to those of a non-help-seeking normal population (PACL), this man comes across as being normal, with a well-defined interpersonal style that may serve him well in his chosen occupation.

I mentioned previously that most clients who present themselves as normal and healthy on the MCMI-III have a limited, stereotyped set of scores. This is due in part to the problem-focused nature of the items and to the fact that the test was developed and normed on patients in the initial stages of help-seeking. Results of the PACL can also be swayed in a positive direction, but clinical experience indicates that many who successfully avoid revealing themselves on the MCMI-III give a more accurate and varied personality portrait on the PACL. Although research is needed to confirm this impression, the effect may occur as a function of normal social desirability that is accounted for in the scores of the PACL normative sample. In other words, normal persons usually present themselves in a positive light, as they wish to make a positive impression on others. This tendency is recorded and normalized on the PACL so that the effect of an extraordinary effort to be self-biasing is not as strongly noted on the PACL as on the MCMI-III.

REFERENCES

American Psychiatric Association. (1987). *Diagnostic and statistical manual of mental disorders* (3rd ed., rev.). Washington, DC: Author.

American Psychiatric Association. (2000). *Diagnostic and statistical manual of mental disorders* (4th ed., text rev.). Washington, DC: Author.

Butcher, J. N. (2001). *MMPI-2 revised personnel system user's guide* (3rd ed.). Minneapolis, MN: University of Minnesota Press.

Butcher, J. N., Graham, J. R., Ben-Porath, Y. S., Tellegen, A., Dahlstrom, W. G., & Kaemmer, B. (2001). *MMPI-2 manual for administration, scoring, and interpretation* (Rev. ed.). Minneapolis, MN: University of Minnesota Press.

Choca, J. P., & Van Denburg, E. (1997). *Interpretive guide to the Millon Clinical Multiaxial Inventory* (2nd ed.). Washington, DC: American Psychological Association.

Craig, R. J. (2002). Essentials of MCMI-III assessment. In S. Strack (Ed.), *Essentials of Millon inventories assessment* (2nd ed., pp. 1–51). New York: Wiley.

Craig, R. J., Kuncel, R., & Olson, R. E. (1994). Ability of drug abusers to avoid detection of substance abuse on the MCMI-II. *Journal of Social Behavior and Personality, 9*, 95–106.

Daubert, S. D., & Metzler, A. E. (2000). The detection of fake-bad and fake-good responding on the Millon Clinical Multiaxial Inventory III. *Psychological Assessment, 12*, 418–424.

Horowitz, L. M., Alden, L. E., Wiggins, J. S., & Pincus, A. L. (2000). *Inventory of interpersonal problems*. San Antonio, TX: Psychological Corporation.

Horton, A. D., & Retzlaff, P. D. (1991). Family assessment: Toward *DSM-III-R* relevancy. *Journal of Clinical Psychology, 47*, 94–100.

Loevinger, J. (1957). Objective tests as instruments of psychological theory. *Psychological Reports, 3*, 635–694.

McCann, J. T., Flens, J. R., Campagna, V., Collman, P., Lazzaro, T., & Connor, E. (2001). The MCMI-III in child custody evaluations: A normative study. *Journal of Forensic Psychology Practice, 1*, 27–44.

Millon, T. (1981). *Disorders of personality*. New York: Wiley.

Millon, T. (1983a). *Millon clinical multiaxial inventory manual* (3rd ed.). Minneapolis, MN: National Computer Systems.

Millon, T. (1983b). *Modern psychopathology*. Prospect Heights, IL: Waveland Press. (Original work published 1969)

Millon, T. (1986a). A theoretical derivation of pathological personalities. In T. Millon & G. L. Klerman (Eds.), *Contemporary directions in psychopathology: Toward the* DSM-IV (pp. 639–670). New York: Guilford Press.

Millon, T. (1986b). Personality prototypes and their diagnostic criteria. In T. Millon & G. L. Klerman (Eds.), *Contemporary directions in psychopathology: Toward the* DSM-IV (pp. 639–670). New York: Guilford Press.

Millon, T. (1987). *Manual for the MCMI-II* (2nd ed.). Minneapolis, MN: National Computer Systems.

Millon, T. (1990). *Toward a new personology.* New York: Wiley.

Millon, T. (1994). *Millon index of personality styles manual.* San Antonio, TX: Psychological Corporation.

Millon, T. (1996). *Disorders of personality* (2nd ed.). New York: Wiley.

Millon, T. (1997). *MCMI-III manual* (2nd ed.). Minneapolis, MN: National Computer Systems.

Millon, T. (1999). *Personality-guided therapy.* New York: Wiley.

Millon, T. (2004). *MIPS-R manual.* Minneapolis, MN: Pearson Assessments.

Millon, T., & Davis, R. D. (1994). Millon's evolutionary model of normal and abnormal personality: Theory and measures. In S. Strack & M. Lorr (Eds.), *Differentiating normal and abnormal personality* (pp. 79–113). New York: Springer.

Millon, T., & Davis, R. D. (2000). *Personality disorders in modern life.* New York: Wiley.

Pincus, A. L., & Wiggins, J. S. (1990). Interpersonal problems and conceptions of personality disorders. *Journal of Personality Disorders, 4,* 342–352.

Retzlaff, P. D., & Gibertini, M. (1987). Factor structure of the MCMI basic personality scales and common-item artifact. *Journal of Personality Assessment, 51,* 588–594.

Robbins, B. (1998). *WinPACL 2.0 user's guide.* South Pasadena, CA: 21st Century Assessment.

Sperry, L. (2003). *Handbook of diagnosis and treatment of* DSM-IV-TR *personality disorders* (2nd ed.). New York: Brunner-Routledge.

Strack, S. (1987). Development and validation of an adjective checklist to assess the Millon personality types in a normal population. *Journal of Personality Assessment, 51,* 572–587.

Strack, S. (1991a). *Comparison of PACL PI scale elevations in samples of psychiatric patients and normal adults.* Unpublished manuscript.

Strack, S. (1991b). Factor analysis of MCMI-II and PACL basic personality scales in a college sample. *Journal of Personality Assessment, 57,* 345–355.

Strack, S. (1991c). *Manual for the personality adjective checklist (PACL), Revised* South Pasadena, CA: 21st Century Assessment.

Strack, S. (1993). Measuring Millon's personality styles in normal adults. In R. J. Craig (Ed.), *The Millon clinical cultiaxial inventory: A clinical research information synthesis* (pp. 253–278). Hillsdale, NJ: Erlbaum.

Strack, S. (1994). Relating Millon's basic personality styles and Holland's occupational types. *Journal of Vocational Behavior, 45,* 41–54.

Strack, S. (1997). The PACL: Gauging normal personality styles. In T. Millon (Ed.), *The Millon inventories: Clinical and personality assessment* (pp. 477–497). New York: Guilford Press.

Strack, S. (Ed.). (1999). Millon's evolving personality theory and measures [Special series]. *Journal of Personality Assessment, 72*(3), 323–456.

Strack, S. (2002). *Essentials of Millon inventories assessment* (2nd ed.). New York: Wiley.

Strack, S. (in press). Measuring normal personality the Millon way. In S. Strack (Ed.), *Handbook of personology and psychopathology*. New York: Wiley.

Strack, S., & Guevara, L. F. (1999). Relating PACL measures of Millon's basic personality styles and MMPI-2 scales in patient and normal samples. *Journal of Clinical Psychology, 55,* 895–906.

Strack, S., & Lorr, M. (1990). Three approaches to interpersonal behavior and their common factors. *Journal of Personality Assessment, 54,* 782–790.

Strack, S., Lorr, M., & Campbell, L. (1989, August). *Similarities in Millon personality styles among normals and psychiatric patients.* Paper presented at the annual convention of the American Psychological Association, New Orleans, LA.

Strack, S., Lorr, M., & Campbell, L. (1990). An evaluation of Millon's circular model of personality disorders. *Journal of Personality Disorders, 4,* 353–361.

Strack, S., Lorr, M., Campbell, L., & Lamnin, A. (1992). Personality and clinical syndrome factors of MCMI-II scales. *Journal of Personality Disorders, 6,* 40–52.

Wiggins, J. S., & Pincus, A. L. (1989). Conceptions of personality disorders and dimensions of personality. *JCCP: Psychological Assessment, 1,* 305–316.

Wiggins, J. S., & Pincus, A. L. (1994). Personality structure and the structure of personality disorders. In P. T. Costa & T. A. Widiger (Eds.), *Personality disorders and the five-factor model of personality* (pp. 73–93). Washington, DC: American Psychological Association.

CHAPTER 5

Issues in the Assessment of Personality Disorders and Substance Abusers with the MCMI

PATRICK M. FLYNN

SINCE ITS introduction in the 1970s, the original and all subsequent versions of the MCMI have been routinely used as diagnostic and screening tools with substance-abusing populations to assess for personality and symptom characteristics. The importance of identifying co-occurring disorders has recently come to the forefront in the study of addictions. Because of its correspondence with *DSM* Axis I and II disorders, the MCMI has become an increasingly popular instrument for assessing clinical populations. Major strengths of this inventory are its ability to differentiate between various psychiatric problems and its utility in producing both diagnostic and dynamic profiles for use in clinical decision making (e.g., suggesting diagnoses, treatment planning). It is one of the few theoretically based psychopathology assessment tools with a strong research base that has been developed over the past three decades. These studies provided evidence of psychometric properties that support the clinical utility of the MCMI.

This chapter is based on and revisits issues presented in an earlier article (Flynn, McCann, & Fairbank, 1995). The author (Flynn) recognizes the contributions of his earlier co-authors, particularly those of Joseph T. McCann, Psy.D., J. D. who wrote a presentation on this topic for the first American Psychological Association (APA) MCMI symposium. This presentation was given by Flynn at that annual APA meeting (August 1991), and it included many of the key issues covered in this chapter.

The purpose of this chapter is to describe current and ongoing issues surrounding the use of the MCMI with substance abusers. Suggestions are offered to help answer some questions and manage concerns arising from clinical applications that may present unclear, conflicting, or ambiguous interpretations of patient profiles among problem substance users. These issues include categorical classifications and the use of prototypical (i.e., face-valid) items in assessing substance use disorders, cut-off scores, and formulating diagnostic recommendations. Several operating characteristics and functions affecting research, particularly outcome studies, are also discussed in detail. Considerations and recommendations for using the MCMI with substance users are presented as closing comments for issues related to each major topic area.

CATEGORICAL CLASSIFICATIONS

Historically, categorical labels and classification systems were developed in response to a need for designations to help communicate relevant clinical information among health care professionals about their patients. There was a clear need for information that uniformly described presenting problems in a standard nomenclature that could be understood by other practitioners. These categorizations have also been important and standard constructs for researchers in their quest to understand disorders and treatment responses. To fulfill this need, the official *Diagnostic and Statistical Manual of Mental Disorders* (*DSM*) nomenclature was adopted in the field of mental health science. This system is also a public health tool for aggregating and conveying statistical information regarding disorders among varying populations (American Psychiatric Association, 1994).

With each new generation of the MCMI (Millon, 1977, 1982, 1987), and more so in the latest version, items and scales have been constructed to reflect *DSM* criteria and correspond with the American Psychiatric Association's officially recognized disorders (Millon, Davis, & Millon, 1997). Indeed, each corresponding MCMI manual also has evolved in its presentation of this correspondence. The most recent edition included tabular presentations of *DSM* criteria with their corresponding MCMI prototypical items for each of the personality disorder scales. These charts map how individual items tap the clinical attributes and criteria associated with specific *DSM* disorders, as well as their relation to the personality constructs in Millon's theory of personality and psychopathology. The maps, coupled with other material, provide considerable detail in regard to personality prototypes. Flynn and McMahon (1997) extended this itemization to the Alcohol and Drug Dependence scales to illuminate the role of prototypical items and their counterparts, the more subtle and less face-valid items (i.e., items that have minimal scale loadings but are prototypical for other disorders).

Despite acceptance as objective tools, some degree of fallibility is associated with all assessment instruments because their psychometric properties are always less than perfect. The more subjective clinical methods used to obtain patient information when constructing diagnoses and planning the course of treatment are also prone to inaccuracies. Undeniably, when making clinical decisions, the best course involves principles of concentricity wherein full information methods are used to determine overlap among indicators constructed from various sources and strategies used to identify presenting symptoms. More dynamic profiles of patients and their immediate characteristics can be developed by relying on information gleaned from more than one set and source of indicators. Thus, traditional clinical staffings, in which data are presented from clinical interviews, observations, and collateral sources, as well as those from screening and diagnostic instruments, will always provide a richer clinical perspective than a sole-source decision. Clinicians in private and solo practices, outside of health care centers staffed with mental health professionals from multiple disciplines, can also avail themselves of some of these methods by further studying all available information and looking for convergence of indicators.

The MCMI is only one of many tools available for classifying patients. Results can be used to identify hypotheses that help guide treatment. Because of its comprehensive nature, the Millon inventory can be a key source of data in building a confident and dynamic understanding of issues surrounding each patient's problems. When the MCMI is used to classify patients, whether for research or clinical purposes, such as communicating to colleagues or third-party payers, it is recommended that all available information be used. Additional data should be obtained in the presence of few data sources. Thus, at least two or more corroborating sources should be used in determining a patient's fundamental problem(s).

ASSESSING SUBSTANCE USE DISORDERS

MCMI research and development has been ongoing for almost 30 years since its introduction and the publication of the first manual (Millon, 1977). As others have noted (e.g., Flynn & McMahon, 1997), the scales measuring alcohol and drug problems have changed over the years (1977, Alcohol Misuse and Drug Misuse; 1982, Alcohol Abuse and Drug Abuse;

1987 and 1997, Alcohol Dependence and Drug Dependence). These revisions have included efforts to improve correspondence with the *DSM* and its routine modifications as it also evolved to its current version IV. The latest scales included in the MCMI-III for assessing substance use disorders are labeled Alcohol Dependence and Drug Dependence. Their content, correspondence with *DSM* criteria, and item weights have been mapped and presented in some detail in another publication (Flynn & McMahon, 1997).

Research has examined various versions of the substance dependence scales, and in general, some studies supported their utility (see Craig, 1997; Craig & Olson, 1998; Flynn & McMahon, 1983, 1984). However, other studies have raised caution and questioned the validity and utility of these scales (e.g., Bryer, Martines, & Dignan, 1990; Calsyn, Saxon, & Daisy, 1990, 1991; Craig & Weinberg, 1992a, 1992b). Because results have been inconclusive, these indicators should be used in conjunction with other measures of dependence when possible, even when the scales show considerable elevations (e.g., base rates [BRs] of 75 or higher). Other clinical evidence (e.g., interviews, records, reports, collateral reports) is often necessary when determining whether a substance problem is present and needs attention in the therapeutic plan.

When faced with unconvincing information, another recommended approach involves a closer scrutiny of item-level responses. McCann and colleagues (McCann, Flynn, & Gersh, 1992) suggested that item-level analyses (e.g., prototypical item endorsements compared with BR cut-offs) could be used to improve the diagnostic efficiency of MCMI scales. This methodology was used in a later study to examine the MCMI-II Drug Dependence scale (Flynn et al., 1997). Results demonstrated that prototypical item cut-offs had higher levels of diagnostic and positive predictive power in identifying regular drug users than the traditional BR cut-off scores, which encompassed the entire scale. Although this alternative method of determining cut-offs increased scale sensitivity or the probability of detecting dependence when it was present in the study sample, sensitivity was still less than perfect. However, this alternative cut-off configured from prototypical items did discriminate substance dependence better than the BR cut-off. More recently, Blais and colleagues (Blais et al., 2003) used this same approach with other scales and found that prototypical items from the MCMI Anxiety scale also had better discriminant validity than the present Anxiety scale. They speculated that these findings may have been due to the prototypical and face-valid items being more directly related to anxiety, the construct assessed by the scale.

Because of the questions surrounding the validity and utility of the Dependence scales and the caveats about their use, a closer examination of items and their scale loadings offers a practical approach to problem solving when faced with conflicting or inconclusive Dependence scale scores. Sufficient evidence exists to support the use of item-level analyses in clinical decision making. A reasonable surrogate for the traditional Dependence scale BR cut-offs when using the MCMI with known substance abusers is to configure a set of prototypical items as an alternative marker. The Dependence scale items (Scale B, Alcohol; Scale T, Drug Dependence) are few and brief, and it would not take more than several minutes of a clinician's time to review patients' responses after becoming familiar with these items. After establishing procedures to have available MCMI responses to these critical items for closer inspection when needed, an alternative indicator of dependence could be easily and readily available to inform decision-making processes.

Another issue pertinent to collecting information from substance users involves the source or type of report. Self-reports among substance-using populations have been routinely questioned, and debates about the validity of self-reported drug use have been ongoing for a number of years. Some of the issues involve demand characteristics for reporting socially undesirable behaviors (see Embree & Whitehead, 1993) and situation-specific requirements (e.g., the need to show evidence of recent opioid use for admission to methadone treatment). Others involve limitations associated with natural recall, as well as recall that is affected by chemical agents. Even though more research is needed to determine methods to improve these self-reports, it is clear that the most efficient means of determining substance use is through self-report (Harrison & Hughes, 1997). Because the MCMI is self-administered and involves self-reports, users should be familiar with these caveats and use caution when results are less than conclusive.

In summary, if situations arise where traditional scale scores do not indicate a substance problem or dependence, but other clinical data may indicate such problems, it is best to examine all available information. Information should be obtained from corroborating sources and evaluated whenever possible. Biological specimens are often obtained and tested in conjunction with self-reports from substance abusers. Also, a simple inspection of item-level responses may provide additional data for use in determining whether or not a substance use problem exists and needs to be addressed in therapy. For example, some responses to prototypical items that have face-valid content (e.g., item 13: "My drug habits have gotten me into a good deal of trouble in the past") may prove to be more direct problem indicators and may be a more valuable source of information than exceeding a BR scale cut-off. The Drug and Alcohol Dependence scales each have 6 prototypical items. As recommended by the instrument's author and developers, "Clinicians may still choose to inspect the prototypal items of each scale as so-called critical items when seeking support for particular criteria and when making diagnostic judgments" (Millon et al., 1997, p. 2). For all possible substance dependence cases, prototypical items should be considered critical items, and responses to these should be carefully weighed. It is recommended that both corroborating and disputing information be examined and at least two data sources be used when specifying drug or alcohol dependence.

CUT-OFF SCORES

A major strength of the MCMI is in its structural ability to provide not only dimensional indicators but also diagnostic or categorical recommendations about personality and other clinical disorders. Despite the DSM's widely used and accepted approach to diagnostic classification, one that uses criterion endorsements to make clinical classifications, much has been said and written regarding the need for dimensional measures of psychopathology. Research has shown that dimensional measures can be better predictors of treatment retention (Broome, Flynn, & Simpson, 1999), and use of such measures clearly adds clinical relevance to diagnostic classifications. In determining a clear picture of a presenting patient's problems, clinicians hope to develop a dynamic understanding or dimensional view of symptoms, characteristics, cognitive styles, interpersonal behaviors, and so forth. Even though there is a clear and convincing need for nonnominal measures, diagnoses are still necessary to communicate information to insurers, colleagues, and researchers. Standardized nomenclature is used to define and articulate a relevant representation of psychiatric problems for which treatment will be tailored and planned accordingly. Because of the distinguishing measurement features of the MCMI and its correspondence with DSM diagnoses, a rich source of dimensional and diagnostic data can be provided from this objective psychological instrument. The inventory's profiles can both complement and supplement other clinical, and perhaps sometimes more subjective, sources of information.

Initially, MCMI cut-offs for suggesting diagnostic assignments were focused on key *presence* (BR 75 to 84) or *prominence* (BR 85+) markers. Too often, during its earlier years, the focus of routine use was on single scale indicators. More recently, because prototypical cases are a rarity (e.g., those represented by a single scale only elevation), the focus is now on code types, where elevations occur on two or more scales (McCann & Seuss, 1988). Millon, Davis, and Millon (1997) refer to this approach as *configural interpretation* and note the importance of the highest scale elevation in relation to secondary or tertiary scale elevations. These patterns can often indicate patient characteristics other than just those found in single scale indications and will require blended interpretations.

MCMI cluster analytic research with substance-abusing populations has paralleled this approach in its identification of key scale subclusters. In their review of the literature, Flynn and McMahon (1997) identified and described four recurring clusters based on scale elevations or profile peaks. The first of these was characterized as interpersonally dominant, manipulative, and exploitive, with substance use likely related to self-pleasure and excitement. The second cluster represented users with severe pathology characterized by pessimism, irritability, paranoia, mood swings, irregular behaviors, and unconstrained actions. Substance use for this group was likely to be associated with an attempt to manage interpersonal feelings. Cluster 3 was characterized by social avoidance, dependence, hesitance, ineptness, anguish, depression, and anxiety, and the likely use of substances was also for dealing with feelings, as suggested in cluster 2. The fourth and last cluster was labeled subclinical because scale elevations indicated less pathology and fewer problems than those found among the other clusters identified in the research.

Because substance-using clinical populations have been found to have high levels of co-occurring disorders (Havassy, Alvidrez, & Owen, 2004; Onken, Blaine, Genser, & Horton, 1997; Zimmerman, Sheeran, Chelminski, & Young, 2004), including personality disorders, prevalence rates should also be carefully considered when using cut-off scores in diagnostic processes. Antisocial Personality Disorder (ASP) is one of the most frequently found Axis II disorders among substance users (Ziedonis, 1992). Results from a national study of drug abusers in treatment showed the ASP level in a sample of treatment clients to be approximately 40% (Flynn, Craddock, Luckey, Hubbard, & Dunteman, 1996). High prevalence rates of this disorder are unique to this population, which diverges considerably from the MCMI validation sample. Every consideration possible should be given to developing local and/or substance user norms when routine practice involves assessing substance-using populations.

The operating characteristics of the MCMI are dependent on various factors, including the prevalence of disorders assessed by the instrument's scales. The MCMI-III validation sample included an Antisocial prevalence rate of approximately 6%, which is considerably lower than might be expected in a drug-abusing sample. Research reported in the literature indicates that this prevalence rate is likely to be 30% or more in known substance-using populations. Flynn and McMahon (1997), using a formula from Gibertini and colleagues (Gibertini, Brandenburg, & Retzlaff, 1986), showed that, for screening purposes, the base rate cut-off of

85 using MCMI standardization sample data would indicate a considerably lower probability for suggesting an ASP diagnostic assignment than if the higher prevalence data for ASP among substance-using populations were used. Thus, it is recommended that prevalence data be carefully considered when screening for disorders in substance-using populations because expected and obtained rates of certain disorders are typically different from those found in the instrument's validation sample.

A related issue, but of equal importance, identified by McCann (1990) involves statistical bias due to less than perfect sensitivity and specificity. Because these operating characteristics are imperfect (<1.0), adjustments can be made to allow for this bias when using the MCMI to determine prevalence rates of disorders in both clinical and research populations. McCann also showed how methods developed by Rogan and Gladen (1978) can be used to improve prevalence estimates and offered a formula for making these adjustments.

It should be recognized that cut-off scores might be misleading when patient samples diverge from those used to develop and validate the MCMI. Configural interpretations that consider patterns beyond single scale elevations will provide a richer and more complete portrayal of presenting problems. Finally, always recognize an instrument's foibles without losing sight of its strengths and utility. In regard to the MCMI, the wealth of dynamic and diagnostic information far outweighs some of its minor weaknesses, which are also found in most other inventories.

It is recommended that clinicians working with known substance-using populations supplement BR cut-offs by developing alternative and local norms. Adjustments to help control for biases due to less than perfect operating characteristics should also be made as indicated when using the MCMI to determine prevalence rates in clinical populations.

DIAGNOSTIC RECOMMENDATIONS

Clinical interviews such as the Structured Clinical Interview for *DSM* (SCID; First, Spitzer, Gibbon, & Williams, 1995), interviews for nonclinical staff such as the Diagnostic Interview Schedule (DIS; Robins, Helzer, Croughan, & Ratcliff, 1981), and inventories such as the MCMI and other similar assessment tools, as well as some unstructured interview techniques used by clinicians all have associated decision-making rules. However, in contrast to the codified diagnostic guides used in SCID and DIS types of assessments, diagnostic decision-making rules for configural interpretations of the MCMI are less strict and often more subjective.

These require an ability to integrate and synthesize a considerable amount of data. As cautioned in the MCMI manual and interpretive reports, diagnostic decisions should be made only in combination with other clinical data such as biographical, observational, interview, test results, and other knowledge of current circumstances (Millon et al., 1997).

The best rule of thumb in using the MCMI as an aid in clinical diagnoses is to look for convergence of information sources, beginning with at least two indicators to confirm a clinical hypothesis (e.g., interview data and MCMI profile). In ideal situations, all sources (e.g., biographical, observational, interview, MCMI, collateral such as reports from significant other/family/friends) generate similar hypotheses and decisions are clear-cut. In the least favorable, data sources are inconsistent and contradictory, requiring further assessment and knowledge to formulate a diagnostic assignment. These situations, in which there is considerable data disagreement, are comparable to a weather vane in a severe storm, when the wind is changeable and inconstant, giving no direction to the vane other than constant spinning. However, in *most* clinical cases, there will be some overlapping indicators with a majority of consistent data and few discrepancies that warrant further examination. Faced with inconsistent indications, item-level examinations of prototypical, as well as some of the more subtle items may help resolve these discrepancies. When presented with a lack of evidence from various sources to support a diagnostic hypothesis, it may be necessary to obtain additional information. This is of particular importance if clinical record data is sparse and other sources are equally limited.

More than one source of information obtained through different methods is the recommended and logical approach to clinical decision making. Configural interpretations, where MCMI patterns indicated by multiple scale elevations are interpreted and corroborated with other sources, should be used when making diagnostic assignments. Information must be integrated and then synthesized to minimize both false positives and false negatives. The MCMI is one of several inventories that can be used in the process of clinical assessment. But, as do all other assessment tools, it has imperfect operating characteristics (e.g., sensitivity and specificity), and it should not be used as a sole source for diagnostic determinations. When coupled with other clinical information, however, it can provide important dynamic input for classifying patients and identifying disorders that need immediate attention. Because this chapter focuses on assessing substance users and personality disorders, procedures are suggested herein for identifying potential diagnostic assignments. To illustrate this point, specific examples are provided for determining if ASP and substance dependence (SD) are presenting problems.

Certain pathways can be followed depending on whether information from clinical intakes is consistent with and supports MCMI results, or whether there is disagreement between the sources. In situations where clinical records for an adult may or may not indicate behavioral patterns suggesting ASP, and where a subsequent MCMI profile supports or refutes an ASP diagnosis, a review of responses to MCMI prototypical items may help to clarify this discrepancy and serve as an aid in decision making. On the one hand, positive responses to such prototypical items that ask about troubles with the law, impulsivity, and behaving without forethought of effects on others may prove to be better indicators of ASP characteristics than using the entire scale 6A Antisocial. For example, responses to more subtle items such as those that ask whether responders like to flirt or if they are moral and proper are also included in the scale and its score. These responses, combined with other scale items, may be contributing to a score inconsistent with clinical intake reports. On the other hand, negative responses to the direct and face-valid items may be an indication of denial or faking. In this case, the nonprototypical items (i.e., items that are indirectly related to a scale without obvious content association) that were endorsed may provide some insight into discrepancies between indicators derived from different data sources. By using this information, it may be possible to determine which and whether clinical record data or scale score data are either false positive or false negative, and clinicians will then be in a better position to specify the presenting problem(s). Also, as described earlier, close examination of item-level responses may yield information with greater specificity for clinical decision making.

Similarly, when substance dependence information from scales B (Alcohol Dependence) and T (Drug Dependence) and clinical record/intake interview data do not agree, an examination of item-level responses may help to answer questions. Consider a scenario where scale B or T is sufficiently elevated to indicate dependence and the clinical records do not indicate a history or problem in this area. It is highly likely that patients will have endorsed at least several of the prototypical items, such as those that ask directly about an alcohol problem or use of illegal drugs. These items may offer reasons why a dependence scale was elevated and stimulate questions about the absence of this information in clinical records. Such situations may also suggest some probes for future patient sessions to begin to explore problematic substance use.

To summarize briefly, at times, MCMI profiles may not agree with other sources of data. When this happens, a close examination of item-level responses may help to resolve such a discrepancy and further inform clinical decisions. It is recommended that unless all sources of information have some overlap and indicate a clear diagnostic assignment, clinicians should look beyond scale scores and profiles to item-level indicators, particularly those prototypical items weighted most heavily in generating BR scores.

OPERATING CHARACTERISTICS AND OUTCOME STUDIES

Temporal stability of research measures is an important consideration in outcome studies, particularly when using MCMI-like instruments over time in repeated research designs. Transitory symptoms targeted by therapeutic approaches are frequently the focus of outcome research, but often other associated problems also are of interest as potential outcomes. On the one hand, at least in theory, personality scale scores that measure enduring characteristics should remain generally stable in the short run unless a specific, tactical, and efficacious intervention for a particular personality disorder is being used to directly address the problem. On the other hand, reducing less enduring symptoms that are more amenable to change—ones that are typically measured at clinically relevant intervals—is often a goal in determining the efficacy of therapeutic strategies used in treatment. Whether the goal is a change in symptoms or personality, stability of measures needs to be examined before a change in outcomes is assessed.

Further complicating stability of measures are conceptual considerations that have been recently challenged regarding the acute or transient states of *DSM* Axis I and the chronic or enduring characteristics of Axis II personality disorders. Shea and Yen (2003) question temporal stability as a distinguishing feature between axes. As they indicate, some Axis I disorders are chronic and enduring. Their analyses of large data sets suggest that stability is not a clinically meaningful discriminator between axes. Despite these issues, temporal stability has a considerable role in statistical analyses and interpretations in the study of therapeutic outcomes.

As Hsu and his colleagues (Hsu, Maruish, & Moreland, 1992) noted, scale stability is an important issue when examining treatment effects. They offered an excellent discussion of scale stability in regard to the MCMI-II that is every bit as relevant for all versions of the MCMI. Their monograph describes how stability coefficients operate as *linear standard scores* and how they should function independently from change scores if a targeted treatment uniformly affects all patients. The assumption is that scale score stability should continue to be a linear function such that the treatment has an estimated equal effect on all individuals. Scores from pre- and postadministrations should remain stable but yet lower after the intervention (Hsu et al., 1992).

For example (assuming appropriate research methods such as random-ization, sufficient subjects, etc.), with significant group changes and uniform reductions in MCMI scores across all patients over time after participation in a cognitive-behavioral treatment (CBT), stability coeffi-cients should remain high if the changes are associated with CBT. How-ever, if significant group changes with low stability are found, it would be unclear whether the changes were attributable to CBT or some other factor, such as differential intervention effects for patient subgroups. The assumption is that the stability of scores should continue to be a lin-ear function if CBT has a somewhat equal effect on participating pa-tients; repeated MCMI measures should remain stable but yet lower at subsequent administrations if the effects are to be associated with the intervention. Given these characteristics, the recommendation when ex-amining MCMI outcomes is to calculate and report stability coefficients and consider these data when interpreting changes associated with a therapeutic intervention.

CONCLUSION

Issues involved in the use of the MCMI to assess substance users and per-sonality disorders have been presented and recommendations offered to address five key concerns. First, categorical classifications are necessary elements of clinical nomenclature guided by standard *DSM* criteria. In making diagnostic judgments, clinicians should rely on more than just MCMI profiles or BR scores. At least two sources of data should be used to identify patient problems, and the MCMI should be recognized as just one of several tools in this process.

Second, self-reports among substance-using populations are suscepti-ble to different demand characteristics that may affect responses to in-ventories such as the MCMI. Face-valid or prototypical items may provide a keener insight into dependence issues than the overall BR scores from these scales. These critical items should always be considered when formulating diagnostic judgments.

Third, a major strength of the MCMI is its ability to provide both di-mensional and diagnostic indicators of personality and symptom disor-ders. MCMI users should be familiar with the patient samples used to develop and validate the MCMI and recognize that substance-using popu-lations will likely vary considerably from those used to transform raw scores into base rates. Thus, alternative norms and adjustments for bias may be needed for some applications with known substance abusers.

Fourth, clinicians must synthesize and integrate all sources of data rather than rely on a simple indicator. Configural interpretations are preferable to single scale determinations when formulating clinical decisions. Critical or prototypical items may yield considerable confirmatory verification for diagnostic hypotheses.

Finally, MCMI users should become familiar with the inventory's operating characteristics. Understanding these psychometric properties will help to promote sound clinical and research decisions.

REFERENCES

American Psychiatric Association. (1994). *Diagnostic and statistical manual of mental disorders* (4th ed.). Washington, DC: Author.

Broome, K. M., Flynn, P. M., & Simpson, D. D. (1999). Psychiatric comorbidity measures as predictors of retention in drug abuse treatment. *Health Services Research, 34,* 791–806.

Blais, M. A., Holdwick, D. J., McLean, R. Y. S., Otto, M. W., Pollack, M. H., & Hilsenroth, M. J. (2003). Exploring the psychometric properties and construct validity of the MCMI-III Anxiety and Avoidant personality scales. *Journal of Personality Assessment, 81,* 237–241.

Bryer, J. B., Martines, K. A., & Dignan, M. A. (1990). Millon Clinical Multiaxial Inventory alcohol abuse and drug abuse scales and the identification of substance-abuse patients. *Psychological Assessment: A Journal of Consulting and Clinical Psychology, 4,* 438–441.

Calsyn, D. A., Saxon, A. J., & Daisy, F. (1990). Validity of the MCMI drug abuse scale with drug abusing and psychiatric samples. *Journal of Clinical Psychology, 46,* 244–246.

Calsyn, D. A., Saxon, A. J., & Daisy, F. (1991). Validity of the MCMI drug abuse scale varies as a function of drug choice, race, and Axis II subtypes. *American Journal of Drug and Alcohol Abuse, 17,* 153–159.

Craig, R. J. (1997). Sensitivity of MCMI-III scales T (drugs) and B (alcohol) in detecting substance abuse. *Substance Use and Misuse, 32,* 1385–1393.

Craig, R. J., & Olson, R. (1998). Stability of the MCMI-III in a substance-abusing inpatient sample. *Psychological Reports, 83,* 1273–1274.

Craig, R. J., & Weinberg, D. (1992a). Assessing alcoholics with the Millon Clinical Multiaxial Inventory: A review. *Psychology of Addictive Behaviors, 6,* 200–208.

Craig, R. J., & Weinberg, D. (1992b). Assessing drug abusers with the Millon Clinical Multiaxial Inventory: A review. *Journal of Substance Abuse Treatment, 9,* 249–255.

Embree, B. G., & Whitehead, P. C. (1993). Validity and reliability of self-reported drinking behavior: Dealing with the problem of response bias. *Journal of Studies on Alcohol, 54,* 334–344.

Flynn, P. M., Craddock, S. G., Luckey, J. W., Hubbard, R. L., & Dunteman, G. H. (1996). Comorbidity of antisocial personality and mood disorders among psychoactive substance-dependent treatment clients. *Journal of Personality Disorders, 10,* 56–67.

Flynn, P. M., & McCann, J. T. (1991, August). *Issues and Dilemmas in Clinical Diagnosis Using the MCMI-II*. Symposium and paper presented by P. M. Flynn at the 99th Annual Convention of the American Psychological Association, San Francisco, CA.

Flynn, P. M., McCann, J. T., & Fairbank, J. A. (1995). Issues in the assessment of personality disorder and substance abuse using the Millon Clinical Multiaxial Inventory (MCMI-II). *Journal of Clinical Psychology, 51,* 415–421.

Flynn, P. M., McCann, J. T., Luckey, J. W., Rounds-Bryant, J. L., Theisen, A. C., Hoffman, J. A., et al. (1997). Drug Dependence Scale in the Millon Clinical Multiaxial Inventory. *Substance Use and Misuse, 32*(6), 733–748.

Flynn, P. M., & McMahon, R. C. (1983). Stability of the drug misuse scale of the Millon Clinical Multiaxial Inventory. *Psychological Reports, 52,* 536–538.

Flynn, P. M., & McMahon, R. C. (1984). An examination of the drug abuse scale of the Millon Clinical Multiaxial Inventory. *International Journal of the Addictions, 19,* 459–468.

Flynn, P. M., & McMahon, R. C. (1997). MCMI applications in substance abuse. In T. Millon (Ed.), *The Millon inventories: Clinical and personality assessment* (pp. 173–190). New York: Guilford Press.

First, M. B., Spitzer, R. L., Gibbon, M., Williams, J. B. W. (1995, June). The Structured Clinical Interview for *DSM-III-R* Personality Disorders (SCID-II): Part I. Description. *Journal of Personality Disorders, 9*(2), 83–91.

Gibertini, M., Brandenburg, N. A., & Retzlaff, P. D. (1986). The operating characteristics of the Millon Clinical Multiaxial Inventory. *Journal of Personality Assessment, 50,* 554–567.

Harrison, L., & Hughes, A. (Eds.). (1997). *The validity of self-reported drug use: Improving the accuracy of survey estimates.* (NIDA Research Monograph 167; NIH Publication No. 97-4147). Rockville, MD: National Institute on Drug Abuse.

Havassy, B. E., Alvidrez, J., & Owen, K. K. (2004). Comparisons of patients with comorbid psychiatric and substance use disorders: Implications for treatment and service delivery. *American Journal of Psychiatry, 161,* 139–145.

Hsu, L. M., Maruish, M. E., & Moreland, K. L. (1992). *Conducting publishable research with the MCMI-II: Psychometric and statistical issues.* Minneapolis, MN: National Computer Systems.

McCann, J. T. (1990). Bias and Millon Clinical Multiaxial Inventory (MCMI-II) diagnosis. *Journal of Psychopathology and Behavioral Assessment, 12,* 17–26.

McCann, J. T., Flynn, P. M., & Gersh, D. M. (1992). MCMI-II diagnosis of borderline personality disorder: Base rates versus prototypic items. *Journal of Personality Assessment, 58,* 105–114.

McCann, J. T., & Seuss, J. F. (1988). Clinical applications of the MCMI: The 1-2-3-8 codetype. *Journal of Clinical Psychology, 44,* 181–186.

Millon, T. (1977). *Millon Multiaxial Clinical Inventory Manual.* Minneapolis, MN: National Computer Systems.

Millon, T. (1982). *Millon Clinical Multiaxial Inventory-II Manual.* Minneapolis, MN: National Computer Systems.

Millon, T. (1987). *Millon Clinical Multiaxial Inventory-II Manual.* Minneapolis, MN: National Computer Systems.

Millon, T., Davis, R., & Millon, C. (1997). *Millon Clinical Multiaxial Inventory-III Manual* (2nd ed.). Minneapolis, MN: National Computer Systems.

Onken, L. S., Blaine, J. D., Genser, S., & Horton, A. M. (Eds.). (1997). *Treatment of drug-dependent individuals with comorbid conditions.* (NIDA Research Monograph 172; NIH Publication No. 97-4172). Rockville, MD: National Institute on Drug Abuse.

Robins, L. N., Helzer, J. E., Croughan, J., & Ratcliff, K. S. (1981). National Institutes of Mental Health Diagnostic Interview Schedule: Its history, characteristics, and validity. *Archives of General Psychiatry, 38,* 381–389.

Rogan, W. J., & Gladen, B. (1978). Estimating prevalence from the results of a screening test. *American Journal of Epidemiology, 107,* 71–76.

Shea, M. T., & Yen, S. (2003). Stability as a distinction between Axis I & Axis II disorders. *Journal of Personality Disorders, 17*(5), 373–386.

Ziedonis, D. M. (1992). Comorbid psychopathology and cocaine addiction. In T. R. Kosten & H. D. Kleber (Eds.), *Clinician's guide to cocaine addiction* (pp. 335–358). New York: Guilford Press.

Zimmerman, M., Sheeran, T., Chelminski, I., & Young, D. (2004). Screening for psychiatric disorders in outpatients with *DSM-IV* substance use disorders. *Journal of Substance Abuse Treatment, 26,* 181–188.

CHAPTER 6

International Uses of the MCMI: Does Interpretation Change?

GINA ROSSI AND HEDWIG SLOORE

IN THE United States, the domain of psychopathology and abnormality is strongly influenced by the *DSM*-taxonomic system (*Diagnostic and Statistical Manual of Mental Disorders, DSM-IV-TR*; American Psychiatric Association [APA], 2000). The same can be said about the European situation: Both research in the domain of psychopathology and clinical practice are strongly influenced by the same taxonomy. Nevertheless, the *ICD* taxonomy (*International Classification of Diseases*; World Health Organization, 1992) is also frequently used, especially in the southern part of Europe. The classification systems are not that different and are typical products of our Western way of thinking.

In the past several decades, a lot of attention has been paid to the possible influence of culture on the taxonomies, on the processes of psychological assessment, and on the process of psychotherapy. Shiraev and Levy (2004) point to the fact that there are at least five areas in which culture can affect psychological disorders. What is considered to be a psychological problem can vary a lot from culture to culture. This is a problem of subjective experience and culturally determined definitions. The second area has to do with culture-based idioms: the ways clients express and explain complaints. The third problem concerns the influence of culture on diagnoses. To put it differently, is the use of questionnaires, projective techniques, and so on accepted in the same way in different countries? The fourth and fifth areas have to do with therapy: Are the ways people try to overcome psychological problems similar, and are the criteria for treatment outcome and evaluation the same?

In the domain of psychopathology and culture, one of two perspectives may be adopted: the relativist perspective or the universalist perspective. In the former, all psychological phenomena are considered to be relative and influenced by specific circumstances and cultural factors. The proponents of this approach are in favor of the use of *emic* methods, or the use of diagnostic instruments that are culture-specific. The second perspective considers psychological phenomena to be universal. The proponents of the universal perspective are in favor of the use of *etic* methods, which means that existing instruments (most of the time developed in the United States) are translated into other languages and adapted for use in other cultures. Psychopathology, as described by *DSM-IV-TR* (APA, 2000), is considered to be universal and mostly invariable across different countries and cultures. This is not the place to discuss this problem in detail, but as more and more disorders and syndromes seem to have a biological component or basis, a universalist view seems the most evident. However, we should accept that certain aspects of diseases and especially behaviors associated with the different forms of psychopathology can vary as a function of cultural circumstances.

There is already a rather substantial body of literature on cross-cultural research in the field of psychopathology. The absolute majority of studies in the domain of psychiatry and psychopathology have focused on U.S. groups of patients, and we assume that these results apply in the same way to European patients and are true for most cultural groups. An important part of these studies is looking, for instance, at differences between Western and Asian cultures, between specific populations such as Hispanics and Blacks and Caucasians, or studying very specific and small cultures (an interesting list of specific culture-bound syndromes can be found in Shiraev & Levy, 2004, pp. 244–246). In the context of the internationalization of our clinical practices and the globalization of our world, all these studies are of great importance. This literature suggests that psychological differences between populations in the United States and most of the European countries are nonexistent, or at least of no importance. Indeed, in clinical practice in European countries, we do not encounter many problems using the *DSM*-classification system and the diagnostic tools associated with this taxonomy. However, the fact that the *DSM* taxonomy and the *ICD* taxonomy have been developed and are used side by side in Europe shows that many European psychiatrists and psychologists are not that happy with the "American" classification system.

Still, the major U.S. questionnaires to measure psychopathology are used in most European countries. Particularly in the past several decades, international rules for translating questionnaires have been established and, in most cases, are followed rather strictly. These rules determine translation procedures, back-translations, item endorsement research, research on factor structure, and so on.

The main problem when using translations of questionnaires is the question of their equivalence. Different forms of equivalence have been distinguished by Van de Vijver and Poortinga (1982). *Conceptual equivalence* has to do with the question of the universality of the concepts of the taxonomy. *Functional equivalence* concerns the problem of variation in the empirical expression or the concrete manifestations of the syndromes across different cultures. *Metric equivalence* concerns the similarity of the psychometric properties of an instrument across different cultures. *Scalar equivalence* presumes, for instance, that a base rate score of 76 on the scale Narcissistic Personality Disorder (5) of the MCMI-III (Millon, Davis, & Millon, 1997) is indicative for approximately the same degree of narcissism in different countries. In a more recent article, Van de Vijver and Tanzer (1997) point out that three kinds of measurement bias can be distinguished:

1. Construct bias: occurs when the construct measured is not identical across cultural groups
2. Method bias
3. Item bias or differential item functioning

Cross-cultural research on the MMPI-2 has shown that a fairly good equivalence can be achieved when specific procedures are followed during the translation and validation process (Butcher, 1996). The MCMI-III has been translated into Dutch/Flemish taking into account the guidelines described by Butcher, namely, using a combined committee approach and a translation–back-translation procedure. More details about the translation procedure used in Belgium/The Netherlands can be found in *Issues in the international use of psychological tests* (Derksen & Sloore, 2005).

In translating the MCMI-III (Sloore & Derksen, 1997), a new and specific problem arises: The transformation of raw scores is based on the base rate of the different syndromes and personality disorders in a given population or country. Although it has been shown repeatedly that, for instance for the MMPI-2 (Butcher, 1996), the mean values and standard deviations for the scales obtained in different countries are very similar, this may not be true for the MCMI-III, where base rates are used instead of T-scores.

Questionnaires using normalized scores are relatively easy to adapt after translation: A comparable norm group is tested, and new mean values and standard deviations are calculated. However, the use of base rates presents the researcher with more important problems. We cannot presume that the base rates of different clinical syndromes or personality disorders are the same in different cultures and countries. Can we, for example, take for granted that the base rate of the Narcissistic Personality Disorder is the same in the United States, Sweden, Belgium, Spain, and countries such as China, the Philippines, and Tasmania? Van de Vijver and Tanzer (1997) come to the following conclusion: "It can not be taken for granted that scores obtained in one culture can be compared across cultural groups" (p. 276). However, such statements refer most of the time to comparisons over different cultures (e.g., United States versus China) or to minority groups in a given society. U.S. culture is considered to be very similar to the cultures of most European countries. This similarity is accepted blindly; it should be examined and proven.

Preliminary research on the MCMI-I (Millon, 1982b), done in Belgium in the 1980s, was not that successful (Sloore & Derksen, 1997). As we were in the possession of a standardized clinical evaluation for 358 patients in terms of Millon's theory and the MCMI, we tried to construct our own base rates. We used two types of information to determine the 75 and 85 base rates: The total prevalence rate of each personality type or syndrome disorder and the most salient prevalence rate. The former represents the percentage of patients who were judged by the clinicians to display some of the characteristics of the syndrome, regardless of whether that syndrome was primary, secondary, or tertiary. The latter rate represents the percentage of patients who were judged to present the syndrome under study as primary. As described in the manual (Millon, 1982b), we calculated the median values for the different scales.

This procedure was revealed to be problematic: For 13 of the 20 scales, the median values of the BR 85 group were lower than the median values of the BR 75 group. The phenomenon was less pronounced on the female subsample (8 out of 20 scales), although this group was smaller ($n = 153$) than our male group ($n = 267$).

Van den Brande (2002) was the first researcher in Belgium to do research on the MCMI-III (Millon, 1997). The results made it clear that there was a need for local base rates because the differences between the Belgian results and the U.S. results could not always be explained in terms of cultural differences.

Rossi (2004) examined the advantages of criterion referencing over norm referencing. Criterion and norm referencing are two possible ways to standardize tests (Millon, 1983, 1987, 1994; Millon, Davis, & Millon, 1997). However, norm referencing, converting raw scores into standardized scores, can lead to problems when used with personality questionnaires. Standardized scores imply normal distributions and comparable frequencies with regard to the characteristics that are measured. According to Thorndike (1982), personality styles or disorders and clinical syndromes are neither normally distributed nor evenly spread throughout patient populations. These scales mostly have skewed distributions (Craig, 2001). In a previous study (Rossi, Hauben, Van den Brande, & Sloore, 2003), we confirmed that indeed personality disorders do not show comparable frequencies and have different prevalence rates. This implies that the distribution of the scores varies from scale to scale. Kolmogorov-Smirnov tests (with Lilliefors significance correction; Lilliefors, 1967; Massey, 1951) revealed clearly that, in the current data set, all the MCMI-III-scales, for men as well as for women, were significantly different from normality ($p < .05$). Criterion referencing resolves the problems (Retzlaff, 1996). It is important to do criterion referencing in a way that is relevant for diagnostic decisions. Millon et al. (1997) made use of base rates. Craig (1999) defines a base rate score as a transformed score that selects that point in a distribution of scores whereby a patient has all the features of the disorder or syndrome on a diagnostic level. Millon et al. anchored a cut-off score for each scale to the real prevalence ratio of the characteristic in a specific population. In contrast, a standardized score is linked to a fixed percentile of the norm group and ignores the different scale distributions.

Anchoring scale elevations to the exact prevalence rate of the disorder assumes that patients with that particular disorder obtain the highest scores on this scale. In reality, this is not always the case. Especially personality disordered individuals fail to describe themselves accurately on self-report instruments. They often have very limited insight into their intrapsychic and interpersonal patterns (Hynan, 2004). In these cases, a direct connection of the scores to the prevalence percentage can yield problems for some of the scales. For this reason, we decided to use receiver operating characteristic curve (ROC) analyses.

The area under the receiver operating characteristic curve (AUC) is a measure that considers the distribution of the scores between a population with and one without disorders. It determines the probability that a randomly selected person from the population with disorders will have a higher score on the scale than a randomly selected person from the population without disorders (Hanley & McNeil, 1983; Hsu, 2002; McFall & Treat, 1999; Swets, 1973). Consequently, this measure estimates whether the scale can accurately differentiate the disordered population from the population without the specific disorders (ratio $>.50$). Therefore, use of the measure is recommended in recent clinical literature (e.g., Gardner, Lidz, Mulvey, & Shaw, 1996; Grissom, 1994, 1996; Hsu, 2002; McFall & Treat, 1999; McGraw & Wong, 1992; McNiel, Lam, & Binder, 2000; Swets,

Dawes, & Monahan, 2000). Moreover, the associated curve represents the ratio of sensitivity and specificity, according to the raw score or anchor point used to differentiate the populations with and without disorders. *Sensitivity* is the probability of a test being positive if a disorder is present, or the true positive cases, and *specificity* is the probability of a test being negative in the absence of any disorder, or the true negative cases (Gibertini, Brandenburg, & Retzlaff, 1986). Derogatis and DellaPietra (1994) define sensitivity and specificity as the most fundamental validity indexes of a screening test. Good scales have a sensitivity and specificity of 70% or more; 50% to 69% is still relatively good. Scales with values below 50% are weak (West & Finch, 1997).

Nurnberg et al. (2000) applied ROC analyses to the development of a clinical screening instrument for the presence of a personality disorder. They emphasize that the choice between restricting the impact of false negatives (type I error) or false positives (type II error) is very important. We tried to optimize the ratio between sensitivity and specificity when determining base rates by choosing an anchor point so that sensitivity and specificity were above 70%. When optimization was not possible, we gave priority to sensitivity because in Europe, the MCMI-III is most often applied as a screening instrument. Therefore, the test has to be effective in identifying persons with disorders in a group. In other words, the emphasis lies on avoiding false negatives rather than avoiding false positives. Screening implies that features present according to the test scores are further explored with more specific diagnostic evaluations. Features that the test indicated as absent are mostly not taken into account in the further diagnostic process (Derogatis & DellaPietra, 1994).

MCMI-III results and clinical judgments were collected for 535 patients (Rossi, 2004). Because no golden standard exists to evaluate personality disorders (Perry, 1992; Spitzer, 1983), we developed our own rating system to enhance the reliability of the clinical ratings (Rossi & Van den Brande, 1998). It was mainly based on the system of Millon (1982a) and the rating form published in Millon et al. (1997, p. 93). A thorough description is given in Rossi et al. (2003) and Rossi (2004). Personality disorders (styles) and clinical symptoms were evaluated as present or absent. When a personality disorder was present, the degree was determined on a scale from 1 (trait) to 9 (extreme disorder). Important anchor points for the ROC analyses are 1 (trait) and 5 (disorder). Definitions for these anchor points can be found in Millon et al. (p. 91, figure 4.33). The definition of disorder, for example is as follows: "The personality pattern is sufficiently problematic to justify a clinical diagnosis. Characteristics definitively impair life functioning, resulting in periodic, but significant adaptive difficulties. Outpatient treatment is indicated." For the clinical syndromes, too, the degree to which a symptom was present was rated on a scale from 1 (slight) to 9 (extreme syndrome). Clinical evaluations were retained only in cases of a minimum of 4 hours of clinical contact. The evaluation was done at the end of the assessment procedure. In this way, a complete understanding of the personality of the patient was possible. The clinical rating was made independently of the MCMI-III test results. If possible, a LEAD (longitudinal expert evaluation that uses all data) standard was used (Millon, 1983). The MCMI-III was considered invalid when 12 or more answers were missing or double-marked, or if $V \geq 2$, or if the raw score of scale X was ≤ 34 or ≥ 178.

The whole procedure resulted in a final data set consisting of 524 patients, 255 males and 269 females. The average age was 36.6 years (range 18 to 73, $SD = 11.6$). The majority of the subjects were coming from different clinical settings ($n = 438$, or 83.6%). A smaller group came from forensic settings ($n = 86$, or 16.4%). To be able to compare the efficiency of base rates using prevalence percentages or ROC analyses, both were calculated.

We did not follow Millon et al. (1997) completely with regard to the determination of the anchor points. This means the following: raw score 0 equals BR 0, and the maximum possible raw score on a scale equals BR 115. BR 115 also equals the percentile that got a score of 9 on the evaluation. As a result, each scale range is BR 0 to BR 115. In contrast, in Millon et al., the maximum score on scale 4 for men, for example, is BR 84, which imposes that men can never have a Histrionic Personality Disorder. For the personality disorder scales as well as for the clinical syndrome scales, BR 75 equals the raw score that is the cut-off between individuals with a rating of 0 and those with a rating of 1 or more. BR 85 equals the raw score that is the cut-off between individuals with a rating of 5 or more and those with a rating smaller than 5. Using prevalence base rates, the percentiles determine the cut-off; using ROC analyses, the raw score that optimizes the sensitivity and specificity ratio determines the cut-off. Unlike Millon et al., we did not work with primary and secondary elevations, but always took the severity (rating 1 or 5) into account. If, for example, a rating of 1 is given on Anxiety, we always include the individual in the group to define BR 75. If the individual has no higher ratings on clinical syndromes, Millon et al. would classify this person in the group as defining BR 85 (primary syndrome). BR 60 equals the median value of the distribution of the raw scores for that scale. This anchor point is not applied in cases where the median equals a raw score that is greater than the raw score that is linked to BR 75 or 85. Similar to Millon et al., linear interpolation was used to assign BR scores to raw scores between the five anchor points.

Table 6.1
AUC of Scale 3 for BR 75

Area	Standard Deviation*	Asymptotic Significance	95% Reliability Interval	
			Lowest Border	Highest Border
.742	.042	.000	.660	.824

*Under nonparametric assumption.
Note: p values can never equal 0, but they are shortened to 3 decimals. If significance = .000, this means *p* < .0005.

Concerning the scales X, Y, and Z, we used the same approach as Millon et al. (1997) did. We linked BR 85 to the highest 10% of the patient population, BR 75 to BR 84 to the following 15%, BR 35 to 74 to the middle 60%, and BR 0 to 34 to the lowest 15%. Between the anchor points, linear interpolation was applied. In contrast to Millon et al., the base rates for scale X were separately calculated for men and women because scale X raw scores are significantly different for men and women ($p < .0001$).

As an example of the method using ROC analyses, we present the calculation of the base rates of the Dependent Personality Disorder in men. Table 6.1 shows that a randomly selected person with dependency traits (rating of 1 or more) will, in 74.2% of the cases, score higher on scale 3 of the MCMI-III than a randomly selected person without dependency traits. Anchoring BR 75 on raw score 11 (see Table 6.2 on p. 152) places the sensitivity of this scale for the personality traits, calculated on the basis of the raw score, between 67% and 74% and the specificity between 62% and 67%. As can be deduced from Table 6.3 on page 153, a randomly selected person with a Dependent Personality Disorder will, in 78.8% of the cases, score higher on scale 3 of the MCMI-III than a randomly selected person without a Dependent Personality Disorder. By anchoring BR 85 to a raw score of 13, the sensitivity of this scale, which is calculated on the basis of the raw score for the personality disorder (rating of 5 or more), is positioned between 70% and 73% and specificity between 72% and 76% (see Table 6.4 on p. 154). On the basis of the cumulative percentage of the raw scores of scale 3, the median lies on raw score 9 and is anchored on base rate 60. Based on linear interpolation between the anchor points, this leads to the base rates displayed in Table 6.5 on page 155.

In the same way, base rates were calculated for all the MCMI-III scales. Table 6.6 on page 156 compares the sensitivity of base rates for our data set, using ROC analyses, with the base rates of the Millon et al. (1997) system.

We can clearly conclude that the base rates using ROC analyses perform better than the prevalence base rates. This is the case on trait level

Table 6.2
Coordinates for the Curve of Scale 3 for Rating ≥ 1

Positive if Greater Than or Equal To*	Sensitivity	1 − Specificity
−1.00	1.000	1.000
0.50	1.000	.911
1.50	1.000	.869
2.50	1.000	.789
3.50	.905	.723
4.50	.857	.657
5.50	.833	.592
6.50	.810	.531
7.50	.786	.488
8.50	.786	.455
9.50	.762	.418
10.50	.738	.376
11.50	.667	.329
12.50	.643	.282
13.50	.619	.235
14.50	.595	.197
15.50	.476	.150
16.50	.357	.094
17.50	.310	.075
18.50	.238	.056
19.50	.143	.033
20.50	.095	.014
21.50	.095	.005
22.50	.048	.000
24.00	.000	.000

*The smallest cut-off value is the minimal observed test value minus 1, and the greatest cut-off value is the maximal observed test value plus 1. Every other cut-off value is the mean of two subsequent observed test values.

as well as disorder level. For trait and symptom levels, there was a good to very good sensitivity for all scales. As far as the disorder level is concerned, the sensitivity remains weak on three personality scales (2B, 8B, and S). The difference between BR 75 and 85 was often very small for the personality disorder scales: Frequently, the difference was just 1 raw score. For example, BR 75 from the Dependent Personality Disorder scale

Table 6.3
AUC for Scale 3 for Rating ≥ 5

Area	Standard Deviation*	Asymptotic Significance	Asymptotic 95% Reliability Interval	
			Lowest Border	Highest Border
.788	.043	.000	.704	.871

*Under nonparametric assumption.
Note: *p* values can never equal 0, but they are shortened to 3 decimals. If significance = .000, this means *p* < .0005.

corresponds to raw score 11 and BR 85 to raw score 13. In view of this small difference, we advise avoiding interpretations about the distinction between trait and disorder level on the basis of the MCMI-III. Strictly speaking, this would even be contradictory to the continuum thinking of Millon. This implies that the MCMI-III has to be seen as a screening instrument, where scores above BR 75 indicate a certain presence of traits/symptoms. Higher scores increase the probability of the existence of a disorder, but a diagnosis can be made only on the basis of supplementary information.

Very important to clinicians, but often missing in the test manuals, is solid information on the diagnostic validity of the test. Classic measures in clinical literature studying the diagnostic efficiency of a test usually focus on sensitivity, specificity, positive predictive power (PPP), and negative predictive power (NPP; Baldessarini, Finklestein, & Arana, 1983; Daubert & Metzler, 2000; Gibertini et al., 1986; Griner, Mayewski, Mushlin, & Greenland, 1981; Hsu, 2002; Mausner & Bahn, 1974). Furthermore, Hsu (2002) defines some important supplementary measures that verify the increasing validity of a test or the difference between pretest and posttest probabilities: the increasing PPP (IPPP), the increasing NPP (INPP), Cohen's kappa (Cohen, 1988), Cohen's greatness effect d, and the AUC.

In the MCMI-III manual, Millon (1994) published a first validity study. This study was characterized by certain methodological problems (Millon, 1994; Retzlaff, 1996). A lot of questions remained about the reliability of the clinical evaluations. Some of the diagnoses were made after only one clinical contact (e.g., merely an intake interview), and minimal diagnostic criteria were forehanded (no descriptions or no formal interview). As a result, the second validity study (Millon et al., 1997) explicitly demanded that clinicians evaluate only those patients about whom they had sufficient information. Clinicians were even

Table 6.4

Coordinates for the Curve of Scale 3 for BR 85 in Men

Positive if Greater Than or Equal To*	Sensitivity	1 − Specificity
−1.00	1.000	1.000
0.50	1.000	.914
1.50	1.000	.874
2.50	1.000	.797
3.50	.939	.725
4.50	.879	.662
5.50	.879	.595
6.50	.879	.532
7.50	.848	.491
8.50	.848	.459
9.50	.848	.419
10.50	.818	.378
11.50	.758	.329
12.50	.727	.284
13.50	.697	.239
14.50	.667	.203
15.50	.576	.149
16.50	.424	.095
17.50	.364	.077
18.50	.273	.059
19.50	.182	.032
20.50	.121	.014
21.50	.121	.005
22.50	.061	.000
24.00	.000	.000

* The smallest cut-off value is the minimal observed test value minus 1, and the greatest cut-off value is the maximal observed test value plus 1. Every other cut-off value is the mean of two subsequent observed test values.

encouraged to evaluate patients that already had an MCMI-III profile. On top of this, the scores had to be filled in on the evaluation form, which leads to a new methodological problem: Foreknowledge of the test results when making the clinical rating (which should be done blindly or at least independently). Moreover, there is a possibility that the clinician will remember the actual base rates, thus potentially

Table 6.5

Distribution of Frequencies of Raw Scores of Scale 3
(Dependent Personality) and Matching Base Rate Scores in Men

		Frequency	Cumulative %	BR Anchor Points and Linear Interpolation	Round Numbers or Final BR
Valid	0	19	7.50	**0**	0
	1	9	11	6.67	7
	2	17	17.60	13.34	13
	3	18	24.70	20.01	20
	4	16	31	26.68	27
	5	15	36.90	33.35	33
	6	14	42.40	40.02	40
	7	10	46.30	46.69	47
	8	7	49	53.36	53
	9	9	5.50	**60**	60
	10	10	56.50	67.50	68
	11	13	61.60	**75**	75
	12	11	65.90	80	80
	13	11	70.20	**85**	85
	14	9	73.70	88	88
	15	15	79.60	91	91
	16	17	86.30	94	94
	17	6	88.60	97	97
	18	7	91.40	100	100
	19	9	94.90	103	103
	20	6	97.30	106	106
	21	2	98	109	109
	22	3	99.20	112	112
	23	2	100	**115**	115
	24	0	100	**115**	115
	Total	255			

Note: Anchor points appear in boldface.

unconsciously relying on non-MCMI-III information with an affirmative bias, consistent with the exceptional increases on the MCMI-III (Garb, 1998; Hsu, 2002).

These methods probably resulted in an underestimation of the diagnostic validity statistics from the 1994 study and an overestimation in the 1997 study. Table 6.7 on page 157 gives an overview and compares the study of Rossi (2004) with the 1994 and 1997 validity studies. Mean diagnostic validity statistics over the different scales are given.

Table 6.6

Comparison of Sensitivity of ROC Base
Rates and Prevalence Base Rates

	Sensitivity Prevalence Base Rates % BR ≥ 85	Sensitivity ROC Base Rates % BR ≥ 85	p Value ≠ n = 524	Sensitivity Prevalence Base Rates % BR ≥ 75	Sensitivity ROC Base Rates % BR ≥ 75	p Value ≠ n = 524
1 Schizoid	12	**67.86**	.00	16.28	**74.42**	.00
2A Avoidant	16.67	**51.39**	.00	16.48	**68.09**	.00
2B Depressive	5.56	**33.33**	.00	12.33	**62.96**	.00
3 Dependent	25	**59.78**	.00	36.75	**73.50**	.00
4 Histrionic	27.03	**55.41**	.00	31.96	**68.04**	.00
5 Narcissistic	36	**60**	.00	43.43	**74.75**	.00
6A Antisocial	32.65	**67.35**	.00	30	**74.29**	.36
6B Aggressive	41.67	66.67	.50	31.58	**84.21**	.50
7 Compulsive	11.91	**66.67**	.00	32.84	**79.11**	.00
8A Negativistic	6.82	53.19	.12	14.29	**76.19**	.00
8B Masochistic	0	**14.29**	.00	0	**52.50**	.00
S Schizotypal	5	25	.50	6.90	**55.17**	.00
C Borderline	33.61	60.50	.25	47.97	**65.54**	.00
P Paranoid	16.13	67.74	.10	29.17	**68.75**	.00
A Anxiety Disorder	51.84	69.27	.00	75.39	75.39	.00
H Somatoform Disorder	51	**59.00**	.00	85	71.01	.00
N Bipolar: Manic Disorder	10.71	64.52	.01	11.11	**68.06**	.05
D Dysthymic Disorder	41.84	72.34	.16	55.80	**70.09**	.00
B Alcohol Dependence	60.35	73.28	.00	62.64	**79.89**	.00
T Drug Dependence	53.85	80.77	.00	53.85	**78.57**	.00
R PTSD	35	71.25	.37	44.80	**74.40**	.50
SS Thought Disorder	15.22	**60.87**	.50	26.79	**63.39**	.36
CC Major Depression	63.31	75.74	.00	67.83	72.09	.01
PP Delusional Disorder	22.86	**57.14**	.00	25.68	**60.81**	.23

Note: The highest sensitivity value appears in boldface if there is a significant difference between the prevalence and ROC base rates, with $p < .01$.

Table 6.7

Comparison of the Mean Diagnostic Validity Statistics over Three Studies

Diagnostic Validity Statistic	Rossi (2004)	Millon (1994)	Millon et al. (1997)	Differences Rossi (2004) Millon (1994)	Differences Rossi (2004) Millon et al. (1997)
Sensitivity	.705	.275	.670	.430	.035
Specificity	.558	.860	.968	−.302	−.410
PPP	.283	.223	.640	.060	−.357
NPP	.869	.887	.964	−.018	−.095
IPPP	.073	.102	.549	−.029	−.476
INPP	.078	.014	.055	.064	.023
Cohen's k	.161	.128	.610	.033	−.449
Cohen's d	.569	.588	2.362	−.019	−1.793
AUC	.669	.653	.937	.016	−.268

Source: Hsu (2002, p. 418); Rossi (2004, p.94)

As expected, the diagnostic validity statistics from our study are, in general, weaker than in the 1997 study and higher than in the 1994 study. Sensitivity was highest in Rossi (2004), but specificity was lowest compared to the other studies. This is logical because we gave priority to avoiding false negatives. The mean NPP was lower in our study compared to the 1994 study. In the 1994 study, 19 scales had an NPP above 90%, three scales an NPP above 80%, and two scales showed a low NPP: Anxiety Disorder (scale A) at 30% and Dysthymic Disorder (scale D) at 62%. In Rossi (2004) 11 scales had an NPP above 90%, 11 scales an NPP above 80%, the Anxiety Disorder scale an NPP of 58%, and the Dysthymic Disorder scale an NPP of 69%. We consider the results comparable: 22 scales also have an NPP above 80%, and the scales with the lowest sensitivity values (A and D) showed higher values. Mean IPPP and Cohen's d values are lower than in the 1994 study. Nevertheless, this does not imply a lower diagnostic validity. In Rossi (2004), all scales have positive values, which implies that all scales consistently perform better than guessing. In the study of 1994, four scales had a negative INPP and three scales a negative Cohen's d. This means that in five cases, guessing was better than using scale information.

CONCLUSIONS

The most important conclusion we have drawn from our research is that interpretation of the MCMI-III results changes in an important way. The higher sensitivity values in Rossi (2004), compared to the 1994 and 1997 studies, make the MCMI-III an excellent screening device. The lower specificity measures constrain its diagnostic use. Present personality patterns and clinical symptoms, according to scale scores, are very hypothetical and should be further investigated before making diagnostic decisions.

Millon et al. (1997) considered the positive predictive ratio (PPP divided by the prevalence rate) to be the most useful diagnostic validity statistic. In contrast to Rossi (2004), their priority was to avoid false positives. Especially in the area of U.S. forensic evaluations, this can be an important goal (Goodman-Delahunty, 1997). The question of whether the MCMI-III meets the Daubert criteria remains unanswered (Dyer & McCann, 2000; McCann & Dyer, 1996; Retzlaff, 2000; Rogers, Salekin, & Sewell, 1999, 2000). Therefore, we are convinced that clinicians should have all possible diagnostic validity statistics available when using a test. This is the only way to have knowledge about how to interpret scale scores. Notwithstanding, these statistics are seldom applied to evaluate tests (Hunsley & Meyer, 2003) and therefore are not often available to clinicians.

The main advantage of ROC base rates is that the ratio of sensitivity to specificity can, in part, be controlled. We gave priority to avoiding false negatives, whereas Millon et al. (1997) considered the ability of the test to avoid false positives an important issue.

Another possible approach is to search for an optimal cut-off whereby the probability on false negatives and positives is in balance. According to Nurnberg et al. (2000), this cut-off value equals the highest hit ratio (HR). Following the method of Meehl and Rosen (1955), for each possible cut-off value in a scale, the HR is calculated by summing two products. The first product is determined by multiplying the true positive rate by the prevalence rate, and the second product by multiplying the true negative rate by 1 minus the prevalence rate.

Overall, we want to emphasize the importance of deciding whether to give priority to avoiding false positives or false negatives during standardization of the test and to the necessity of evaluating to what extent the test meets this objective.

REFERENCES

American Psychiatric Association. (2000). *Diagnostic and statistical manual of mental disorders* (4th ed., text rev.). Washington, DC: Author.

Balderassini, R. J., Finkelstein, S., & Arana, G. W. (1983). The predictive power of diagnostic tests and the effect of prevalence of illness. *Archives of General Psychiatry, 40,* 569–573.

Butcher, J. (Ed.). (1996). *International adaptations of the MMPI-2.* Minneapolis, MN: University of Minnesota Press.

Cohen, J. (1988). *Statistical power analysis for the behavioural sciences* (2nd ed.). Hillsdale, NJ: Erlbaum.

Craig, R. J. (1999). Overview and current status of the Millon Clinical Multiaxial Inventory. *Journal of Personality Assessment, 72,* 390–406.

Craig, R. J. (2001). Millon Clinical Multiaxial Inventory-III (MCMI-III). In W. I. Dorfman & M. Hersen (Eds.), *Understanding psychological assessment* (pp. 173–186). New York: Kluwer Academic/Plenum Press.

Daubert, S. D., & Metzler, A. E. (2000). The detection of fake bad and fake good responding on the Millon Clinical Multiaxial Inventory. *Psychological Assessment, 12,* 418–424.

Derksen, J., & Sloore, H. (2005). Issues in the international use of psychological tests. In S. Strack (Ed.), *Handbook of Personology and Psychopathology* (Chapter 22). New York: Wiley.

Derogatis, L. R., & DellaPietra, L. (1994). Psychological tests in screening for psychiatric disorder. In M. E. Maruish (Ed.), *Testing for treatment planning and outcome assessment* (pp. 23–49). Hillsdale, NJ: Erlbaum.

Dyer, F. J., & McCann, J. T. (2000). The Millon Clinical Inventories, research critical of their forensic application, and Daubert criteria. *Law and Human Behavior, 24,* 487–497.

Garb, H. N. (1998). *Studying the clinician: Judgement research and psychological assessment.* Washington, DC: American Psychological Association.

Gardner, W., Lidz, C. W., Mulvey, E. P., & Shaw, E. C. (1996). Clinical versus actuarial predictions of violence in patients with mental illness. *Journal of Consulting and Clinical Psychology, 64,* 602–609.

Gibertini, M., Brandenburg, N. A., & Retzlaff, P. D. (1986). The operating characteristics of the Millon Clinical Multiaxial Inventory. *Journal of Personality Assessment, 50,* 554–567.

Goodman-Delahunty, J. (1997). Forensic expertise in the wake of Daubert. *Law and Human Behavior, 21,* 121–140.

Griner, P. F., Mayewski, R. J., Mushlin, A. I., & Greenland, P. (1981). Selection and interpretation of diagnostic tests and procedures: Principles and applications. *Annals of Internal Medecine, 94,* 557–593.

Grissom, R. J. (1994). The probability of superiority of one treatment over another. *Journal of Applied Psychology, 79,* 314–316.

Grissom, R. J. (1996). The magical number .7 ± .2: Meta-meta-analysis of the probability of superior outcome in comparisons involving therapy, placebo, and control. *Journal of Consulting and Clinical Psychology, 64,* 973–982.

Hanley, J. A., & McNeil, B. J. (1983). A method of comparing the areas under receiving operator characteristic curves derived from the same cases. *Radiology, 148,* 839–843.

Hsu, L. M. (2002). Diagnostic validity statistics and the MCMI-III. *Psychological Assessment, 14,* 410–422.

Hunsley, J., & Meyer, G. J. (2003). The incremental validity of psychological test-ing and assessment: Conceptual, methodological, and statistical issues. *Psychological Assessment, 15*, 446–455.

Hynan, D. J. (2004). Unsupported gender differences on some personality disor-der scales of the Millon Clinical Multiaxial Inventory-III. *Professional Psychology: Research and Practice, 35*, 105–110.

Lilliefors, H. W. (1967). On the Kolmogorov-Smirnov test for normality with mean and variance unknown. *Journal of the American and Statistical Association, 64*, 399–402.

Massey, F. J., Jr. (1951). The Kolmogorov-Smirnov test for goodness of fit. *Journal of the American and Statistical Association, 46*, 68–78.

Mausner, J. S., & Bahn, A. K. (1974). *Epidemiology: An introductory text.* Philadel-phia: Saunders.

McCann, J. T., & Dyer, F. J. (1996). *Forensic assessment with the Millon inventories.* New York: Guilford Press.

McFall, R. M., & Treat, T. A. (1999). Quantifying the information value of clini-cal assessments with signal detection theory. *Annual Review of Psychology, 50*, 215–241.

McGraw, K. O., & Wong, S. P. (1992). A common language effect size statistic. *Psychological Bulletin, 111*, 361–365.

McNiel, D. E., Lam, J. N., & Binder, R. L. (2000). Relevance of interrater agree-ment to violence risk assessment. *Journal of Consulting and Clinical Psychology, 68*, 1111–1115.

Meehl, P. E., & Rosen, A. (1955). Antecedent probability and the efficiency of psychometric signs, patterns, or cutting scores. *Psychological Bulletin, 52*, 194–216.

Millon, T. (1982a). *Millon Clinical Multiaxial Inventory: Clinical judgement study in-structions booklet.* Unpublished manuscript. Coral Gables, FL: Institute for Advanced Studies in Personology and Psychopathology.

Millon, T. (1982b). *Millon Clinical Multiaxial Inventory Manual.* Minneapolis, MN: National Computer Systems.

Millon, T. (1983). *Millon Clinical Inventory Manual* (3rd ed.). Minneapolis, MN: National Computer Systems.

Millon, T. (1987). *Millon Clinical Multiaxial Inventory-II: Manual for the MCMI II.* Minneapolis, MN: National Computer Systems.

Millon, T. (1994). *MCMI-III manual.* Minneapolis, MN: National Computer Systems.

Millon, T., Davis, R. D., & Millon, C. (1997). *MCMI-III: Manual* (2nd ed.). Min-neapolis, MN: National Computer Systems.

Nurnberg, H. G., Martin, G. A., Somoza, E., Coccaro, E. F., Skodol, A. E., Oldham, J. M., et al. (2000). Identifying personality disorders: Towards the develop-ment of a clinical screening instrument. *Comprehensive Psychiatry, 41*, 137–146.

Perry, J. C. (1992). Problems and considerations in the valid assessment of per-sonality disorders. *American Journal of Psychiatry, 149*, 1645–1653.

Retzlaff, P. D. (1996). MCMI-III diagnostic validity: Bad test or bad validity study? *Journal of Personality Assessment, 66*, 431–437.

Retzlaff, P. D. (2000). Comment on the validity of the MCMI-III. *Law and Human Behavior, 24,* 499–500.

Rogers, R., Salekin, R. T., & Sewell, K. W. (1999). Validation of the Millon Clinical Multiaxial Inventory for Axis II disorders: Does it meet the Daubert standard? *Law and Human Behavior, 23,* 425–443.

Rogers, R., Salekin, R. T., & Sewell, K. W. (2000). The MCMI-III and the Daubert standard: Separating rhetoric from reality. *Law and Human Behavior, 24,* 501–506.

Rossi, G. (2004). *Interpersoonlijk uit balans: Empirische validatie van de MCMI-III en de theorie van Millon met betrekking tot de afhankelijke, narcistische, theatrale en antisociale persoonlijkheid* [Interpersonally imbalanced: Empirical validation of the MCMI-III and the theory of Millon considering the dependent, narcissistic, histrionic and antisocial personality]. Unpublished manuscript PhD thesis. Brussel, Belgium: Vrije Universiteit Brussel.

Rossi, G., Hauben, C., Van den Brande, I., & Sloore, H. (2003). Empirical evaluation of the MCMI-III personality disorder scales. *Psychological Reports, 92,* 627–642.

Rossi, G., & Van den Brande, I. (1998). MCMI-III: Klinische beoordelingen [MCMI-III: Clinical ratings]. Unpublished manuscript. Brussel, Belgium: Vrije Universiteit Brussel.

Shiraev, E., & Levy, D. (2004). *Cross-cultural psychology: Critical thinking and contemporary applications.* Boston: Pearson Education.

Sloore, H., & Derksen, J. (1997). Issues and procedures in MCMI translations. In T. Millon (Ed.), *The Millon Inventories: Clinical and personality assessment* (pp. 286–302). New York: Guilford Press.

Spitzer, R. L. (1983). Psychiatric diagnosis: Are clinicians still necessary? *Comprehensive Psychiatry, 24,* 399–411.

Swets, J. A. (1973). The relative operating characteristic in psychology. *Science, 182,* 990–1000.

Swets, J. A., Dawes, R. M., & Monahan, J. (2000). Psychological science can improve diagnostic decisions. *Psychological science in the Public Interest, 1,* 1–26.

Thorndike, R. M. (1982). *Data collection and analysis.* New York: Gardner Press.

Van den Brande, I. (2002). *Empirische validering van de theorie van Th. Millon m.b.t. de persoonlijkheidsstoornissen* [Empirical validation of Th. Millon's theory concerning personality disorders]. Unpublished manuscript PhD thesis. Brussel: Vrije Universiteit Brussel.

Van de Vijver, F., & Poortinga, Y. (1982). Cross-cultural generalization and universality. *Journal of Cross-Cultural Psychology, 13,* 387–408.

Van de Vijver, F., & Tanzer, N. (1997). Bias and equivalence in cross-cultural assessment: An overview. *European Review of Applies Psychology, 47,* 263–279.

West, S. G., & Finch, J. F. (1997). Personality measurement: Reliability and validity issues. In R. Hogan, J. Johnson, & S. Briggs (Eds.), *Handbook of personality psychology* (pp. 143–164). San Diego, CA: Academic Press.

World Health Organization. (1992). *International statistical classification of diseases and related health problems* (10th ed.). Geneva, Switzerland: Author.

PART II

Newer Applications with the MCMI-III™

CHAPTER 7

Using the MCMI-III™ for Treatment Planning and to Enhance Clinical Efficacy

JEFFREY J. MAGNAVITA

THE MILLON Clinical Multiaxial Inventory (MCMI) was developed to provide an instrument that would offer a practical, objective tool with which to assess personality and clinical syndromes. In developing this instrument, Theodore Millon sought to further establish a scientific personology (Strack, in press). He emphasizes that the crucial aspect of advancing clinical science is the ability of a system of classification, theory, and instrumentation to cohere. Thus, personality and psychopathology, the latest developments in psychiatric classification, and instrumentation supported by research findings would be logically derived and able to measure the constructs of the system (Millon et al., 1996). Millon (1990; Millon, Grossman, Meagher, Millon, & Everly, 1999) has developed such a theoretical metapsychology, which uses an evolutionary model to depict psychopathological adaptations, personality structure-organization-function, and a "synergistic" system of therapy. The MCMI-III (Millon, 1994) is an instrument that has considerable clinical utility for those providing mental health treatments. In this chapter, I review some of the ways this instrument can be effectively utilized to enhance clinical practice. A case is presented using the MCMI in a process-oriented manner useful in conceptualizing personality functioning and orienting the treatment for a couple with complex clinical syndromes. The scope of settings where the MCMI is used is discussed in the following section.

UTILITY OF THE MCMI-III IN
CLINICAL PRACTICE SETTINGS

There are a number of settings where the MCMI-III can be advantageous and can enhance clinical practice by enabling the clinician to rapidly gather vital data that will assist in treatment planning. Unfortunately, in many settings, the MCMI is underutilized, even though it offers considerable utility for diagnostics and in treatment planning. Hopefully, this can be rectified as more clinicians become familiar with the application of the MCMI in various settings. The range of settings and uses of the MCMI are briefly reviewed here, and many are explained in greater detail and depth in this volume.

PSYCHIATRIC AND MEDICAL HOSPITAL PRACTICE

The use of the MCMI-III in a medical or psychiatric hospital offers the treatment team the ability to rapidly attain diagnostic information that will be useful for treatment planning and establishing a differential diagnostic profile. The MCMI is used in some Veteran Administration hospitals as well as general medical facilities when a qualified person is on staff to administer and interpret the findings. In the past, the length of hospitalization for psychiatric treatment tended to be long, months or even years, which afforded the clinical treatment team a leisurely approach to completing a diagnostic workup. Often during the course of treatment, a full psychological battery, including an intellectual assessment, full projective and objective personality measures, such as the Rorschach, Thematic Apperception Test, Sentence Completion Tests, and MMPI, was administered. Along with these, a careful psychiatric history and diagnostic interviews were conducted. Findings were traditionally presented in multidisciplinary treatment team meetings and were used for diagnosis and treatment planning. As the length of hospitalization was dramatically reduced in the past 20 years, due to cost containment issues and managed care influences, extensive in-depth psychological and psychiatric evaluation was no longer reimbursed, nor was there time to conduct these. In many institutions, psychodiagnostic assessments became a lost art. In many hospitals, the length of stay was reduced to days, or weeks in extreme cases. Often, there was no time for extensive evaluation, which requires large blocks of time to administer and to prepare a narrative report. The time required for these evaluations usually resulted in the treatment team's receiving a copy of the report weeks after the patient was discharged.

As the length of hospitalization continued to be reduced, the pressure on the treatment team to diagnose and stabilize patients became enormous. Many hospitals sought alternatives to the costly and time-consuming standard psychological battery that had always been the bulwark of psychological diagnosis. The MCMI began to fill the void for many reasons. The MCMI was designed to make administration as practical as possible by limiting the number of items so that most patients, even the most disturbed, could successfully complete the instrument (Millon et al., 1996). The development of computer technology and complicated software allowed most facilities the option of rapidly processing the results in house. Using scanning and computer scoring, the report could be generated shortly after administration at a reasonable cost. Given the increased need for rapid assessment data to guide treatment planning for the ever-decreasing length of hospitalization, the MCMI offers a great advantage. Having accurate information with a rapid turnaround is extremely important to the treatment team, who are faced with short admission and discharge cycles.

COMMUNITY MENTAL HEALTH CENTERS

The community mental health system treats patients who generally cannot afford to be treated by private practitioners. Often, the patients seen in these settings tend to be those suffering from chronic psychiatric disorders, many of which were previously treated in the state hospital system. As the pressure to reform the state hospital system gained momentum in the early 1960s, the need for a community-based system to provide treatment for these patients was mandated. Unfortunately, many of the patients discharged from the state hospital system fell through the cracks and became lost members of society, living as street people in major metropolitan areas and smaller communities.

In many community mental health centers, because of funding challenges psychologists often were not included in the staff composition, which tends to be primarily dominated by clinical social workers and, more recently, licensed mental health counselors. As a result, diagnostic testing was not available for most clinicians. If psychologists are on staff, their heavy caseloads often preclude time-intensive and costly psychodiagnostic assessment. In many agencies, psychological testing is not available to the clinical treatment team. This has serious drawbacks, as the level of complexity of the cases seen is often quite high and the refractory nature of many of these conditions could benefit from careful diagnostic evaluation. In one community mental health center that I have been a consultant for, there is no psychologist on staff who can provide the treatment team with psychodiagnostic assessment. Often, clinicians who staff these community mental health centers have only recently received their training and are faced with trying to treat the most difficult and complex patients, with comorbid clinical syndromes (a combination of personality dysfunction and multiple Axis I disorders; Magnavita, 2000a). The MCMI can offer an alternative and cost-effective solution to many of these underfunded community mental health centers. Unfortunately, because of a lack of awareness, many administrators and clinicians are not aware of the utility and cost-effectiveness of the MCMI, so this population remains underserved in many areas. Even in the major metropolitan area where I practice, the local community mental health center was not informed of the existence or the potential benefit of the MCMI to rapidly gather essential clinical data to be used in treatment decision making.

PRIVATE PRACTICE

The MCMI has a wide range of application for the private practice clinician. The clinician in private fee-for-service practice, whether in a group or solo clinical practice, is often quite solitary. This is especially the case for those in rural practices, who may not have access to other mental health and medical specialists. For these clinicians, cost-effective, time-efficient psychodiagnostic assessment can be a valuable asset. Psychologists can easily utilize the available computer technology and software to do rapid in-office assessments; those who do not want to invest in the computer system can send the answer sheet in by mail for scoring. In a private practice setting, the MCMI can be utilized in various ways: It can serve a diagnostic function, be used in case conceptualization, offer treatment planning strategies, and be used for strategic interventions with individuals and couples who are in treatment. Although in some cases, the MCMI may be used strictly for diagnostic purposes when the clinician is unclear about diagnosis, it can serve multiple functions to enhance the treatment process.

FORENSIC SETTINGS

The MCMI is also a useful instrument for forensic settings, such as prison and court evaluations. The MCMI offers forensic psychologists and psychiatrists a method to attain a rapid and cost-effective assessment and clinical profile of inmates and those being evaluated for various forensic issues. In addition to psychotherapeutic planning, as a psychodiagnostician, I have used the MCMI for collaborative support along with clinical interviewing in fitness-for-duty evaluations, and the results have been quite useful. The format that I have developed is to use the assessment information in a process-oriented fashion, discussed later in the chapter.

This entails administering the MCMI-III and reviewing the findings during a clinical interview. The benefit of this method is that one can then see how the person being evaluated handles the information, providing another window into the client's functioning. I am particularly interested in the portions of the evaluation that clients agree with or fit and those that don't seem to fit. It is also valuable to see how they explore and either reject or try to understand the information, especially if it is getting at something of which they are unaware.

THE IMPORTANCE OF ASSESSMENT FOR TREATMENT PLANNING

Accurate diagnostic formulation and case conceptualization is the bulwark of clinical treatment and is guided by one's theoretical system. "Theory does so by providing a guide for viewing the organization, structure, and process of complex systems and offering organizing principles from which to make sense of the phenomena" (Magnavita, 2004b, p. 56). The MCMI is based on an integrative theory, blending many elements of the domain systems of human functioning, and thus is useful to clinicians from various theoretical schools. Theory determines the manner in which treatment is conceptualized and delivered. The development of effective *treatment packages* (TPs; Magnavita, 2004c) requires a comprehensive understanding and holonic, or three-dimensional, mapping of the patient's personality system using multiple assessment tools (Magnavita, 2000b). This includes intrapsychic, dyadic, triadic, and sociocultural and family processes. A TP is the combination of treatment modalities, type of treatment, and treatment format that the clinician formulates and then recommends to the patient or patient system (couple, family, larger social system). To determine the most efficacious TP, a comprehensive assessment is vital. In addition, a rapid assessment is especially important in the era of brief treatment, which requires much more of the clinician and patient (Magnavita, 1997). In their groundbreaking work on brief treatment, Alexander and French (1946) emphasized the importance of a comprehensive assessment early in treatment. They did not have the luxury of the psychometric advances that were made later in the twentieth century, such as the MCMI. Thus, early clinicians had to rely primarily on diagnostic interviewing as their main psychodiagnostic tool or, if necessary, a standard psychological test battery, which was costly and required a good deal of time.

Cost Considerations versus the Need for Collaborative Data

One of the dilemmas faced by the clinician is the tension between the need for gathering as much information as possible and the time required and additional costs this entails. Clinicians are always making choices about whether additional consultation, psychodiagnostic batteries, or self-report measures are worth the time and additional expense. In the ideal world, we would have extensive diagnostic information on all patients. However, the time involved and costs of ordering additional assessments must be balanced with the potential benefit of more information. Too much information is not likely to be carefully read by the busy clinician, who may read only the summary. The optimal amount of assessment information enables the clinician to conceptualize the core issues of the patient and the broader system in which he or she is embedded and formulate an accurate diagnostic profile. The MCMI is a reasonably cost-effective method considering the amount of valuable data that it generates. The emphasis on depicting the personality configuration of the patient is of major importance to the therapist who realizes the value of understanding personality functioning that is unique to each of us.

The Personality System as the Guide to Treatment Conceptualization and Formulation

Millon's career has been devoted to bringing the personality system back to clinical psychology and psychopathology (Strack, in press). His theoretical work has had substantial impact on the development of the field and has reinforced what early psychoanalytic workers knew from clinical experience: that personality or character is the key to effective treatment (Magnavita, 2002a). Millon's theoretical model places personality at the center of the clinical process. He believes that effective therapeutic work takes place when the function of the personality of the patient is understood and interventions are tailored to the patient's configuration (Millon et al., 1999). Millon has written extensively on personality-guided therapy and has been generating a number of volumes in his personality-guided series by authors who appreciate the value of this perspective.

The personality system can be conceptualized as a number of embedded subsystems that, at the microscopic level, involve intrapsychic processes integrally intertwined at increasingly macroscopic levels with dyadic, triadic, and sociocultural structures and processes (Magnavita, 2004c, 2005). In this regard, personality and clinical syndromes can be thought of as integrally connected. Anxiety, depression, psychotic process, relational dysfunction, and so forth emanate from vulnerabilities within an individual's intrapsychic system expressed and mutually shaped by dyadic, triadic, familial, and sociocultural processes. As such, the MCMI and its subsequent revisions keep this vital interrelationship at the forefront of the test construction and evolution. Clinical syndromes do not emerge randomly but out of the matrix of personality and thus must be conceptualized and measured in consideration of this fact. As a part of the assessment process, the MCMI-III is useful in obtaining valuable information about the way the personality and clinical symptom constellations coexist. When the personality system is stressed, each of us will respond in a different manner based on our vulnerabilities. For example, the patient with an obsessive personality configuration often becomes dysthymic under the constant pressure of constricting affect. When stress increases further, there may be explosiveness of affect, like a capacitor that is slowly charged and then releases its energy in a burst. Sexual dysfunction is another expression of vulnerability due to the demands that intimacy/closeness exert on the obsessive personality. Often due to the level of emotional constriction and difficulty with anger, any conflict in the dyadic configuration can be expressed in sexual dysfunction, such as lack of libido. A narcissistic personality configuration may be susceptible to substance abuse and Major Depression when there is a major narcissistic injury that the intrapsychic system cannot endure. A patient with a dependent or avoidant personality configuration might be prone to Somatization Disorder; if the family constellation is reinforcing, he or she may also eventually develop severe Agoraphobia. These are but a few of the common vulnerabilities seen in clinical practice.

Understanding personality structure, function, and organization alerts the clinician to the vulnerabilities and possible pathways of symptomatic expression. The MCMI-III provides the clinician with an overview of the terrain that requires further investigation and understanding.

USING THE MCMI-III TO FORMAT TREATMENT FOR OPTIMAL EFFICACY

The development of differential therapeutics was a major advance for clinical science. It proposes that certain treatments and treatment formats are appropriate in some cases and not in others (Frances, Clarkin, & Perry, 1984). Prior to this era, there was little consideration given to making the optimal match among the array of treatment and patient variables. Also, as clinical science matured, more modalities of treatment were developed. The delivery of the most effective treatment occurs when there is an optimal match among the characteristics of a patient system and various components of treatment with some of the following considerations:

1. *Type of therapy:* Psychopharmacological, psychoeducational, cognitive, cognitive-behavioral, psychodynamic, relational, integrative, unified, and so on. Concomitant with the type of therapy an individual uses, there is a theory of personality and psychopathology,

which explains how dysfunction occurs and the developmental factors that lead to personality disturbance and clinical syndromes.

2. *Modality of treatment:* Individual, couples, family, group, multifamily, ecological, multiple modalities of therapy, and so on. Each modality of treatment has a specialized set of methods and techniques that are used to restructure and modify process and structural components of the personality system.

3. *Treatment format:* Length of sessions, frequency of sessions, intervals between sessions.

Treatment selection can be optimized and TPs formulated when careful formulation of the patient's or patient system's dynamical forces can be rapidly attained. The MCMI-III can offer data useful in determining important aspects of the TP. The following considerations illustrate some of the treatment formulation decisions.

Type of Therapy

The type of therapy selected is a complex choice influenced by many factors, including the clinician's training, preferences, and knowledge of clinical literature and empirical evidence to support a particular type of therapy for a certain clinical presentation. The MCMI-III offers an orienting guide to more effectively inform these clinical decisions. For example, in cases where *severe personality pathology* is high, the clinician should be concerned with a treatment approach that offers adequate structure and potency to deal with frequent acting-out and crises that are an inevitable part of the treatment process. Treatment approaches such as dialectic behavior therapy (Linehan, 1993) or transference-focused therapy (Clarkin, Yeomans, & Kernberg, 1999) might be selected or elements of these integrated into one's therapeutic approach. Also, the clinician should closely evaluate patients who score high on Thought Disorder, Major Depression, and Delusional Disorders on the Severe Syndromes scales and on Bipolar: Manic on the Clinical Syndromes scale, as such patients often are in need of psychopharmacological treatment due to the biological insufficiencies that these patients are suspected of having. Hospitalization or a structured day treatment program offering psychoeducational, family, and supportive therapies is often warranted.

Modality of Treatment

Various modalities of treatment have been developed that, when used alone, in combination, or sequentially, can maximize the potency of treatment. There is little empirical literature to guide these types of selection issues, and much of one's ability is derived from clinical experience. The modality or combinations of modalities of treatment should be selected to maximize the fit between the patient's presenting symptoms and his or her personality configuration. In cases where there are elevations on the Clinical Personality scales, for example, the clinician might want to augment therapy by combining treatment modalities for best effect. For example, a patient who is married and suffering from depression and has elevated Personality scale scores may need a multimodal combination of psychopharmacology, individual psychotherapy, and marital therapy. Clinical and research evidence suggests that depression and marital dysfunction often go hand in hand, so that marital intervention may be optimal when combined with a standard treatment protocol. In other cases, sequential delivery of treatment might be more practical and cost-effective. For example, a couple with marital conflict may begin with a phase of marital therapy; after examining the MCMI-III and finding a significant elevation of the Alcohol scale, this may be followed by a phase of individual therapy with the alcohol abuser and concomitant attendance at Alcoholics Anonymous meetings. It should be underscored that it is best to emphasize a collaborative approach with patients and to assume a flexible stance. Patients often see clinicians who rigidly give prescriptions as controlling, authoritative, and noncollaborative.

Treatment Format

The treatment format has various components that need to be considered:

- *Length of sessions:* Although it is fairly standard procedure to offer most treatment modalities in 45- to 50-minute segments, there is scant evidence to suggest that this is the most efficacious way to deliver treatment. In fact, there is accumulating clinical and anecdotal evidence to suggest that one of the more robust ingredients of treatment may be the length of session (Magnavita, 1997; Mahoney, 2003). Extended sessions of 2 to 3 hours seem to afford the therapist and patient an optimal length of time in which to complete a through assessment, develop a therapeutic alliance, and mobilize affective processes so vital to the change process. Sometimes, briefer sessions are beneficial to patients who need support and a consistent attachment to monitor their progress and alter treatment if a relapse is eminent.
- *Frequency of sessions:* The most effective frequency for sessions is another aspect of the TP that has little empirical validation. Some patients seem to require regular weekly appointments or, in some severe cases, daily appointments to function at their optimal level of adaptive capacity. Yet others seem to benefit when sessions are spaced at longer intervals to allow for metabolizing of feelings and to provide sufficient time to practice

the new skills and patterns they are trying to develop. There is little in the research or clinical literature to inform clinicians about how to proceed in this regard. A general rule of thumb is that increasing the frequency or length of sessions intensifies the treatment. A caveat is necessary, however, as some patients with a high degree of defensive resistance to the process may actually experience a reduction in benefit. For example, increased frequency might be detrimental in a patient with an elevated Dependent scale score who uses the attachment with the therapist to avoid the anxiety associated with changing interpersonal patterns by becoming more autonomous. A determination of the frequency of sessions should be made in collaboration with the patient, taking into consideration how quickly he or she wants to work, logistical concerns (i.e., distance needed to travel, ability to carve out time), financial status, clinical assessment, and ability to benefit from more or less intensive treatment.

• *Short-term, intermittent, or long-term treatment:* Another aspect of the treatment format is how the treatment is conceptualized. Many patients can benefit enormously from a brief treatment, and in fact, most treatment delivered today is brief. Generally speaking, patients without elevated clinical syndromes who do not demonstrate elevations in Personality scales or Severe scales are likely candidates for a briefer treatment. As scores on the Severe scales increase, it is likely that the patient will require intermittent treatment delivered over a long span of time or ongoing long-term therapy. Of course, the treatment format in this case should be modified as the patient's needs and situation change.

CLARIFYING COMPLEX DIAGNOSTIC ISSUES IN THE INDIVIDUAL

The complexity of psychopathological conditions seen in clinical practice varies enormously from setting to setting. Inpatient hospital settings often are faced with a range of chronic relapsing patients who have more severe psychopathological adaptations and acute crises that can be stabilized and referred to appropriate outpatient treatment. The MCMI-III provides an excellent tool for sorting out complex clinical presentations and offering treatment recommendations. It is often very difficult to understand the interrelationships among overlapping clinical syndromes and personality dysfunction. The MCMI-III can assist in this process and confirm or rule out various constellations that a patient may present. For example, Panic Disorder in a patient with an elevated Severe Personality Profile is going to present a greater challenge than a patient whose score is lower. In the former, the patient's panic is less likely to be related to conflict and repressed affect and more likely to be the result of emotional dysregulation and attachment disturbance, requiring a more stabilizing treatment and less of an uncovering approach. Often, patients who require inpatient hospitalization have personality disorders that exacerbate clinical syndromes and make them more treatment-refractory. Certain clinical profiles are potentially lethal, such as elevated Bipolar and Alcohol Dependence scales, especially in the setting of elevations on the Severe Personality Pathology scales. Reviewing the MCMI-III early in treatment can alert the clinician to this and other profiles that place the patient at risk to harm self or others.

TREATMENT PLANNING AND STRATEGIZING

The MCMI-III offers great utility for the clinician in planning and strategizing various treatment interventions. The profiles often corroborate initial clinical findings, but more often point out other syndromes or personality profiles that have been overlooked and deserve further exploration. The MCMI-III can provide additional support for one's impressions and open up other areas of exploration. Often, patients will not spontaneously provide information that they will report on a paper-and-pencil test. Treatment planning can be more focused when the clinician has more confidence in what he or she is treating. When the clinician feels on more solid ground with the patient, he or she is able to titrate the intensity of treatment at the optimal level of anxiety for the patient (Magnavita, 1997). Methods and techniques that increase anxiety can be applied to the overregulated or constricted patient and those that reduce anxiety to those patients who are more fragile in their structural capacities.

OFFERING A SECOND OBJECTIVE PERSPECTIVE

Another valuable way to incorporate the MCMI-III in clinical practice is to offer a second objective perspective to a patient who has not been open to the diagnostic impressions formulated by the clinician. A report that supports what the clinician has formulated may reduce the patient's resistance. The objectivity of the report is something that is difficult to argue with, although some will. Again the report should be presented as tentative until the findings are either corroborated or disconfirmed by interview, collateral material, history, and observation. Often, patients are impressed with the accuracy of the findings and feel more at ease knowing that what they are suffering with is something others suffer with, and that it is being studied and treated by other clinicians and researchers. Sometimes patients have a strong need to understand what their condition or syndrome is and what it is called. To this end, the MCMI-III can be an effective psychoeducational aid. Patients then may want to read scientific and other literature that educates them and can increase their sense of hopefulness.

PROCESS-ORIENTED ASSESSMENT

Assessment is an ongoing process that should be seamlessly integrated with treatment. As new information is gathered and a deeper appreciation of the patient is developed, treatment can be modified as necessary. Assessment is never a static event. No assessment instrument or interview can hope to capture the complexity of human experience, resilience, and capacity for change. Any assessment device is a tool that requires clinical experience and sophistication to use correctly. Clinicians need to be familiar with the test and, in the case of the MCMI-III, need also to be conversant with psychopathology, personality theory, and psychodiagnostics. Assessment data are optimized when they become part of the clinical process and are utilized in a way that most benefits the patient. *Process-oriented assessment* is based on the assumption that the process generated by the data from an assessment instrument is essential. The clinician uses the information in an ongoing collaboration with the patient about the meaning and relevance of the data.

PROVIDING PROCESS-ORIENTED FEEDBACK

In my experience, when giving feedback to the patient it is best that he or she be told, "The impressions and descriptions of you that have been formulated from the evaluation will have some elements that will fit and some that will not. It is important that we discuss the aspects that fit, as well as those that do not." I often also add, "You know yourself better than anyone, but this is an opportunity to explore some aspects of the way you relate to others and cope with conflict and stress." I modify this based on the patient's level of sophistication, intelligence, and psychological-mindedness. This allows patients to defend themselves from information that may be overwhelming as well as discuss the meaning of the data. Thus, the goal is to create a forum for an open discussion and consideration of the patient's personality system. The clinician then has the opportunity to observe the patient's defensive style *in operation* as he or she deals with what can be a stressful situation. Process-oriented test interpretation uses the findings in a way similar to the way many therapists use dreams, as a way for patients to understand and know themselves (Mahoney, 2003). It is also important to inform the patient that the report is written in clinical terminology for a trained professional audience, so that terms may need to be explained. The test data are not used as a final word about how an individual functions but as a way of opening up a dialogue that can enhance an individual's awareness and focus the treatment on the most prominent issues that are interfering with more adaptive functioning.

Before reviewing the findings with the patient, I suggest that the clinician go over the test and underline aspects that seem important to discuss. It is generally preferable for the clinician to read the findings to the patient in bites small enough for the patient to digest and then stop and explore reactions. Sometimes it is better to paraphrase or translate the material in lay terms. Some patients will request to read the evaluation; in some cases, this is appropriate, and in others, it should be discouraged. If the patient reads the evaluation, it is important that the clinician be present to handle reactions and questions and pace the discussion based on the patient's needs and areas of concern or curiosity. Patients may have questions about technical terms that need to be answered.

Usually, it does not take long for the test findings to be reviewed and then a focus to be found that the patient wants to discuss. This type of process-oriented testing often opens the door for communication and establishes a sense of confidence in the clinician's ability to formulate and explore personality issues and clinical constellations. Sharing the current knowledge in a psychoeducational and compassionate way is often a vital step in developing a positive therapeutic alliance and is a way to frame the treatment as collaborative.

CASE EXAMPLE: MARITAL DYSFUNCTION AND SPOUSAL ABUSE

The couple* consulted the author for severe marital dysfunction, which included a pattern of escalating violence. They presented as two intelligent professionals in their mid-30s, well educated and financially successful. Their relationship began to deteriorate after the birth of their first child about 1 year prior. They described episodes that were triggered by the wife's "not adequately fulfilling her duties as a spouse." When asked to elaborate, she said that if she did not iron his shirt and lay out his clothes, he would erupt into a severe temper tantrum, during which he would scream at her and belittle her, threatening divorce. She often would respond by withdrawing and on some occasions would provoke him verbally or even hit him. On one occasion, things escalated to the point that he smashed their son's crib as she was holding the baby during

---

* The case material presented is based on an actual case, with all identifying information altered so as to obscure the identity of the individuals.

a fight. They both became concerned about the possible effect on their child, for whom they both had strong feelings of affection.

PRESENTATION ON INITIAL CONSULTATION

The couple was seen together for the first few sessions and exuded much hostility in their interaction. The husband tended to be highly sarcastic toward and belittling of his wife and highly critical of her housekeeping and the way she managed their finances. He was resistant to coming to therapy and seemed to be motivated only by his fear of divorce and losing custody of his son, to whom he was very attached. He was also mortified by the thought of how his family would react to his divorcing. The wife seemed unable to stand up for herself and was intimidated and bullied by his verbal assaults on her adequacy. She seemed to become detached as he described her inadequacies. As is the case with many couples that experience this level of dysfunction, personality disturbance was suspected. However, the husband's denial of any personal difficulties and his tendency to externalize and blame others made it difficult for him to commit to treatment. Their circular interactive pattern seemed to almost always lead to a downward spiral, where each of them would display increasingly regressive defenses, increasing their anxiety and stimulating more waves of regressive defending.

   The benefit of a couple's therapy modality is that it allows the clinician to actually observe the dyadic processes as they occur in vivo during the couple's communication with one another and the clinician. A careful evaluation and cataloguing of the husband's and the wife's defensive constellations was undertaken (Magnavita, 1997). Establishing the constellation of defenses and the rapidity with which each of them regresses to a more primitive level of defenses is crucial in making a determination about the intensity and pace of treatment they can tolerate.

THE FIRST OBSTACLE: THE HUSBAND'S EXTERNALIZATION

It quickly became apparent that the treatment was in danger of collapsing because of the husband's reliance on the defense of externalization, whereby he blamed all his symptoms and difficulties on his wife's inadequacy. This, along with his tendency to project, rationalize his behavior, and blame, were his primary defenses. He also used ancillary defenses such as sarcasm and argumentativeness and would sulk and distance. During each of the early sessions, he complained of having to attend therapy and felt that his wife should be the focus of treatment because of her problems. Individual sessions with each of them were offered as a way of detoxifying their dyadic interactions and attempting to establish a positive therapeutic alliance. The treatment was in danger of being swamped by his resistance.

As a way of establishing a clearer picture of the levels of psychopathology each contributed to the disturbed dyadic processes, they were each offered the opportunity to take the MCMI-III for diagnostic clarification and treatment planning. They both readily agreed to this out of their frustration and possibly as a way to prove the other the sicker one in need of treatment. They each completed the MCMI-III, and a session was scheduled with both of them to review the results. They agreed to do this together as a way of gaining a better appreciation for the other.

Test Results and Utilization for Optimizing Treatment Efficacy

The husband and wife both completed the MCMI-III, and the results were manually entered into a computer and a profile and interpretive report generated. The couple granted their informed consent regarding the clinical nature of the findings, and both agreed to be present during the interpretations. A couple therapy session was held, during which the findings were summarized and parts of the report were read verbatim. Both profiles were valid.

The Husband's Profile

The husband's profile revealed a number of significant elevations in the clinical personality patterns, which is not atypical (Millon, 1994), as there tends to be overlap among the personality disorder categories (Magnavita, 2004a). In fact, it is often the case that clinicians diagnose two or three personality disorders. In this case, the patient had significant elevations on five scales: Schizoid, Avoidant, Depressive, Dependent, and Passive-Aggressive. There were three notable elevations in three clinical syndromes: Anxiety Disorder, Dysthymic Disorder, and Alcohol Dependence.

The findings seemed to capture the patient's most prominent features, and both he and his wife were amazed at how well the interpretive report characterized his behavior and personality. Because this patient was a well-educated professional, the intellectual aspect of the evaluation and explanation was something that intrigued him. He was surprised by the test's ability to capture and describe aspects of his personality and intrapsychic functions. His level of ego-syntonicity (identification with defenses, a lack of awareness about his impact on others, and emotional disconnection) made it difficult for him to take any constructive feedback from his wife, which would have helped him mature and modulate his affect and behavior. The report confirmed many of the things that she said and some of the feedback he received by the clinician observing his behavior in session with his wife. This intervention seemed to be a remarkable breakthrough in his externalization and denial of his personality dysfunction, which was robbing his life of all that he had worked so hard for and threatening to destroy his family.

The Wife's Profile

The wife's profile was equally illuminating and helpful to the clinical process. Her profile showed a significant elevation on the Posttraumatic Stress clinical scale. Discussing this finding, she disclosed that she had been the victim of traumatic physical and emotional abuse as a child. Although she had previously been in treatment, she was unhappy with the therapist's approach and discontinued because of an incident of physical contact that she felt uncomfortable with. The husband responded with a surprising degree of empathy when she described what she had experienced. The symptoms of PTSD were explained to them both, and he then began to see how the way she reacted was the result of being retraumatized by his emotionally abusive behavior and not because she was deficient and inferior to him.

The Interrelationship of the Individual Personality Systems and Impact on Dyadic and Triadic Functions

The way the individual personality system of each partner interrelates can be seen in dyadic and often in triadic processes, whereby an unstable dyad attempts to draw in a third party to stabilize their relationship. In this case, the couple's son was the obvious third corner of the triad and was in danger of being overwhelmed and traumatized by their behavior. We discussed how each of the spouses entered into recursive reenactment patterns that led to downward spiraling. The wife's PTSD, which included symptoms of dissociation, made her exceptionally vulnerable to conflict and anxiety aroused in the couple when issues of intimacy and closeness became overwhelming. The husband was not aware of how his behavior was triggering flashbacks to early violence, when she either froze or fought for her life in any way she could. Problems with intimacy and closeness were a major theme in their relationship. His typical pattern of passive-aggressive responding took its toll on her feelings toward him, as it always does in those in relationships with people with a passive-aggressive style. His dependency strivings were constantly frustrated because he expected her to act as his mother did; she used to indulge and pamper him, which would stimulate his passive-aggressive style of relating, increasing tension and conflict in the dyad.

Given the cantankerous nature of their relationship, the feedback session went surprisingly well, with each of them demonstrating a greater level of understanding and empathy for the other. The husband's chronic depression (dysthymia and depressive personality combination) and low self-esteem was revealed directly. He realized that no matter how successful he was, he was never happy and always felt like he was working in the "coal mine," in spite of substantial professional and financial success. He also discussed his inability to spend money commensurate with his social class, describing how he was unable to buy himself a new car or take his family on vacation. The clinician, explaining the impact of personality dysfunction on an individual and family life, took a psychoeducational stance, to which the husband responded well. The fact that the husband admitted that he had suffered all his life was the first acknowledgment of the potential need for professional help. The importance of a zero tolerance for violence agreement was explained, and they both participated in strategies for de-escalating an escalating conflict. Re-traumatization of the wife was not something the husband realized he was creating, and he made a commitment to stop.

TREATMENT PLANNING AND RECOMMENDATIONS

This couple was in extreme distress and headed for a major catastrophe or divorce unless treatment were accepted. Given the complexity of the case and the corroborative data from the MCMI-III, it was determined that before they proceeded with couple's therapy, each of them should have individual treatment. The focus of treatment with the husband was on his passive-aggressive personality, dysthymia, and anxiety, which were interrelated. The wife's treatment was to focus on the PTSD and her ability to begin to appropriately stand up for herself instead of withdrawing or attacking. She decided she would see a therapist who specialized in treating women with PTSD, and a referral was made. The husband was offered the opportunity to do some intensive short-term dynamic psychotherapy (Magnavita, 1993), which, along with family-oriented interpersonal psychotherapy (Smith Benjamin & Cushing, 2004), can be effective with passive-aggressive personalities. In addition, it was recommended that they have conjoint marital therapy on a monthly basis until they were each prepared for more intensive work on their marriage.

The use of multiple modalities of treatment with patients suffering from personality dysfunction can augment the therapeutic process (Magnavita, 2000b; Magnavita & MacFarlane, 2004). The corroboration of the presence of passive-aggressive personality was important in treatment planning, as these patients can be treatment-refractory and sabotage the therapy as their need to win is expressed in self-destruction (I will be more powerful by showing how ineffective the therapist is). Indications from the clinical literature and from experience treating these disorders shows that extended sessions are essential to break through the defensive barrier and begin a restructuring of the patient's personality (Magnavita, 1997). These patients often respond much better when extended sessions of 3 hours are offered at the beginning of treatment. Once some restructuring of the defenses has occurred, it is still beneficial to see the patient for 90-minute sessions as their defenses can reconsolidate rapidly, making them refractory to standard formats.

In this case, the husband made considerable progress in identifying the early contributions to his personality dysfunction. He identified never being able to please a highly narcissistic father who continually criticized and outdid him and who still overwhelmed him. He was able to restructure many of his passive-aggressive defenses so as to be able to relate to others in a more direct and honest manner. The marital relationship slowly improved and treatment was terminated with moderate improvement.

SUMMARY AND CONCLUSIONS

The MCMI-III is a valuable asset to the mental health clinician in a variety of settings. Clinicians' access to accurate diagnostic material that is cost-effective and has a rapid turnaround is essential but under-utilized in many clinical settings. There are a number of ways the MCMI-III can be utilized to enhance treatment efficacy. Using the MCMI-III to more efficiently construct treatment packages crafted to each patient's unique personality system requires the clinician to be conversant with the multiple aspects of the treatment package so that the best fit can be found with the many aspects of treatment that are within the control of the clinician, such as modality of treatment, treatment format, type of treatment, and whether treatment is delivered in multiple or sequential modalities. This is still very much a clinical art as there is little empirical evidence to suggest how these elements of treatment need to be arranged and delivered. There is accumulating clinical evidence that personality functioning is crucial in understanding the unique interplay of dynamical forces that lead to clinical syndromes. The MCMI-III is one of the most useful objective instruments that enable clinicians to map the topography and internal workings of the personality system.

REFERENCES

Alexander, F. G., & French, T. M. (1946). *Psychoanalytic therapy: Principles and applications.* New York: Ronald Press.

Clarkin, J. F., Yeomans, F. E., & Kernberg, O. F. (1999). *Psychotherapy for borderline personality.* New York: Wiley.

Frances, A., Clarkin, J., & Perry, S. (1984). *Differential therapeutics in psychiatry: The art and science of treatment selection.* New York: Brunner/Mazel.

Linehan, M. M. (1993). *Cognitive-behavioral treatment of borderline personality disorder.* New York: Guilford Press.

Magnavita, J. J. (1993). The treatment of passive-aggressive personality disorder: A review of current approaches (Pt. 1). *International Journal of Short-Term Psychotherapy, 8*(1), 29–41.

Magnavita, J. J. (1997). *Restructuring personality disorders: A short-term dynamic approach.* New York: Guilford Press.

Magnavita, J. J. (2000a). Integrative relational therapy of complex clinical syndromes: Ending the multigenerational transmission process. *Journal of Clinical Psychology/In Session: Psychotherapy in Practice, 56*(8), 1051–1064.

Magnavita, J. J. (2000b). *Relational therapy for personality disorders.* Hoboken, NJ: Wiley.

Magnavita, J. J. (2002a). Psychodynamic approaches to psychotherapy: A century of innovations. In F. W. Kaslow (Series Ed.) & J. J. Magnavita (Vol. Ed.), *Comprehensive handbook of psychotherapy: Psychodynamic/object relations.* (Vol. 1, pp. 1–12). Hoboken, NJ: Wiley.

Magnavita, J. J. (2002b). *Theories of personality: Contemporary approaches to the science of personality.* Hoboken, NJ: Wiley.

Magnavita, J. J. (2004a). Classification, prevalence, and etiology of personality disorders: Related issues and controversy. In J. J. Magnavita (Ed.), *Handbook of personality disorders: Theory and practice* (pp. 3–23). Hoboken, NJ: Wiley.

Magnavita, J. J. (2004b). The relevance of theory in treating personality dysfunction. In J. J. Magnavita (Ed.), *Handbook of personality disorders: Theory and practice* (pp. 56–77). Hoboken, NJ: Wiley.

Magnavita, J. J. (2004c). Toward a unified model of treatment for personality dysfunction. In J. J. Magnavita (Ed.), *Handbook of personality disorders: Theory and practice* (pp. 528–553). Hoboken, NJ: Wiley.

Magnavita, J. J. (2005). *Personality-guided relational therapy: A unified approach.* Washington, DC: American Psychological Association.

Magnavita, J. J., & MacFarlane, M. M. (2004). Family treatment of personality disorders: Historical overview and current perspectives. In M. M. MacFarlane (Ed.), *Family treatment of personality disorders: Advances in clinical practice* (pp. 3–39). New York: Haworth Press.

Mahoney, M. J. (2003). *Constructive psychotherapy: A practical guide.* New York: Guilford Press.

Millon, T. (1990). *Toward a new personology: An evolutionary model.* New York: Wiley.

Millon, T. (1994). *Millon Clinical Multiaxial Inventory-III manual.* Minneapolis, MN: National Computer Systems.

Millon, T., Davis, R. D., Millon, C. M., Wenger, A., Van Zuilen, M. H., Fuchs, M., et al. (1996). *Disorders of personality* DSM-III *and beyond* (2nd ed.). New York: Wiley.

Millon, T., Grossman, S., Meagher, S., Millon, C., & Everly, G. (1999). *Personality-guided therapy.* Hoboken, NJ: Wiley.

Smith Benjamin, L., & Cushing, G. (2004). An interpersonal family-oriented approach to personality disorder. In M. M. MacFarlane (Ed.), *Family treatment of personality disorders: Advances in clinical practice* (pp. 41–69). New York: Haworth Press.

Strack, S. (Ed.). (in press). *Handbook of personology and psychopathology: Essays in honor of Theodore Millon.* Hoboken, NJ: Wiley.

CHAPTER 8

Use of the MCMI-III™ with Other Personality Inventories

ROBERT J. CRAIG

WHILE PROJECTIVE tests have long been presented as part of an integrated psychodiagnostic test battery, examples of a similar process with objective tests (i.e., self-report inventories) are absent in the literature. This is true despite the fact that objective personality tests are also used as part of a test battery, but the literature generally presents interpretive principles for these tests as if they were used as a single instrument. This chapter presents a case report illustrating how objective personality tests (i.e., MMPI-2, MCMI-III, Sixteen Personality Factors [16PF]; Adjective Check List [ACL]) can be used as part of an integrated and refined interpretation of personality.

The personality literature is replete with examples of how to integrate projective and objective personality tests into the interpretive process. This approach has a long history (Rapaport, Gill, & Shafer, 1968) and continues to the present time (Finn, 2003). For example, discussions and demonstrations continue to appear in the literature on how to integrate the Rorschach with the MMPI (Acklin, 1993; Archer & Krishnamurthy, 1993; Finn, 2003; Ganellen, 1996; Lovitt, 1993; Weiner, 1993). Similar examples of interpreting objective personality tests as a test battery are absent from the literature. The most recent text on teaching personality assessment includes a plethora of chapters on how to interpret individual

This test material was collected prior to the recent APA Ethical Code revision (2002), which requires patients' written consent to publish test data, and the patient was lost to follow-up.

tests but does not contain a chapter on test integration (Handler & Hilsenroth, 1998).

There have been some attempts to demonstrate how the Millon Clinical Multiaxial Inventory (MCMI; Millon, 1983, 1987) can be used to refine interpretations from MMPI code types (Antoni, 1993; Antoni, Levine, Tischer, Green, & Millon, 1986, 1987; Antoni, Tischer, Levine, Green, & Millon, 1985a, 1985b; Levine, Tischer, Antoni, Green, & Millon, 1985), but these reports do not illustrate how to integrate the information. Rather, they suggest ways that Millon's theory and instrumentation can be used in conjunction with some MMPI code types. A few studies have reported on the use of two objective personality tests with the same population (Hyer, Woods, Boudwyns, Harrison, & Tamkin, 1990), but they have not illustrated how to integrate the tests (in this case, the MCMI and the 16PF) into a single, integrated interpretation.

Because objective personality tests, particularly those that produce a computerized narrative report, have become increasingly popular with psychologists (Butcher & Rouse, 1996), the purpose of this chapter is to illustrate how to integrate these tests into a refined interpretation as an objective test battery. By test integration, I am referring to a situation where more than one objective personality test is used with the same patient. Clinically, such tests would be more commonly used in a test battery that includes projective tests and tests of cognitive ability, but for purposes of illustration, I demonstrate only how objective personality tests, emphasizing self-report methodology, can be used in an integrated manner to refine the interpretive process. It is understood that most psychologists reading this chapter will have a good sense of this skill, but graduate students in psychology courses on assessment have essentially no literature that can serve as an example of how this integration is to be done.

CASE HISTORY

The patient is a 40-year-old, divorced, White male who was self-referred for outpatient psychotherapy for postdivorce adjustment problems, primarily depression and guilt over the fact that his drinking caused his divorce. He is in the construction trades and drinks 4 to 5 beers a day and several shots of vodka at lunch and 8 to 10 shots of vodka at night. He had one prior 28-day inpatient treatment episode for alcohol and remained abstinent for 6 months, but relapsed following the death of a close friend. He has been drinking continually now for several years. He also had been abusing marijuana and was unable to father a child due to low sperm count, which was probably related to his chronic marijuana use, which is now in remission. This added to his marital problems, and his wife filed for divorce. She has since remarried and now has a child, which further adds to his feelings of guilt and blame.

Despite these sincere emotions, he reports no desire to stop drinking and has set up enabling relationships to foster his drinking: (1) His supervisor at work is a recovering alcoholic, "understands" the patient's problems, is "supportive," and doesn't hassle him about his two-hour daily lunches and chronic drinking, especially as the employee does not appear drunk and gets the work done; (2) he has a girlfriend who knows about his drinking but never pressures him to stop; he alleges that she drinks occasionally but does not have an alcohol problem; (3) upon setting treatment goals, the patient vehemently asserted that he did not want his therapist to deal with his drinking and wants "no intervention" (a concept in addiction therapy whereby those who are intimately involved with the patient meet with the patient and communicate their feelings about the patient's past behavior). Subsequently, the patient did allow me to contact his personal physician to ascertain health status, where I learned that the patient has a fatty liver—the first signs of liver disorder associated with heavy drinking. He was quite adamant about stating that his goals in therapy were to help him improve his mood and to deal with his interpersonal problems; he did not want substance abuse counseling. (When asked how likely it was that he would stop drinking on a scale from 1 [never] to 10 [as soon as possible], he said 5 [reflecting his ambivalence] and then spontaneously said "No, 3").

The patient has a history of poor judgment and impulsivity associated with his drinking. He reported that once he was at a stoplight and when the light turned green, Puerto Rican teens spit on his face and then ran away. He alleged this was unprovoked. He was able to impulsively grab one of them by the head and then stepped on the gas, intending to drag him to his death, but the youth slipped out of the hold. He said if he had a gun, he would have killed him. The patient was probably legally drunk at the time. He made a U-turn and began chasing after them. By now, they had gotten into a car and the chase was on. They turned into an alley, where he pursued them. They then stopped and jumped out of the car (there were four of them), brandishing long-blade knives. He then realized the predicament he was in and quickly reentered his car and backed out of the alley. He had been drinking his usual amount that day.

My initial impression was of a patient who was filled with denial and rationalizations, anxiety manifested by nervous tension and humor designed to protect his current behavior, and chronic depression (dysthymia) manifested mostly by low self-esteem and with negative cognitions associated with guilt over his behavior causing dissolution of the marriage as well as a possible alcohol-related mood disorder. Underlying personality structure appeared to be combinations of passive-aggressive and self-defeating behaviors. He has gamma (alcohol-dependent) alcoholism.

The patient was given initial cognitive and personality tests as part of the workup. He tested in the average range of intelligence. Memory and neurological tests revealed deficits in visual-motor information processing, visual reproduction, associative learning, and short-term auditory memory and concentration. Because he subsequently always came to the sessions after work and after his usual amount of drinking, and because he drank several hours prior to testing, I was unable to determine if these deficits were due to acute or chronic drinking, but told him I would readminister these tests when he came to a session after several days of abstinence. His objective personality test protocols appear in the appendix.

TESTS ADMINISTERED

Minnesota Multiphasic Personality Inventory 2 (MMPI-2; Butcher, Dahlstrom, Graham, Tellegen, & Kaemmer, 1989)

Millon Clinical Multiaxial Inventory III (MCMI-III; Millon, 1994)

Sixteen Personality Factors Questionnaire (16PF; Institute for Personality and Ability Testing, 1991)

Adjective Check List (ACL; Gough & Heilbrun, 1983)

These tests were selected based on both clinical and empirical considerations. The MMPI-2 was selected because there is a vast literature on its use with substance-abusing populations (Craig & Olson, 1992; Graham & Strenger, 1988; Moss & Werner, 1992; Sutker & Archer, 1979). The MCMI-III was selected because this test has become a frequently used clinical test (Butcher & Rouse, 1996; Piotrowski & Zalewski, 1993), because a personality disorder was suspected in this particular patient, and because we have substantial empirical knowledge of how substance abusers score on this test (Craig, 1988; Craig & Olson, 1992; Craig & Weinberg, 1992a, 1992b). The ACL was selected because it is able to assess a person's basic psychological needs and because there is a research base on how substance abusers score on the ACL (Craig, 1988). The 16PF was selected to ascertain nonclinical personality traits and as a complement to the ACL.

SOME GENERAL INTERPRETIVE PRINCIPLES

Before presenting an analysis of this case, I first present some general principles in interpreting objective personality tests using an integrated approach:

1. The multitrait-multimethod approach, so highly recommended in establishing construct validity, is the method of choice in integrating psychological test interpretations from multiple data sources and test indicators. Using multiple tests for an individual assessment should not only tap general traits extant across tests, but should also refine interpretations for each individual test, perhaps by revealing traits, characteristics, and issues that are identified by one of the tests but not revealed or not addressed by the others.

2. Behaviors, traits, and symptoms seen across all tests are likely to be an essential component of the patient's present psychological functioning.

3. Behaviors, traits, and symptoms seen in only one of the tests may be present but not tapped by the other tests, or may be inaccurate to the extent that they are a false positive finding. Sometimes there are contradictory findings among tests and the clinician needs to evaluate the reason for the discrepancy.

4. At the conclusion of this process, the psychologist integrates findings that appear across all tests, integrates a finding from one test that is not detected by the others and that is considered applicable in the individual case, and does not interpret a test sign if the examiner concludes that it is not applicable or relevant to the assessment question(s).

CASE ANALYSIS

I first provide a brief interpretation of each individual test and then demonstrate how to integrate the material across tests (Craig, 1999).

MMPI-2

The patient's MMPI-2 code type (26'437+8-190: 1:6:13) is somewhat atypical among patients with alcoholism (Graham & Strenger, 1988; Hodo & Fowler, 1976) and suggests a person who is moody and depressed and tends to overreact to criticism. He can be described as bitter, angry, resentful, argumentative, and touchy—a kind of a person with a "chip on the shoulder" attitude. He is quite vulnerable to threat and has the potential for explosive behavior, though most of the time, when criticized, patients with this code type become passive. Because they harbor long-lasting resentments, they will occasionally erupt in expressions of anger, hostility, and resentment toward those who have aggrieved them (Over-controlled Hostility [OH]), and he appears to have a chronic tendency to misunderstand the motives of others (Paranoia [Pa]). The elevations in Psychopathic Deviate (Pd) and Pa along with low score on Masculinity/Femininity (Mf) (465 passive-aggressive V) also indicates that, in general, he is passive-aggressive, though irritable and tense with undue suspicions, malevolent projections, and rigidity of thought.

Primary symptoms include depression (Dep, DEP; Subjective Depression [D1]; Brooding [D5]; Lassitude-Malaise [Hy3]), hopelessness, poor memory, poor concentration (Variable Response Inconsistency [VRIN]; Lack of Ego Mastery, Cognitive [Sc4]), self-alienation (Pd5), chronic anger (ANG), and admitted family problems (Pd1, FAM). His substance abuse is apparent (Pd, MacAndrews Alcoholism Scale-Revised [MAC-R]; Addiction Admission Scale [AAS], Addiction Potential Scale [APS]). Although his Social Introversion scale is average, his elevated scores on several scales measuring depression suggests that he is emotionally withdrawing from people, if not in actual withdrawn behavior. Content analysis indicated that he endorsed no items pertaining to suicide.

The MMPI-2 suggests the presence of an Affective Disorder, Substance Abuse Disorder, and Personality Disorder (Craig, 1999; Greene, 1991). Patients with elevations on Pd find it difficult to change, though his Negative Treatment Indicators (TRT) scale is average.

MCMI-III

The patient's MMCMI-III code type is often seen among alcoholics (Craig & Weinberg, 1992a), and Millon has described this personality disorder subtype as "abrasive negativistic." The pattern is characterized by significant elevations on Passive-Aggressive (Negativistic) and Aggressive personality disorder scales and suggests a conflict between dependency and self-assertion, which dominates his life (code type). Millon views this intrapsychic conflict as whether one should seek gratification primarily from oneself or from others, which leads to this ambivalent pattern. Although they feel an intense need for acceptance, their feelings of mistrust about others lead them to expect negative outcomes in their relationships with others (Millon & Davis, 1996). This patient has a mixture of compliance at one moment and negativistic and oppositional behavior at the next. Angry, irritable, hostile, mistrusting, grumbling, and pessimistic, disillusionment permeates his personality. He vacillates between passive dependency and stubborn contrariness. This unstable pattern demoralizes others and keeps those closest to him constantly on edge, as they are uncertain how he will react. He often feels guilty and contrite after these outbursts, but he is unable to control his erratic emotionality (Borderline PD scale). He is in chronic distress

(Anxiety, Dysthymia), and it is unknown if he is using substances (Alcohol, Drug) to help him cope with these emotions, or whether these emotions are the result of his chronic substance abuse. He also has a number of antisocial features associated with his personality, but these may be explained by his substance abuse (Alcohol, Drug), as the patient's history shows little evidence of antisocial behavior and an absence of criminality (Craig, 1993, 1999).

The MCMI suggests the presence of an Anxiety Disorder, an Affective Disorder, substance abuse, and a Personality Disorder.

16PF

On the 16PF, the patient reports significant anxiety, restlessness, and irritability (Global factor: Anxiety +; factor Q4: Tense, Driven +). Because of this anxious insecurity (factor L: Suspicious +), it is probable that he does not relate well to others. He seems to lack interpersonal warmth and is more on the reserved side (factor A: Warmth −). Low scores on this factor suggest a person who tends to be more submissive, retiring, passive, and withdrawn and who has difficulty expressing anger. These patients tend to sulk, suppress their feelings, and also become obstructionistic and difficult to relate to and work with. Low scores here also suggest a person who has much difficulty gratifying underlying dependency needs.

On the other hand, he does show evidence of a need for dominance and assertiveness (factor E: Dominance +). High scores on this factor usually suggest a person who is demanding, aggressive, overreactive, and independent and who shows hostility. When restricted, these people tend to become emotional and impulsive (factor Q3: Self-Disciplined −) and project emotions onto others (factor L: Suspicious +). He tends to dwell on his suspicions and feels that people are talking about him behind his back. Accordingly, he is quick to become oppositional. To help him cope with this conflict, he seems to prefer more solitary activities and tends to be too direct with other people (factor N: Shrewd −).

The interaction of a high score on factor E (Dominant) and a low score on factor L (Suspicious) characterizes persons with a passive-aggressive personality style. They tend to express their anger in indirect ways, thereby denying they are angry. They assume that those people closest to them will feel resentful if this anger is directly expressed, and this makes them even angrier (Craig, 1999).

Although this description may seem at times contradictory, it actually highlights his essential conflict, which is asserting his independence versus gratifying his dependency needs. Test results suggest that he finds it difficult to change (factor Q1: Experimenting +; Craig, 1999).

ADJECTIVE CHECK LIST

The ACL is interpreted by describing psychological needs in terms of their need pattern, hierarchy, or degree of salience. Then behavioral projections are made based on that need pattern. This patient's need pattern consists of high needs for Aggression, Achievement, Succorance (Dependence), Autonomy, and Exhibition, and low needs for Affiliation, Nurturance, Deference, and Intraception (i.e., the ability to understand one's behavior and the behavior of others).

This need hierarchy suggests a patient who is prone to engage in behaviors that hurt others, either emotionally or physically, and one who maintains a fiercely independent and controlling demeanor (Aggression [Agg], Autonomy [Aut]), yet a person who also leans on others for support and care (Succorance [Suc]). He is quite critical of others, and his aggressiveness, displayed when he feels slighted, would make him difficult to live with. Deficient in affiliating and nurturing behaviors (Affiliation [Aff], Nurturance [Nur]), he lacks self-control (SCn), shows a discrepancy between the way he is and the way he would like to be (ISS), and is maladjusted (Personal Adjustment [PAdj]). His high score on counseling readiness (CR) may suggest a desire and willingness to pursue counseling or, more likely, is yet another manifestation of a willingness to place himself in a dependent relationship with his therapist. Despite this—which is probably a transference reaction to authority—change is questionable (Cha; Intraception [Int]).

TEST INTEGRATION

I ask students to make a chart of salient traits, behaviors, and symptoms, particularly those that are relevant to the referral question and those that pertain to treatment recommendations. The chart should contain a column that stipulates the areas to be assessed and/or test findings on a particular measure and one that cites those test scales for each issue that pertains to the assessment question and test finding, along with the raw data. A structural summary is available for the MMPI-2 interpretation (Greene & Nichols, 2003), but similar approaches for within-test interpretation have not been published for the other tests used in this assessment. Accordingly, Table 8.1 presents a sample chart for this case that will help to integrate the information.

One should look first as those symptoms, behaviors, and traits that are consistently expressed across all or most of the tests. Reference to Table 8.1 indicates that the patient is in a significant amount of psychological distress, characterized by anxiety and depression. His affective disturbance

Table 8.1

Test Signs across Tests for 40-Year-Old White Male

Trait	MMPI-2	MCMI-III	ACL	16PF
Anxiety	Pt (66), A (65) ANX (65)	Anx (78)	NA	Q4 (10)
Depression	Dep (74) DEP (77)	Dys (88) MDep (60)	NA	
Anger/Aggression	ANG (78)	Agg (112)	nAgg (9)	
Suspiciousness	Pa (72)			L (8)
Dominance	Do (58)		nDom (7)	E (9)
Narcissism	Pd (67)	Narc (71)		
Hostility	OH (35) TPA (56)			L (8)
Substance Abuse	MAC-R (29) AAS (80) APS (73)	B (93) T (87)	NA	NA
Health Concerns	Hs (59) HEA (48)	Soma (50)	NA	NA
Dependency	Dep (74)	Depend (21) Agg/ASPD*	nDom (9) nAut (8) nSuc (8) nDef (3)	
Thought Disorder	Sch (62) OBS (59) BIZ (63)	Thgt (87)	NA	NA
Emotional Stability Impulsivity			Padj (2)	C (6)
Acting Out	Pd (67) ASP (51)	ASPD (83) AGG (112) COMP (34)		
Family Problems	FAM (74) Pd1 (65)			
Nurturance			nNur (3) NAff (2)	
Treatment Indicators	TRT (56) Code type	Code type	nCha (5) CR (8)	

* Millon's classification of these two styles is called "active-independent."

appears to be of moderate intensity and most likely is Dysthymia, based on several lines of evidence. First, Major Depression can be diagnosed with or without psychotic manifestations. The patient shows little evidence of psychotic symptoms on this test (MMPI code type; Schizophrenia [Sc] 62, Obsessive Thinking [OBS] 59, Bizarre Mentation [BIZ] 63). Although the

MCMI at 87 suggests the presence of a Thought Disorder, this scale has been shown to be problematic in diagnosing psychosis (Craig, 1997). Second, this diagnosis requires the presence of vegetative signs, and the patient is not reporting any of these symptoms (MMPI-2: Dep < 75, DEP 77, Hypochondriasis [Hs] 59, Health Concerns [Hea] 48; MCMI Dys 88, Maj. Dep 60, Somataform [Soma] 50). His anxiety also appears to be mild to moderate in intensity (three of four test signs).

The next area of consistency is the presence of a substance abuse problem, which is clearly indicated on both the MMPI-2 and MCMI-III, and of severe intensity. While the test evidence also indicates the likelihood of acting-out tendencies (MMPI Pd 67; MCMI ASPD 83, AGG 112, Compulsive [Comp] 34 [the latter suggesting a lack of controlled behavior]), such tendencies will tend to be in the area of substance abuse and emotional expressions of underlying anger and hostility, as opposed to criminal behavior. The following evidence leads to that conclusion: While the MMPI Antisocial Practices scale is average, the ASP Content Component scale Antisocial Attitudes was elevated and the Antisocial Behaviors scale was in the average range (not shown in the table). Next, Millon's Antisocial Personality Disorder scale can be elevated with or without antisocial or criminal behavior. The clinical interview indicated an absence of arrests and criminal behavior by patient self-report. Hence, the preponderance of evidence suggests acting-out expressed in terms of substance abuse.

The next area of acting-out is at the emotional level, especially anger, which is of moderate to above moderate emotional intensity (MMPI Anger [ANG] 78, OH 35; MCMI code type, Agg 112; ACL nAgg 9), accompanied by unfettered hostility (OH 35). His interpersonal relationships are likely to be quite strained (MMPI FAM 74, Pd1 65; 16PF: factor A Warmth–, factor L Suspiciousness +).

All tests, in one way or another, find this patient manifesting passive-aggressive personality traits characterized by negative, resentful, irritable, and oppositional behavior at one moment, and contrite, passive, and compliant behavior at the next moment. All except the ACL found this patient to feel easily slighted, with undue suspiciousness and externalization of blame (i.e., projections), who overreacts to perceived slights, and who maintains his resentments and then is prone to erupt in quick episodes of anger. It can be theorized that his alcoholism, in part, serves to quell and control these resentments. When not drinking, his main coping device seems to be emotional withdrawal.

What might this patient be so angry about? An apparent inconsistency brings us to the nub of the issue: This patient is psychically struggling with problems in satisfying his underlying dependency needs (MMPI Dep 74; ACL nSuc 8, Counseling Readings [CR] 8, nDef 3) combined with a moderate to high need for autonomy and independence (MCMI code type reflecting an independent personality classification, Depend 21; ACL nDom 9). It is an underlying struggle between dependence and independence at the psychological level. He has strong needs for surgency and assertiveness yet feels an equally strong need for control and fears independence.

The test results also provide us with an opportunity to make treatment predictions. Most of the evidence is problematic for positive behavioral change. Elevated scores on MMPI Pd (and MCMI Pass/Agg, Agg, Aspd) generally reflect poor response to treatment and an increased likelihood of treatment noncompliance and subsequent dropout, unless treatment is coerced. Treatment goals include the need to (1) reduce manifestations of anxiety and depression, (2) help the patient to move toward independence without using alcohol, (3) motivate the patient to pursue alcohol detoxification and rehabilitation, and (4) help him understand the reasons for his behavior under stress so that he can more consciously develop alternative ways of behaving. It is understood that progress toward these goals is likely to be slow, especially if the therapist moves too fast regarding the need to stop drinking.

With these salient facts, the clinician can now write a more comprehensive report, integrating these essential features into a refined interpretation.

DISCUSSION

This case demonstrates the value of using multiple objective (self-report) personality tests to produce a more accurate and more refined interpretation and one that leads to clearly stated treatment goals. The process of integrating objective tests into a test battery is essentially identical to the process of integrating projective tests or using a combination of objective and projective tests and presenting integrated findings.

In the case example, a clinical history was taken together with a factual statement surrounding the events. Tests were selected based on the nature of the referral question and the adequacy of a literature base for the assessment issues at hand. Objective personality tests using self-report methodology were selected, administered, and interpreted, and the results were integrated using the multitrait-multimethod assessment methodology by interpreting the results from the clinical interview, test findings, and known facts from history. The patient's main conflicts and treatment goals were then established that would lead to an individualized treatment plan.

In clinical situations, it is most likely that cognitive, objective, and projective tests constitute the more typical test battery. My purpose here was to demonstrate how objective personality tests can be integrated as a test battery that can lead to more valid and refined assessments. On the other hand, with continued pressure from HMOs and managed care, psychologists may find the need to use more efficient and time-saving methods to address referral and treatment questions. Objective self-reports and personality tests seem to conform to these requirements.

Clinicians need to determine what kinds of and which specific tests should be selected to answer a given assessment question. Teachers of personality assessment should acquaint students with the integration process and include objective personality tests in such learning modules. Having examples, such as that contained here, should facilitate this learning process. Researchers need to study the incremental validity resulting from adding additional tests to a test battery. Policy makers need to convince third-party payers of the value, clinical utility, and necessity of such assessment practices.

APPENDIX

Test Scores of Sample Case

MMPI-2

Validity Scales			Clinical Scales		
L	T	39	Hypochondriasis	T	59
F	T	55	Depression	T	74
K	T	45	Hysteria	T	66
F(b)	T	XX	Psychopathic Deviate	T	67
F(p)	T	XX	Masculinity/Femininity	T	46
TRIN	T	XX	Paranoia	T	72
VRIN	T	XX	Psychasthenia	T	66
Mean Profile Elevation			Schizophrenia	T	62
Goldberg Index			Hypomania	T	56
			Social Introversion	T	51

Content Scales			Supplemental Scales		
Anxiety	T	65	Factor A	T	65
Fears	T	45	Factor R	T	47
Obsessive Thinking	T	59	Ego Strength	T	40
Depression	T	77	Dominance	T	58
Health Concerns	T	48	Responsibility	T	50
Bizarre Mentation	T	63	Overcontrolled Hostility	T	35
Anger	T	78	PTSD–Keane	T	73
Cynicism	T	48	MacAndrew's Alcohol-R	R	29
Antisocial Practices	T	51	Addiction Admissions	T	80
Type A Personality	T	56	Addiction Potential	T	73
Low Self-Esteem	T	53			
Social Discomfort	T	50			
Family Problems	T	74			
Work Interference	T	67			
Negative Treatment Indicators	T	56			

MCMI-III

X (Disclosure)	BR 77	Schizotypal	BR 64
Y (Desirability)	BR 25	Borderline	BR 93
Z (Debasement)	BR 80	Paranoid	BR 65
Schizoid	BR 74	Anxiety	BR 78
Avoidant	BR 78	Somatoform	BR 55
Depressive	BR 60	Bipolar: Manic	BR 58
Dependent	BR 21	Dysthymia	BR 88
Histrionic	BR 61	Alcohol	BR 93
Narcissistic	BR 71	Drug	BR 87
Antisocial	BR 83	PTSD	BR 60
Aggressive	BR 112	Thought Disorder	BR 87
Compulsive	BR 34	Major Depression	BR 66
Passive-Aggressive	BR 111	Delusional Disorder	BR 50
Self-Defeating	BR 73		

Adjective Checklist (ACL)

Needs	Sten Score	Needs	Sten Score
Achievement	8.2	Exhibition	7.5
Dominance	6.7	Autonomy	7.7
Endurance	4.6	Aggression	8.9
Order	4.1	Change	5.2
Intraception	3.2	Succorance	7.6
Nurturance	2.6	Abasement	4.2
Affiliation	1.6	Deference	2.9
Heterosexuality	6.7		

Topical Scales

	Sten Score		Sten Score
Personal Adjustment	2.4	Counseling	8.4
Self-Control	2.9	Readiness	
Ideal Self	2.3		

16PF Scores

Factors	Sten Score	Global Factor	Sten Score
(A) Warmth	2	Anxiety	8
(B) Abstract	5	Extroversion	5
(C) Emotionally Stable*	6	Independence	7
(E) Dominant	9	Tough-Minded	7
(F) Enthusiastic	6	Self-Control	5
(G) Conscientious	5		
(H) Venturesome	6		

(continued)

197

16PF Scores *Continued*

Factors	Sten Score	Global Factor	Sten Score
(I) Sensitive	5		
(L) Suspicious*	8		
(M) Imaginative	6		
(N) Shrewd	3		
(O) Self-Doubting	6		
(Q1) Experimenting	1		
(Q2) Self-Sufficient	6		
(Q3) Self-Disciplined	4		
(Q4) Tense, Driven	10		

*There are no factors D, J, or K in 16PF 4th edition.

REFERENCES

Acklin, M. W. (1993). Integrating the Rorschach and the MMPI in clinical assessment: Conceptual and methodological issues. *Journal of Personality Assessment, 60,* 125–131.

Antoni, M. (1993). Combined use of the MCMI and MMPI. In R. J. Craig (Ed.), *The Millon Clinical Multiaxial Inventory: A clinical research information synthesis* (pp. 279–302). Hillsdale, NJ: Erlbaum.

Antoni, M., Levine, J., Tischer, P., Green, S., & Millon, T. (1986). Refining personality instruments by combining MCMI high-point profiles and MMPI codes. Part IV. MMPI code 89/98. *Journal of Personality Assessment, 50,* 65–72.

Antoni, M., Levine, J., Tischer, P., Green, S., & Millon, T. (1987). Refining personality instruments by combining MCMI high-point profiles and MMPI codes. Part V. MMPI code 78/87. *Journal of Personality Assessment, 51,* 375–387.

Antoni, M., Tischer, P., Levine, J., Green, S., & Millon, T. (1985a). Refining personality instruments by combining MCMI high-point profiles and MMPI codes. Part I. MMPI code 28/82. *Journal of Personality Assessment, 49,* 392–398.

Antoni, M., Tischer, P., Levine, J., Green, S., & Millon, T. (1985b). Refining personality instruments by combining MCMI high-point profiles and MMPI codes. Part III. MMPI code 24/42. *Journal of Personality Assessment, 49,* 508–515.

Archer, R. P., & Krishnamurthy, R. (1993). Combining the Rorschach and the MMPI in the assessment of adolescents. *Journal of Personality Assessment, 60,* 137–140.

Butcher, J. N., Dahlstrom, W. G., Graham, J. R., Tellegen, A., & Kaemmer, B. (1989). *Minnesota Multiphasic Personality Inventory-2: Manual for administration and scoring.* Minneapolis, MN: National Computer Systems.

Butcher, J. N., & Rouse, S., V. (1996). Personality: Individual differences and clinical assessment. *Annual Review of Psychology, 47,* 87–111.

Craig, R. J. (1988). Psychological functioning of cocaine free-basers derived from objective psychological tests. *Journal of Clinical Psychology, 44,* 599–606.

Craig, R. J. (1993). *Psychological assessment with the Millon Clinical Multiaxial Inventory (II): An interpretive guide.* Odessa, FL: Psychological Assessment Resources.

Craig, R. J. (1997). A selected review of the MCMI empirical literature. In T. Millon (Ed.), *The Millon inventories: Clinical and personality assessment* (pp. 303–326). New York: Guilford Press.

Craig, R. J. (1999). Interpreting personality tests: A clinical manual for the MMPI-2, MCMI-III, CPI-R, and 16PF. New York: Wiley.

Craig, R. J., & Olson, R. (1992). MMPI subtypes for cocaine abusers. *American Journal of Drug and Alcohol Abuse, 18,* 197–205.

Craig, R. J., & Weinberg, D. (1992a). Assessing alcoholics with the Millon Clinical Multiaxial Inventory: A review. *Psychology of Addictive Behaviors, 6,* 200–208.

Craig, R. J., & Weinberg, D. (1992b). Assessing drug abusers with the Millon Clinical Multiaxial Inventory: A review. *Journal of Substance Abuse Treatment, 9,* 249–255.

Finn, E. (2003). Therapeutic assessment of a man with "ADD." *Journal of Personality Assessment, 80,* 115–129.

Ganellen, R. (1996). *Integrating the Rorschach with the MMPI.* Hillsdale, NJ: Erlbaum.

Gough, H. G., & Heilbrun, A. B. (1983). *The Adjective Checklist manual.* Palo Alto, CA: Consulting Psychologists Press.

Graham, J. R., & Strenger, V. E. (1988). MMPI characteristics of alcoholics: A review. *Journal of Consulting and Clinical Psychology, 56,* 197–205.

Greene, R. L. (1991). *The MMPI-2/MMPI: An interpretive manual.* Boston: Allyn & Bacon.

Greene, R. L., & Nichols, D. (2003). *MMPI-2 structural summary.* Odessa, FL: Psychological Assessment Resources.

Handler, L., & Hilsenroth, M. (Eds.). (1998). *Teaching and learning personality assessment.* Hillsdale, NJ: Erlbaum.

Hodo, G. L., & Fowler, R. D. (1976). Frequency of MMPI two-point codes in a large alcoholic sample. *Journal of Clinical Psychology, 32,* 487–489.

Hyer, L., Woods, M. G., Boudewyns, P. A., Harrison, W. R., & Tamkin, A. S. (1990). MCMI and 16PF with Vietnam veterans: Profiles and concurrent validation of MCMI. *Journal of Personality Disorders, 4,* 391–401.

Institute for Personality and Ability Testing. (1991). *Administrator's manual for the Sixteen Personality Factor Questionnaire.* Champaign, IL: Author.

Levine, J. B., Tischer, P., Antoni, M., Greene, C., & Millon, T. (1985). Refining personality assessments by combining MCMI high point profiles and MMPI codes. Part II. MMPI code 27/72. *Journal of Personality Assessment, 49,* 501–507.

Lovitt, R. (1993). A strategy for integrating a normal MMPI and dysfunctional Rorschach in a severely compromised patient. *Journal of Personality Assessment, 60,* 141–147.

Millon, T. (1983). *Millon Clinical Multiaxial Inventory manual* (3rd ed.). New York: Holt, Rinehart and Winston.

Millon, T. (1987). *Millon Clinical Multiaxial Inventory-Manual for the MCMI-II* Minneapolis, MN: National Computer Systems.

Millon, T. (1994). *Millon Clinical Multiaxial Inventory-III: Manual.* Minneapolis, MN: National Computer Systems.

Millon, T., & Davis, R. (1996). *Disorders of personality* (2nd ed.). New York: Guilford Press.

Moss, P. D., & Werner, P. D. (1992). An MMPI typology of cocaine abusers. *Journal of Personality Assessment, 58,* 269–276.

Piotrowski, C., & Zalewski, C. (1993). Training in psychodiagnostic testing in APA-approved PhD and PhD clinical psychology programs. *Journal of Personality Assessment, 61,* 394–405.

Rapaport, D., Gill, M., & Shafer, R. (1968). *Diagnostic psychological testing (rev. ed.)* (R. Holt, Ed.). New York: International University Press.

Sutker, P. B., & Archer, R. P. (1979). MMPI characteristics of opiate addicts, alcoholics, and other drug abusers. In C. Newmark (Ed.), *MMPI: A Clinical and research trends* (pp. 105–148). New York: Praeger.

Weiner, I. B. (1993). Clinical considerations in the conjoint use of the Rorschach and the MMPI. *Journal of Personality Assessment, 60,* 148–152.

CHAPTER 9

Forensic Application of the MCMI-III™ in Light of Current Controversies

FRANK J. DYER

THE MILLON inventories, including the Millon Clinical Multiaxial Inventory II (MCMI-II), Millon Clinical Multiaxial Inventory III (MACI-III), and Millon Adolescent Clinical Inventory (MACI), are mainstream psychological tests that have gained wide acceptance in the psychological community, as reflected in the numerous research and interpretive publications relating to them. One of the most popular applications of the Millon inventories is in the forensic arena, where their self-report format and extensive validity data have led to their adoption in a variety of case types. McCann and Dyer's (1996) remains the only booklength treatment of forensic assessment with the Millon inventories, but many subsequent journal articles and book chapters provide additional information supporting various applications of the inventories in legal matters (Craig, 1997; Craig & Bivens, 1998; Craig & Olson, 1997; Dyce, O'Connor, Parkins, & Janzen, 1997; Dyer, 1997; Flynn & McMahon, 1997; Gondolf, 1999; Kelln, Dozois, & McKenzie, 1998). Guidelines on the use of the MCMI in court-related matters have also been published (Craig, 1999; McCann, 2002). In the past few years, the Millon inventories have been the target of a good deal of critical commentary in journals, books on forensic psychology, and Internet discussions. This chapter relates technical features of the MCMI to current controversies, separating valid from misguided criticism of the forensic utility of the tests.

CRITICISMS AND MISCONCEPTIONS
CONCERNING THE MCMI-II AND MCMI-III

In spite of the fact that the Millon inventories are among the most popular self-report clinical personality measures among forensic psychologists, the tests, especially the MCMI-II and MCMI-III, have incurred heated criticism. There are some blatant misconceptions that have circulated about the practical utility of the inventories, helped along in some cases by statements in publications by senior researchers and practitioners. Two characteristics of the Millon series of tests seem to be responsible for the confusion. These are (1) the standardization of the test on a sample of clients who are either presenting for clinical assessment or treatment and (2) the adoption of base rate (BR) scores rather than T-scores.

Butcher and Miller (1999) and Hess (1998) fault the MCMI-III because it was standardized on a clinical population that did not include so-called normals in the sample. Butcher and Miller state:

> A psychological test like the Millon Clinical Multiaxial Inventory (MCMI) cannot be appropriately used in forensic assessment because it does not provide norms that allow for the discrimination between patients and normals. . . . All persons who are administered the test are assumed to have psychological problems as assessed by the test. The results are therefore considered to be biased toward "finding" problems in the client. (p. 106)

This misconception is echoed in an Internet-published continuing education article on child custody assessments by Brodie (2003): "The MCMI instruments are not based on the presumption of normalcy, but on the assumption that the test respondent belongs to a clinical population. The test will significantly overstate the psychopathology of individuals whose characteristics do not match the standardization sample" (p. 4).

Attorneys, especially those representing litigants in matrimonial cases, have picked up on this criticism of the test. In attempting to impeach witnesses who have evaluated parties to a child custody action using the MCMI-III as part of the battery, they argue that use of the test is inappropriate for their clients because their clients are entirely normal. They assert that the effect of using a test standardized on a clinical population is to make clients appear much more pathological than they actually are. This line of reasoning, which one hears echoed by some psychologists as well, not only rests on an entirely false psychometric proposition, but is inherently flawed from a logical perspective.

In considering the argument that comparison with a clinically disordered standardization population will make normal persons look more pathological than they actually are, anyone with even a smattering of knowledge about the standardization of psychological tests will immediately wonder how this can possibly be so. An example from the field of intellectual assessment will serve to illustrate this point. Imagine that a person of average intelligence is compared with two groups of standardization subjects, one that is a stratified sample of the population including all segments of the IQ spectrum, and the other a selected population restricted to individuals who are highly intelligent. As would be expected, the individual of average intelligence will be found to be nothing more nor less than average when compared with the stratified sample of the general population.

By the logic of the argument concerning the MCMI-III standardization sample, we should expect this person to look far more intelligent than he or she actually is when compared with a standardization group that consists solely of highly intelligent people. In fact, the opposite necessarily holds true. When compared with a standardization sample in which the average IQ is 125, the individual with an IQ of 100 will fall at the extreme lower region of the score distribution and thus earn a significantly lower than average IQ on norms developed on the highly intelligent sample. In that type of standardization sample, an IQ score of 100 is awarded to individuals who have the average IQ of the sample, or 125. Considering the attenuation of the sample standard deviation due to restriction of range, an individual with an IQ of 100 would score more than 2 standard deviations below the sample mean, which would earn that person a score in the retarded range, despite his or her normal intelligence.

This scenario extends to deviation scores for psychopathology developed on a clinical sample, where the frequencies of all psychological disorders are much greater than would be the case in a general population sample (where some estimates place the frequency of having some form of diagnosable mental disorder at 20% anyway). Psychologically normal, that is, genuinely problem-free subjects would be so radically different from a clinical sample that the normal individual would not even begin to approach the mean for that standardization group. If anything, the psychologically normal individual would look much healthier psychologically when compared with an exclusively clinical sample than when compared with a sample composed of other so-called normals.

The MCMI does not purport to make distinctions among examinees on factorially derived traits such as sociability and industriousness. The MCMI-III manual states, "The primary intent of the MCMI is to provide information to clinicians—psychologists, psychiatrists, counselors, social workers, physicians, and nurses—who must make assessments and treatment decisions about individuals with emotional and interpersonal difficulties" (Millon, Davis, & Millon, 1997, p. 5). The manual also makes it clear that use of the MCMI narrative printout should be restricted to individuals who have already been diagnosed as having psychological problems, but that the Profile Report of scale scores is useful as a screening device.

In regard to Butcher and Miller's (1999) assertion that the MCMI "cannot be appropriately used in forensic assessment because it does not provide norms that allow for the discrimination between patients and normals," and that the test is "biased toward 'finding' problems in the client," certain concepts require clarification. In the first place, the MCMI does not contain any sort of general psychopathology scale that differentiates in a global manner between "normals" and "patients." The test assesses the presence or absence of individual disorders, employing individual personality disorder and clinical syndrome scales for this purpose. Thus, even if the MCMI did include a general sample in the standardization in addition to the clinical sample, there would be no way of interpreting an MCMI record in such a way as to discriminate the clinical from the general population groups.

The appropriate way to assess the MCMI as a screening instrument is scale by scale. The question that the test was designed to address is not whether the subject is normal or abnormal in some general sense, but whether or not the subject has one or more of the specific clinical syndromes and personality disorders assessed by the instrument. It should be borne in mind that there are very large segments of the clinical standardization sample that are normal with respect to individual disorders. Schizoid patients will be entirely normal, in the sense of registering well below the clinical threshold, on scales such as Histrionic. Standardization subjects with Antisocial Personality Disorder are highly likely to be normal with respect to anxiety, Compulsive Personality Disorder, and Dependent Personality Disorder. As the great majority of subjects in the clinical sample register elevations on only a few scales, they are normal with respect to most disorders assessed by the MCMI. In this sense, the standardization sample is replete with normals whom the test differentiates very well from clinical cases scale by scale, according to the most recent validity study presenting impressive operating characteristics.

Another concept that needs to be elucidated is that of test bias. This is a term that has a specific meaning in the psychometric literature, which we can relate to the Butcher and Miller (1999) assertion that the test is "biased toward 'finding' problems in the client." Test bias is conceptualized as either a difference in the slope of the prediction equation between subgroups of examinees or a difference in intercepts of a procedure that may be equally valid for both groups but systematically overpredicts or underpredicts for the subgroup (Anastasi & Urbina, 1997). Considering this technical definition, what Butcher and Miller argue is that the MCMI systematically overpredicts psychopathology for normals, in other words, that there are intercept differences. As noted earlier, when considered scale by scale, where large segments of the standardization sample are normal with respect to most measured disorders, the classification efficiency statistics generated in Millon's (Millon, Davis, & Millon, 1997) second validity study of the MCMI-III do not indicate the presence of such bias. Specificities are quite high for all scales, although these statistics were not included in the test manual (Millon, 1996, personal communication). In other words, for each disorder assessed by the test, an extremely high percentage of subjects who were *not* diagnosed by their treating or examining clinician as having the target disorder (in other words, normals with respect to that particular disorder) *were correctly identified by the test as not having it.* By definition, a bias toward overprediction of pathology for normals would result in weak specificity statistics for all scales. The MCMI-II operating characteristics, which do include specificity figures in the manual, also indicate quite strongly that the test does not have a tendency to incorrectly label normals as having a particular disorder. A study by McCann et al. (2001) discussed later also supports the notion that the MCMI-III does not overpredict pathology in normals.

UNIQUENESS OF BASE RATE SCORES AS OPPOSED TO T-SCORES

Separate and apart from the flawed psychometric logic of the overpathologizing criticism just discussed, the argument that the clinical standardization group of the MCMI-III would make a normal subject look excessively pathological assumes that the individual's test score is being compared to the mean of the test scores of the standardization sample. This, of course, would be the case with a T-score procedure, such as that employed in the development of the MMPI-2. As has been repeatedly pointed out in literally scores of workshops and publications that provide an orientation to the MCMI-III, the BR scores in which the test results are presented rest on a completely different psychometric foundation from T-scores. Even though they may have been cast in a metric that has a superficial similarity to T-scores, which may lend substantially to the confusion in this area, BR scores do *not* represent a comparison of the subject's test score with the average test score of the standardization sample.

If anything, BR scores may be considered as representing a form of criterion referencing rather than being deviation scores. This is because BR scores are directly keyed to the frequencies of psychopathology in the standardization sample of the MCMI. In terms of personality disorders, a

BR score of 75 represents that *raw score* point at which treating or evaluating clinicians begin to diagnose clients with traits or features of the target disorder. A BR score of 85 correspondingly represents the *raw score* point at which clinicians begin to diagnose subjects as having the full-blown personality disorder. In theory, then, the test score mean of the standardization sample *is completely irrelevant to the calculation of BR scores*. What matters is at what point in the *raw score* distribution subjects begin to manifest traits or features of the disorder and at what point they begin to manifest the full-blown disorder. Thus, the standardization sample can include relatively few people who have traits and features of the target disorder and relatively few people with the full-blown disorder, or it could be composed almost exclusively of people who have either traits or features of the disorder or the full-blown disorder. *In either case, the treating or examining clinicians would begin to diagnose these people at the same raw score points,* assuming that the particular scale in question has substantial validity. *It is the raw score point at which this occurs, and not the test score mean of the sample, that determines the calibration of BR scores.* This is a concept that has proved extremely difficult for even seasoned clinical and forensic psychologists to grasp, so thoroughly have individuals trained in the 1960s, 1970s, and 1980s been inculcated with a T-score mind-set.

As a further illustration of this concept, consider what a base rate score does: It adjusts for the base rate. Thus, if the base rate of a particular disorder in the standardization sample is 70%, then 70% of the sample will have a BR score of 85 or above on the target disorder. If, on the other hand, the standardization sample is composed of subjects where the base rate for the same disorder is only 20%, then only 20% of records will have a BR score of 85 or above for the target disorder. The BR score ties the point on the raw score distribution to the point at which the diagnosis begins to appear in the sample. BR scores have nothing whatsoever to do with the distance of the subject's individual score from the mean of the group in standard deviation units. The bottom line is that the argument that the clinical standardization sample of the MCMI-III causes the test to overpathologize subjects is entirely spurious *when one considers the BR scores only.* As noted later, there is something of a problem in this area with the computerized narrative report of the test, which has to do with considerations entirely separate and apart from standardization sample characteristics or score format.

Partially in response to the flood of objections from matrimonial attorneys in regard to the purported overpathologizing of the MCMI-III, McCann et al. (2001) undertook a study of 259 child custody examinees obtained from private practice settings in four different states to provide normative data on the MCMI-III. These authors found that the mean base

rate scores were very low for most of the scales. The modal MCMI-III profile in the sample contained an elevation on the Desirability scale and subclinical elevations on the Histrionic, Narcissistic, and Compulsive scales.
There is an additional finding that, with the exception of Histrionic and
Compulsive for females, the frequency of clinically significant elevations
on MCMI-III scales was very low among child custody litigants. The authors concluded that their study provides empirical support for the position that the MCMI-III does not overpathologize child custody examinees.

PROBLEMS WITH THE FORENSIC USE OF THE MCMI-III COMPUTERIZED NARRATIVE REPORT

In spite of the fact that a strong warning against the use of the MCMI-II
computerized narrative report for forensic purposes is to be found in
McCann and Dyer (1996), it is not unusual to find the computerized report appearing in forensic reports, even to the point of being seamlessly
integrated verbatim into the rest of the report without attribution. In
other cases, the computerized narrative report is incorporated into a
forensic evaluation with the disclaimer at the beginning of the printout
preceding the interpretive text. This can lead to considerable confusion in
the minds of attorneys and judges who are called on to make sense of
MCMI-III data, especially appellate court judges, who have nothing to
work from except the expert's report and the transcript of the expert's
trial testimony. An egregious example of such confusion occurs in a New
Jersey Appellate Court's decision *In the Matter of the Guardianship of
D.M.H., C.L.H.W., L.F.H., and R.Q.H., Minors* (1998). In this termination of
parental rights action, the state's psychologist expert used the MCMI-II
and incorporated elements of the computerized narrative report into the
psychological report. The computerized narrative material also includes
the disclaimer, which the appellate court opinion discusses in some detail. The opinion notes that the psychologist expert for the state relied on
MCMI-II to arrive at a negative evaluation of the defendant's psyche. The
court notes:

> The May 24, 1996 report describes it [MCMI-II] as "an instrument designed
> to assess pathological characteristics and dynamics which interfere with
> optimal personal and interpersonal functioning." But the description of the
> test acknowledges that "this inventory does not focus on positive attributes
> and strengths which the individual possesses" and that one "must keep in
> mind the emphasis on pathology, purposefully constructed by the authors
> of the test so as to optimize clinical utility." (p. 12)

In commenting on what they see as a disjuncture between the state's
expert's predictions concerning the defendant's adjustment and the

defendant's actual level of functioning, the appellate court observes that if these predictions were drawn from the test results,

> we wonder how a balanced psychological assessment of such a fundamental issue as a person's parental fitness could be the product of a test that seems to be skewed toward the negative elements of one's psyche and which intentionally omits consideration of the positive attributes and strengths a person may have. (pp. 12–13)

It is apparent from the decision that these appellate court judges held the view that the MCMI-II is an extremely biased instrument that ignores whatever positive attributes an individual may possess and focuses solely on highlighting, or perhaps exaggerating, their pathology. The judges' objections to a psychological test that they see as lacking balance because it intentionally omits consideration of the positive attributes and strengths a person may have seem to reflect the best interests standard that guides psychological evaluations in matrimonial cases. In that particular case type, evaluators often encounter a situation in which both of the contesting parties possess parental fitness and the question is which of them is the better choice as a custodial parent for the child relative to the other spouse, rather than the question of absolute parental fitness per se. In evaluations connected with termination of parental rights actions, however, the model for parental fitness is an absolute rather than a relative one. The paramount question for the evaluator is not a relative assessment of the strengths of the examinees, but the application of a multiple hurdle model to assess whether there is any aspect of the individual's lifestyle, drug status, alcohol status, mental health, personality organization, criminality, or other serious problem that would disqualify that individual from being considered a fit parent. Thus, the wording of the MCMI-II disclaimer included in the state's expert's report opened the door to judicial allegations of bias.

On a more fundamental level, the wording in the narrative urging consumers to "keep in mind the emphasis on pathology, purposefully constructed by the authors of the test source to optimize clinical utility" would frankly suggest bias to just about any judicial authority, regardless of whether matrimonial or termination of parental rights was the frame of reference. The present author's understanding of this disclaimer is that it is guided by both diagnostic and economic considerations. What this disclaimer is actually saying is that, in contrast to the standard interpretation of BR scores given in the MCMI-II or MCMI-III manual, the computerized narrative report lowers the interpretive threshold somewhat in order to augment sensitivity. This lowering of the threshold BR scores to trigger interpretive statements necessarily results in reduced specificity.

If the consumer of the interpretive computerized narrative report bears this in mind, then the statements in the report can be appreciated in the proper perspective as scattershot diagnostic hypotheses resulting from increased sensitivity parameters.

The question of why the interpretive report would deliberately augment the sensitivity for the program's triggering clinical interpretations in response to various BR score configurations is readily understandable in practical economic terms. The cost of a computerized narrative report is roughly three times that of the bare-bones profile report containing only the BR scores without interpretive text. Given that one encounters large numbers of defensive records in practice, especially in forensic practice, keying the interpretive statements according to standard sensitivity parameters would result in a great many computerized narrative reports containing extremely little information about clients in the narrative section. Thus, by augmenting the sensitivity, the authors made certain to increase the amount of text generated by any particular record, which in turn would seem to justify, at least superficially, the much greater expense of the computerized narrative reports relative to the score report alone. Although the claim that the MCMI overpathologizes is a pure myth, *in the case of the computerized narrative reports, it happens to be true.* This is because of the interpretive program's hair trigger for pathology-oriented text, which is at variance with the standard interpretation of the BR score levels as advocated in the test manual.

MCMI-III AND FEDERAL STANDARDS FOR ADMISSIBILITY OF SCIENTIFIC EVIDENCE

The admissibility of scientific evidence in federal courts and in many states has been guided for the past decade by a U.S. Supreme Court decision, *Daubert v. Merrell-Dow Pharmaceuticals* (1993). This decision makes the trial judge the gatekeeper for admissibility based on the scientific procedure's publication in refereed journals, known error rate, falsifiability of results, and general acceptance in the relevant scientific community. In terms of psychometric procedures, this translates into whether there have been sufficient published studies of the instrument in mainstream journals, whether there have been any studies of the instrument's error rate (operating characteristics), whether the research on validity is designed in such a way that the claims of the test developers can be proved false, and whether the test is generally accepted by other psychologists.

In spite of the fact that the Supreme Court's decision in *Daubert v. Merrell-Dow Pharmaceuticals* (1993) was intended to improve the quality of expert testimony by stressing the use of scientifically reliable methods, there is one good example with respect to the MCMI-II and MCMI-III, as well as other procedures, of a judicial ruling that very likely compromised rather than enhanced the validity of the experts' assessments. In an employment discrimination case, *Usher v. Lakewood Engineering & Manufacturing Company* (1994), the plaintiff moved for the issuance of a protective order against the defendant's performing a battery of psychological tests as part of the input for its designated expert to assist in preparing a psychiatrist for trial testimony. Initially, the defendant proposed an all-day testing procedure that would include the administration of the MMPI-2, Rorschach, Thematic Apperception Test, Shipley Institute for Living Scale, Sixteen Personality Factor Inventory, and either the MCMI-II or MCMI-III. The plaintiff objected to the battery partially on factors such as the inapplicability of the Millon for purposes at issue at trial and the "appreciable rate of error of that test." Lakewood retreated by abandoning the Millon test, but proposed to administer the five other tests. The court, in addition to accepting the defendant's abandonment of the MCMI, also ruled that the other five tests were inadequate for the type of evaluation that the defendant proposed. In commenting on its order to grant the defendant's protective order, the court stated, "It is worth observing that this result also has the effect of providing a level playing field for the parties. Usher's psychologist expert will be testifying based upon his clinical evaluation conducted without the disputed testing, and Lakewood's psychiatrist expert will have the identical opportunity." In other words, the court appeared to be saying that on the basis of *Daubert* and the Federal Rules of Evidence, it is preferable to have both of the opposing experts testifying on the basis of interview data that are completely lacking in documented reliability and validity, as opposed to granting either side the opportunity to use a battery of tests that have ample empirical psychometric support. It appears that when the gatekeeper trier of fact is naive to psychometric concepts and research, *Daubert* can be perverted to bar the door to good science rather than junk science.

The impact of the Rogers, Salekin, and Sewell (1999) critique of the MCMI on actual legal proceedings is evident in the arguments advanced in a *Daubert* hearing in *Jeffrey v. Dillard Department Stores and Dillard's Bel Air Mall*, an Alabama employment-related case heard in 2000. This was a hearing on the plaintiff's motion to exclude the defendant's proffered expert witness, a licensed psychologist, from offering opinion testimony as to the psychologist's evaluation of the plaintiff. Among other objections to the proposed testimony by defendant's expert, the plaintiff took exception to the expert's use of the MCMI-III. Citing both the Rogers, Salekin, and Sewell article, as well as the 1996 article by Retzlaff, the defense argued that the MCMI-III yields wrong results in four of five cases (this figure is based on the recalculated data presented in the Retzlaff article).

The motion also states that according to Rogers, Salekin, and Sewell, the MCMI-III "is quite unreliable" and that "less than rigorous standards were used in Millon's criterion-related validity study for the MCMI-III." Indeed, the defendant's motion also points out, on the basis of these articles, that in the original validation study of the MCMI-III,

> Clinicians were asked to make diagnoses when the criteria were unavailable or poorly established. They were not fully informed regarding the purpose of the study, which may have affected their patient selection. The diagnoses were often based on limited contact with unknown reliability and under pressure to get "enough" cases.

Referring to the 1996 article by Retzlaff, the defendant's motion states:

> Dr. Retzlaff calculated a positive predictive power (PPP) for personality disorders based on Millon's research. PPP provides a critical estimate of diagnostic usefulness. It supplies the likelihood that an elevated score correctly identifies the intended disorder. Retzlaff recalculated Millon's data and found that elevated scores are likely to lead to the wrong diagnoses in more than four of five cases.

The motion also notes:

> Defendant's brief establishes that academicians are still debating the accuracy of the MCMI-III. According to Defendant, Millon published a study 5 years ago, in 1994. Retzlaff published an article on Millon's validity study in the first edition of the MCMI-III manual (Millon, 1994) which contended the validity study was flawed. Rogers, Salekin, and Sewell recalculated some portion of Millon's data in light of Retzlaff's comments [Actually it was Retzlaff who performed the recalculation of the Millon data.] and wrote the study Plaintiff found first. Meanwhile, Millon agreed that his original validity study was poorly done and conducted another, published in 1997. Retzlaff's response to Rogers, Salekin, and Sewell will be published in August, 2000. Rogers, Salekin, and Sewell's rebuttal no doubt will be forthcoming: They may feel that the reconfigured test cures the defects they believed existed, or they may not. They may consider further study to be necessary. Others may publish on the subject. Alternate models may be considered. Academic debate may be brief or lingering, but if the matter can be decided by the scientific community before it gains admission into federal court, it should be. The reliability of a particular psychological testing tool is not a question that should be decided by a court, particularly when debate is ongoing in the academic community. The validity of the MCMI-III is a question that should be decided by psychologists before courts entertain its use in litigation.
>
> Even if psychologists everywhere considered the MCMI-III a solid diagnostic tool, that fact alone would not justify its admission into evidence. The

debate about the admissibility of the results of polygraph examinations, for example, remains unresolved even though polygraph examination is nationally accepted by law enforcement officers, who rely on it as a key investigative tool. Yet the results of such tests are not generally deemed not [sic] sufficiently reliable to gain acceptance into evidence under Daubert and Rule 702. . . . The MCMI-III, which is not generally accepted by psychologists, should likewise not be admitted.

The plaintiff's brief also attempts to leverage this critique of the MCMI-III into a complete barring all of the defendant's expert's testimony, citing the expert's statements in deposition that the MCMI-III was necessary to all of that expert's final opinions. The plaintiffs argue that "since the MCMI-III has not gained general acceptance in the scientific community, opinions derived in whole or in part from testing with it ought not be admitted into evidence in federal court." They argue that, therefore, the defendant's expert should not be allowed to testify as to any opinions that were formed on the basis of the MCMI results, and that because all of this expert's opinions rest at least partially on the MCMI-III, as conceded in the expert's deposition, none of them should be admitted.

The trial judge rejected that portion of the plaintiff's motion seeking exclusion of anything related to the MCMI-III on the grounds that the test does not pass muster under Daubert. To the author's knowledge, no court has refused to allow evidence based on the MCMI-III for any reason having to do with the scientific soundness of the instrument, except in the Lakewood case, where the defendants voluntarily withdrew the MCMI-III from consideration prior to the judge's ruling on the remaining instruments.

THE ORIGINAL MCMI-III VALIDITY STUDY DEBACLE

When the MCMI-III was first published in 1994 a group of presenters at the third Millon Inventories Conference in Minneapolis, including the present author, met with Dr. Millon and National Computer Systems staff to voice concerns about the lack of documented empirical support for the test. The principal concern was the absence of validity support for the test against a criterion of clinicians' diagnoses, of the type that had been so impressively presented in the MCMI-II manual in the form of classification efficiency statistics. As Retzlaff (1996) points out, the operating characteristics calculated for the MCMI-III on the basis of standardization/item analysis data were so poor that the publisher did not even include all of the standard classification efficiency statistics in the tables in the MCMI-III manual. According to Retzlaff, who was a participant in the standardization of the MCMI-III, the problem resulted from criterion unreliability. Whereas the clinician raters providing criterion data for the earlier MCMI-II validation study had worked from the Millon Personality Diagnostic Checklist in formulating their diagnoses, which resulted in high criterion reliability, raters for the initial MCMI-III study were simply told to "bubble in" a diagnosis unaided by any type of formal structure (Retzlaff, 1996). This resulted in embarrassingly low sensitivity and positive predictive power statistics for several scales of the test.

It has been axiomatic from the very beginning of criterion-related validity research on psychometric instruments that a study stands or falls according to the adequacy of the criterion. Even a scale that is actually highly valid would fail to register adequate validity coefficients or classification efficiency statistics in a study that lacked a reliable criterion. The authors of the MCMI-III paid scrupulous attention to one of the two main methodological criticisms of early empirical research in clinical psychology, that being the necessity of paying attention to base rates. Inexplicably, however, they ignored the other, even more basic, major criticism of early clinical research. That criticism, which is drummed into the psyche of every first-year graduate student in clinical psychology, is that unaided clinical judgment is notoriously unreliable, a warning that received stunning confirmation in the MCMI-III validation debacle.

Subsequent to the meeting between the Millon presenters and NCS staff, two parallel lines of activity were initiated in regard to the validation problem. On the one hand, Retzlaff (1996) published an article highlighting the deficiencies of the original validation study but generally giving a positive review of the test and noting acceptably high correlations between MCMI-III scales and the corresponding scales of other self-report clinical personality measures, such as the MMPI-2 and SCL-90-R. This article brought the deficiencies of the original MCMI-III validity study to the attention of a number of researchers and practitioners, some of whom reacted sharply to the publication of the latest edition of the MCMI with such poor criterion-related validity in support of the test's claims to provide valuable information to assist in the diagnosis of Axis I and, especially, Axis II disorders.

The second line of activity in response to the meeting between the presenters and NCS staff was a second validity study by Millon and his associates of the MCMI-III against a more structured criterion based on specific *DSM-IV* diagnostic criteria for each disorder and, in the case of Axis II disorders, additionally on Millon's descriptions of the eight clinical domains of personality. This second study is presented in the second edition of the MCMI-III manual and in Millon's edited book on the inventories (Davis, Wenger, & Guzman, 1997).

One potential consequence of the deficiencies in the diagnostic criteria employed in the original MCMI-III item analysis study involves a problem with the calibration of the BR scores, quite separate and apart from any issues bearing on the validity of the test. As noted earlier, the extremely poor validity results presented in the first edition of the MCMI-III manual's classification efficiency statistics resulted from inaccuracies in clinicians' diagnoses of their therapy and assessment clients. Although the subsequent validity study presented in the Millon manual corrected this deficiency to a great extent by substituting reliable diagnostic criteria in which clinicians were asked to follow a very specific structure in assigning diagnostic labels to clients, the improvement in the validity statistics was not accompanied by a simultaneous recalibration of the BR scores based on the new frequencies for the Axis I and Axis II disorders obtained in the second study. Presumably, with greater diagnostic accuracy resulting from the use of a structured guide to assign diagnostic labels, the actual frequencies of the disorders in the clinical sample employed would have been more accurate than the frequencies obtained in the first study. Thus, it may be argued that the BR scores themselves, the very basis of the assignment of numbers to behavior in the Millon inventories, contain a flaw that is just as serious as the original validity problem in the MCMI-III. If the frequencies on which the original BR scores were based are significantly distorted because of diagnostic inaccuracy, then Millon's claim to improve diagnostic accuracy by taking into account base rates for each of the disorders diagnosed by the MCMI-III rests on an inadequate foundation. Hess (1998) states further objections in regard to base rate estimates based on the 998 subjects in the original MCMI-III standardization sample. He characterizes that sample size as a grossly insufficient number from which to derive base rate estimates.

In actual fact, the first objection is only partially applicable. Although the second edition of the MCMI-III manual (referring to the first set of diagnostic ratings with the flawed criterion) states that the target prevalence rates for all of the clinical scales of the instrument were determined by calculating the proportion of times clinicians rated each trait as a client's most prominent problem or as present but not as prominent as the first, this was not the only factor in determining the calculation of base rate scores. The manual goes on to say:

> These empirically derived estimates of population rates were then adjusted to accommodate results from a variety of epidemiological studies of the population prevalence rates of these characteristics. These adjusted percentages became the target prevalence rates from which the base rate transformations were developed. (Millon, Davis, & Millon, 1997, pp. 60–61)

This seems to dispose of the objection by Hess (1998) as well. Although the exact scope of the distortion of base rates used in the development of the MCMI-III BR scores may never be determined, owing to the absence of specifics in the manual concerning the degree to which the item analysis data were relied on, as opposed to the other estimates of population frequency cited in manual, it is the present author's opinion that the degree of distortion is minor. Also to be taken into account is a prior study of the original MCMI conducted in 1981, in which data on 43,218 patients who had taken the MCMI were reviewed. This review resulted in the recalculation and adjustment of the transformation of raw scores to BR scores. Thus, the authors of the MCMI-III had a considerable empirical basis from which to estimate the frequencies of all disorders in a general clinical sample, above and beyond the flawed standardization data from the original MCMI-III study.

In contrast to Retzlaff's (1996) essentially positive view of the MCMI-III, Rogers, Salekin, and Sewell (1997), in a paper presented at the American Psychological Association convention, were far less generous in regard to its utility. They recommended a moratorium on any use of the test apart from research because of the test's low empirical validity. That paper was followed by an article in the journal of the APA Psychology and Law Division, *Law and Human Behavior,* in which Rogers et al. (1999) argued specifically that the purported failure of the MCMI-III to pass muster as admissible scientific evidence under the standards articulated in *Daubert v. Merrell-Dow Pharmaceuticals* (1993) should preclude any forensic use of the test.

In their 1999 article in *Law and Human Behavior,* Rogers, Salekin, and Sewell take exception to some of the conclusions and recommendations regarding the MCMI-II contained in McCann and Dyer (1996). In their response piece, Dyer and McCann (2000) argue that the Rogers, Salekin, and Sewell analysis of the research on the MCMI-II presented an egregious misuse of techniques from meta-analysis and multitrait-multimethod matrix (MTMMM) procedures. Specifically, Dyer and McCann argue that the use by Rogers et al. of a number of the newer personality disorder instruments as criteria against which to evaluate the MCMI-II was arbitrary, as these instruments themselves had been validated against the personality disorder scales of the MCMI-II, suggesting that the authors of the newer scales regarded the MCMI-II as a stable and valid measure of personality disorders that was suitable as a benchmark against which to evaluate their newer instruments. In the Rogers et al. analysis, however, the argument was that if the MCMI-II did not correlate with these newer instruments, then it was the MCMI-II that was deficient. Dyer and McCann also argued that in their attempt to perform a statistical aggregation of those research results, Rogers et al. violated a number of central tenets of meta-analysis, primarily the requirement of including a qualitative assessment of the methodological adequacy of each of the studies being aggregated. We also argued that, because the reliabilities of the many instruments against which Rogers et al. attempted to evaluate the MCMI-II were not factored into their analysis, the correlations were likely to be influenced by the unreliability of some of these criterion variables to an unknown degree.

Dyer and McCann (2000) argued that Rogers et al. (1999) actually misunderstood a central element of the multitrait-multimethod procedure, as reflected in their failure to use multiple methods in conducting their analysis. The Campbell and Fiske (1959) MTMMM procedure asserts that where there are multiple traits being evaluated by multiple methods, there should be a hierarchy of correlations, with the monotrait-heteromethod correlations being the strongest, followed by the heterotrait-monomethod correlations, and then followed by the heterotrait-heteromethod correlations. Campbell and Fiske make the point that validation of an assessment procedure for a single trait by different individuals using the same method can be misleading because of spuriously high correlations resulting from common method variance. What Campbell and Fiske mean by multiple methods is a qualitative difference in format, such as the difference between a self-report scale and supervisory ratings, or the difference between supervisory ratings and peer ratings of the same individual. In the Rogers, Salekin, and Sewell analysis, however, the majority of the instruments used in their aggregate of results were self-report personality inventories. Thus, their analysis violates a central concept of this technique, namely, avoiding spuriously high correlations due to common method variance associated with the use of only a single method. Dyer and McCann also fault the Rogers, Salekin, and Sewell analysis for attempting to assess too large a number of variables in a single analysis and for including an arbitrary criterion for validity, that being that the personality disorder scale's having its highest correlation with the aggregate of other measures of the same personality disorder. In other words, in the Rogers et al. procedure, if a personality disorder such as Avoidant did not correlate highest with the aggregate of other instruments purportedly measuring Avoidant Personality Disorder, then that scale of the MCMI-II was judged to be invalid. This would hold true even if the highest correlation of MCMI-II Avoidant were with the aggregate of other scales purportedly measuring Schizoid Personality Disorder, which is a related disorder, and would in any other system of evaluating results be given at least some credit for establishing the validity of the Avoidant scale. Where the counterpart measure conceptualized the disorder differently from the MCMI-II, causing that scale of the MCMI-II to have its highest correlation with a different scale, Rogers et al. simply interpreted this as indicating that the MCMI-II scale lacked validity.

Further, in regard to the Rogers, Salekin, and Sewell (1999) analysis of the MCMI-II, Dyer and McCann (2000) argue that the arbitrary all-or-nothing criterion of highest correlation with corresponding scale employed in that analysis replaced the commonsense approach advocated by Campbell and Fiske (1959) in their original presentation of the multitrait multimethod procedure. Campbell and Fiske, as well as virtually every other proponent of this method of examining scale validity, advise that the key elements in interpreting an MTMMM are the absolute magnitudes of the correlations and the patterns of correlations. Under that system, a research result in which Avoidant had its highest, and very substantial, correlation with measures of Schizoid Personality Disorder in the hetero-method blocks of the matrix would clearly be interpreted as lending at least partial support for the validity of the Avoidant scale.

Finally, Dyer and McCann (2000) argue that the Rogers et al. (1999) analysis was fatally flawed by their use of a method that by its very nature results in an unreliable criterion. In the matrix of correlations they present, Rogers et al. include only the MCMI-II on the one hand, and on the other hand include an aggregate of 15 other instruments that do not have a particularly high correlation with one another. This in effect creates a criterion variable that has extremely poor internal consistency. In other words, to satisfy the demands of the Rogers et al. analysis, the sum of each individual scale of the MCMI-II would have to correlate simultaneously with the corresponding scales of 15 other measures that do not correlate particularly well with each other. Ironically, it is a situation parallel to the debacle affecting the original validity study of the MCMI-III, in which criterion unreliability caused the study to fail. In the case of the Rogers, Salekin, and Sewell analysis, however, the fault was not naive reliance on unaided clinical judgment, but the use of a method that inherently produced an unreliable criterion, thereby setting up the MCMI-II to fail from the outset.

In regard to the forensic use of the MCMI-III, Rogers, Salekin, and Sewell (1999) conducted a similar analysis but employed the data from the initial validation study of the test, which, as discussed at length earlier, were extremely poor. Even though the subsequent analysis (Millon, Davis, & Millon, 1997) was available to Rogers, Salekin, and Sewell, and in fact had been rather highly publicized by the test publisher, their analysis chose to ignore that study altogether. Dyer and McCann (2000) argue that the later validation study of the MCMI-III, which employed a structured criterion, clearly establishes the validity and utility of the test for forensic use. In the Millon et al. study, the operating characteristics were as good as or better than those of the MCMI-II. In their rejoinder piece, Rogers, Salekin, and Sewell (2000) argue that the sample size of the new study was much smaller than that of the validation study of either the

MCMI-II or MCMI-III, thus limiting its utility. Had Dyer and McCann been extended the courtesy by the editor of *Law and Human Behavior* of being given access to the Rogers et al. rejoinder piece prior to the publication of the series of articles on the topic, we would have commented on their remarks concerning the Millon et al. study. We would certainly have conceded that the relatively smaller sample size makes the Millon et al. validation of the MCMI-III somewhat less impressive than the validation study of the MCMI-II, which one can argue was a model of clinical personality inventory research. Clearly, the psychological community would benefit from further research on the validity of specific scales of the MCMI-III, especially where the numbers of cases representing individual disorders, such as Cluster A personality disorders as cited by Rogers, Salekin, and Sewell, were quite low (the mean sample size being 13.7 cases per confirmed diagnosis in that group). Nonetheless, the study did have 321 participants, which lends it adequate power for the typical effect sizes that are observed in this type of research and reasonably good confidence bounds for the results on most of the MCMI-III scales.

It should be noted as well that convergent-discriminant, or MTMMM, studies of personality disorder measures from the MCMI-II (McCann, 1991) and MCMI-III (Wooley, Dorr, Morgan, & Deselms, 2001) and Morey MMPI-2 PD scales (both studies) and Ben-Porath MMPI-2 PD scales (only in Wooley et al.) found ample evidence of both convergent and discriminant validity for the MCMI and MMPI scales. The one prominent exception, which appeared in both studies, was the Compulsive scale, which appears to be conceptualized differently between the Millon and MMPI systems. As has been the case with virtually every convergent-discriminant validity study that has appeared in the psychological literature, Rogers et al. being the striking exception, the McCann and Wooley et al. studies employed a commonsense criterion, as recommended by Campbell and Fiske (1959). Wooley et al. state:

> The ideology for using this method is that if discriminant validity is to be established, convergent validity coefficients should be significantly greater than other coefficients in the respective row and column in the hetero-trait-heteromethod portion of the matrix . . . as well as the hetero-trait-monomethod triangles in the matrix.

As Dyer and McCann (2000) point out, it is the magnitudes of the validity coefficients as well as the patterns of intercorrelation observed in the matrix that are informative, which was the approach used in these and virtually all other studies of the MCMI employing MTMMM techniques.

In their summary regarding forensic use of the MCMI-III, Rogers, Salekin, and Sewell (2000) state that combining data on diagnostic utility from both the MCMI-II and MCMI-III studies yields sample-weighted positive predictive power figures averaging .31. They then characterize this as "indicating that an MCMI-III Axis II disorder is likely to be wrong two of three times." (p. 505) Although this is technically correct in a very limited context, it is a statement that is readily translated into a gross misrepresentation of the validity of the test that can result in the impeachment of an expert witness who is actually relying on an entirely valid assessment. The key concepts involved include differences between reporting validity information as Pearson product-moment correlations and classification efficiency statistics, as well as the effect of sample preselection in making probability statements.

It is extremely common to find in correlational studies of test validity that correlations in the .20s and .30s are cited as providing clear support for the validity of the test. Even though a correlation of .30 signifies that the criterion and predictor share a modest 9% of variance, statistically significant coefficients of that magnitude are routinely and unquestioningly accepted as demonstrating test validity because they indicate a significantly greater than chance relationship between the two. A positive predictive power of .31 can be conceptualized as being roughly analogous to this modest degree of correlation between test and criterion.

Even though a positive predictive power of 31% is therefore on a par with what is the norm for Pearson product-moment correlation validities, in the hands of a skillful attorney it can turn into a millstone around the neck of the unwary expert witness. Exemplifying the truth of the old adage that a little knowledge is a dangerous thing, the positive predictive power of 31% can be represented to jurors as being a ridiculously poor method of diagnosing clients that is inferior even to what a lay juror could accomplish unaided by psychometrics. As McCann and Dyer (1996) observe, when questioning an expert about an MCMI result for which the positive predictive power is less than 50%, the question "Wouldn't I do better than that by just flipping a coin, Doctor?" can easily make the test appear to be worth less than the quarter that the attorney holds up before the jurors. If the expert displays any hesitation before responding to the further question, "Wouldn't flipping a coin give you fifty-fifty, Doctor?", it will appear that the expert is confused about something that is self-evident to most lay jurors. If the expert insists on defending a 31% correct result against a 50% correct result, then the attorney really does not need to ask anything else along that line. The incompetence, or bias, of the expert is another thing that will then be self-evident to the jury.

Of course, matters are considerably more complex than beating out the MCMI-III by a mere coin flip. The correct answer to the initial question, "Wouldn't I do better than 31% by flipping a coin?", should be a resounding no. This is because the positive predictive power statistic involves only a small part of the sample, namely, that portion that scores above the crite-rion level on the test diagnosing the disorder. It represents the percentage probability that if someone scores above the MCMI cut-off for the target disorder, he or she does in fact have the disorder. The coin-flip method, on the other hand, applies to the entire sample, and its positive predictive power necessarily corresponds to the frequency of the disorder. Thus, if a particular disorder has a frequency (base rate) of 8% in the standardiza-tion sample, as is typical of the personality disorders assessed in the sec-ond MCMI-III validation study (Millon et al., 1997), a coin flip would have a PPP of 8%. Thus, a PPP of 31% would represent nearly a 300% increase in accuracy over the coin-flip method, or chance. A proof of this is given in Dyer (1997).

Rogers, Salekin, and Sewell (2000) do raise an important point in re-gard to the methodology of the second MCMI-III validation study. They correctly point out that instructions to contributing researchers were to select cases of clients whom they would be diagnosing according to a structured procedure and who had taken the MCMI-III. In the instruc-tions to raters, it was explicitly permitted to use cases where the rater had had some prior exposure to the MCMI-III results of particular clients. The instructions stressed, however, that cases were to be ex-cluded when the contributing researcher had a clear recollection of what the subject's MCMI-III profile looked like. If they had seen the subject's MCMI-III record previously, then clinicians were to include only those cases where they could not recall the results and therefore their ratings of the client would not be contaminated by knowledge of the results. Millon (personal communication, 1999) indicates that this affected ap-proximately 20% of cases, largely those of research subjects who were being treated in institutions.

It is not possible to determine with any degree of precision the actual impact of the criterion contamination on the approximately 20% of diag-nostic ratings where there was prior exposure to the subject's test record. The instructions to clinicians printed in the MCMI-III manual stressed that their diagnoses were to be guided by both the *DSM-IV* and Millon's descriptions of the eight clinical domains of personality. In my view, the combination of explicit directions to rely exclusively on the Millon do-main descriptions and *DSM-IV* in making diagnoses, as well as the in-struction to exclude any case where the clinician had a clear recollection of the MCMI-III results would tend to reduce the influence of the criterion contamination to a minimum. Although the inclusion of some cases in which there had been prior exposure to the client's MCMI-III record con-stitutes a flaw in the study that can provide fodder for cross-examination, the practical effect falls far short of even mildly compromising the results.

CONTENT VALIDITY AND THE MCMI-III

Dyer and McCann (2000) point out that criterion-related validity studies of the MCMI-III are not the only factor supporting its use in forensic evaluations. The second edition of the MCMI-III manual also includes a detailed content validity study of the test against specific diagnostic criteria for all personality disorders that appear in *DSM-IV* and two (Self-Defeating and Sadistic) that appeared in *DSM-III-R* but not in *DSM-IV*. Specific *DSM* criteria are listed beside parallel MCMI-III items and are related to the functional processes and structural attributes of Millon's theory of personality. Whereas Rogers et al. (1999) object to what they characterize as a lack of documentation of the procedures for item selection and obtaining of raters' judgments in the content study of the MCMI-III, Dyer and McCann point out that the MCMI-III manual, second edition, gives a detailed account of these procedures. It is noted, however, that Rogers et al. (2000) dismiss this documentation as inadequate. Readers are advised to review Chapter 2 of the MCMI-III manual (Millon, Davis, & Millon, 1997) to form their own independent judgments as to the adequacy of the procedures employed in generating item content.

In terms of forensic applications, McCann and Dyer (1996) argue that *DSM-IV* has assumed the status of the ultimate learned treatise in courts, and that it is the standard against which experts' diagnostic conclusions are judged. It is considered by judges as the official diagnostic reference for psychological disorders, and a favored cross-examination tactic is to challenge the expert's diagnostic conclusions by pointing out areas in which the examinee does not meet *DSM-IV* standards for the disorder. Thus, a clinical personality measure that is directly linked to the *DSM-IV* possesses an inherent advantage as a basis for expert testimony. In addition to citing criterion-related validity evidence in support of MCMI-III test results, experts may also point out that scoring at a clinically elevated level on any of the personality disorder scales of the test necessarily means that the subject has responded in the keyed direction to test questions that are based on the same factors that constitute the standards for a *DSM-IV* diagnosis, the two being presented side by side in the test manual. As of this writing, there is no other mainstream self-report clinical personality measure that offers this type of content validity support.

REFERENCES

Anastasi, A., & Urbina, S. (1997). *Psychological testing* (7th ed.). Upper Saddle River, NJ: Prentice-Hall.

Brodie, L. A. (2003). *Child custody: Issues and techniques (Pt. I).* Available from PsychCredits.com.

Butcher, J. N., & Miller, K. B. (1999). Personality assessment in personal injury litigation. In A. K. Hess & I. B. Weiner (Eds.), *The handbook of forensic psychology* (2nd ed., pp. 104–126). New York: Wiley.

Campbell, D. T., & Fiske, D. W. (1959). Convergent and discriminant validation by the multitrait-multimethod matrix. *Psychological Bulletin, 56*, 81–105.

Craig, R. J. (1997). Sensitivity of MCMI-III scales T (drugs) and B (alcohol) in detecting substance abuse. *Substance Abuse and Misuse, 32*, 1385–1393.

Craig, R. J. (1999). Testimony based on the Millon Clinical Multiaxial Inventory: Review, commentary, and guidelines. *Journal of Personality Assessment, 73*, 290–316.

Craig, R. J., & Bivens, A. (1998). Factor structure of the MCMI-III. *Journal of Personality Assessment, 70*, 190–196.

Craig, R. J., & Olson, R. E. (1997). Assessing PTSD with the Millon Clinical Multiaxial Inventory-III. *Journal of Clinical Psychology, 53*, 943–952.

Daubert v. Merrell-Dow Pharmaceuticals, Inc. 509 U.S. 579 (1993).

Davis, R., Wenger, A., & Guzman, A. (1997). Validation of the MCMI-III. In T. Millon (Ed.), *The Millon Inventories: Clinical and personality assessment* (pp. 327–359). New York: Guilford Press.

Dyce, J. A., O'Connor, B. P., Parkins, S. Y., & Janzen, H. L. (1997). Correlational structure of the MCMI-III personality disorder scales and comparison with other data sets. *Journal of Personality Assessment, 69*, 568–582.

Dyer, F. J. (1997). Application of the Millon Inventories in forensic psychology. In T. Millon (Ed.), *The Millon Inventories: Clinical and personality assessment* (pp. 124–139). New York: Guilford Press.

Dyer, F. J., & McCann, J. T. (2000). The Millon Clinical Inventories, research critical of their forensic application, and Daubert Criteria. *Law and Human Behavior, 24*, 487–498.

Flynn, P. M., & McMahon, R. C. (1997). MCMI applications in substance abuse. In T. Millon (Ed.), *The Millon Inventories: Clinical and personality assessment* (pp. 173–190). New York: Guilford Press.

Gondolf, E. W. (1999). MCMI-III results for batterer program participants in four cities: Less "pathological than expected." *Journal of Family Violence, 14*, 1–17.

Hess, A. K. (1998). *Review of the Millon Clinical Multiaxial Inventory III: Mental Measurements Yearbook.* Lincoln: University of Nebraska Press.

In the Matter of the Guardianship of, D. M. H. C.L. H. W. L.F. H., & R. Q. H., Minors. 309 N. J. Super.179, 706 A.2d 1129 (Decided March 6, 1998).

Jeffrey v. Dillard's Department Stores and Dillard's Bel Air Mall, United States District Court, S.D. AL. 2000. Southern Division.

Kelln, B. R., Dozois, D. J., & McKenzie, I. E. (1998). An MCMI-III discriminant function analysis of incarcerated felons: Prediction of subsequent institutional misconduct. *Criminal Justice and Behavior, 25*, 177–189.

McCann, J. T. (1991). Convergent and discriminant validity of the MCMI-II and MMPI personality disorder scales. *Psychological Assessment, 3*, 9–18.

McCann, J. T. (2002). Guidelines for forensic application of the MCMI-III. *Journal of Forensic Psychology Practice, 2*, 55–69. (III)

McCann, J. T., Campana, V., Flens, J., Campagna, V., Collman, P., Lazzaro, T., et al. (2001). The MCMI-III in child custody evaluations: A normative study. *Journal of Forensic Psychology Practice, 1*, 27–44.

McCann, J. T., & Dyer, F. J. (1996). *Forensic assessment with the Millon Inventories.* New York: Guilford Press.

Millon, T. (1994). *The Millon Clinical Multiaxial Inventory-III manual.* Minneapolis, MN: National Computer Systems.

Millon, T., Davis, R., & Millon, C. (1997). *Manual for the Millon Clinical Multiaxial Inventory-III* (2nd ed.). Minneapolis, MN: National Computer Systems.

Retzlaff, P. D. (1996). MCMI-III diagnostic validity: Bad test or bad validity study? *Journal of Personality Assessment, 66*, 431–437.

Retzlaff, P. D. (2000). Comment on the validity of the MCMI-III. *Law and Human Behavior, 24*, 425–443.

Rogers, R., Salekin, R. T., & Sewell, K. W. (1997). *Validation of the Millon Clinical Multiaxial Inventory for Axis II disorders: Does it meet the Daubert standard?* Paper presented at the 105th Convention of the American Psychological Association, Chicago.

Rogers, R., Salekin, R. T., & Sewell, K. W. (1999). Validation of the Millon Clinical Multiaxial Inventory for Axis II disorders: Does it meet the Daubert standard? *Law and Human Behavior, 23*, 425–443.

Rogers, R., Salekin, R. T., & Sewell, K. W. (2000). The MCMI-III and the Daubert standard: Separating rhetoric from reality. *Law and Human Behavior, 24*, 501–506.

Usher v. Lakewood Engineering & Manufacturing, Inc. No. 93 C 3279. United States District Court, N. D. IL, Eastern Division. (Decided November 10, 1994).

Wooley, M. M., Dorr, D. A., Morgan, C. D., & Deselms, J. P. (2001). *Comparative validity of the MCMI-III and MMPI-2 personality disorder scales.* Poster presented at the 109th annual conference of the American Psychological Association, San Francisco.

PART III

Continuing Controversies

CHAPTER 10

Assessing Response Bias with the MCMI Modifying Indices

R. MICHAEL BAGBY AND MARGARITA B. MARSHALL

ACCURATE ASSESSMENT of personality pathology and symptomatology, particularly with regard to self-report instruments, depends on the respondent's ability and motivation to provide honest responses. Clinicians and researchers have long recognized, however, that scores on these measures may be subject to certain biases as a result of the context in which an individual is assessed. One popular self-report measure of personality psychopathology is the Millon Clinical Multiaxial Inventory (MCMI). The most recent version, the MCMI-III, in addition to assessing symptoms and behaviors of major mental illness, was also developed to provide a means of measuring personality consistent with Millon's (1990; Millon & Davis, 1996) typology of personality psychopathology (Craig, 1999). The MCMI incorporated the terminology of the *Diagnostic and Statistical Manual of Mental Disorders* (*DSM-III-R*; American Psychiatric Association, 1987),[1] and one of the unique strengths of this instrument is that items were selected based on their ability to discriminate general clinical groups from specific diagnostic groups, as opposed to normal samples. Furthermore, standard scores were based on the base rates of diagnoses present in the psychiatric normative sample, as opposed to T-scores that are based on the assumption of a normal distribution of scores, thus taking prevalence rates into account (Craig, 1999).

Although all three versions of the MCMI (MCMI-I, Millon, 1983; MCMI-II, Millon, 1987; MCMI-III, Millon, Millon, & Davis, 1997) include scales designed to detect and correct for potential response biases, the

---

[1] The current version of the MCMI, the MCMI-III, is coordinated with the *DSM-IV* (American Psychiatric Association, 1994).

so-called modifying indices, unlike other measures of psychopathology, such as the Minnesota Multiphasic Personality Inventory 2 (MMPI-2; Butcher, Graham, Ben-Porath, Tellegen, Dahlstrom, et al., 2001) and the Personality Assessment Inventory (PAI; Morey, 1991), there has been comparatively less research addressing the utility of these indices. It is widely accepted that test takers may be motivated for a variety of reasons not to respond honestly or in a straightforward manner to items on instruments measuring psychopathology. Such responding, of course, directly affects scores on the MCMI clinical scales, compromising the interpretative meaning of test results. Detecting such responding, therefore, is an important part of the assessment process.

Two response styles commonly targeted by validity scales, or scales deigned to detect response dissimilation, on measures of psychopathology are underreporting and overreporting; these response styles are also commonly referred to as "faking good" and "faking bad," respectively. Underreporting refers to intentional or unintentional efforts to minimize negative traits or symptoms of psychopathology and exaggerate or claim positive traits; as such, this response style is associated with potential and spurious lower scores on scales designed to assess clinical psychopathology. There are many assessment contexts where respondents may be consciously or unconsciously motivated by personal goals to underreport symptoms of psychopathology. For example, disputing parents undergoing child custody and access evaluation may not report emotional problems they experience, and job applicants in an effort to put their best foot forward may present themselves in an overly favorable light; prisoners seeking parole or early release may exaggerate overall level of adjustment and fail to admit to behavioral problems they might have, and psychiatric inpatients may attempt to disclaim the presence of lingering psychopathological symptoms to secure release from the hospital.

In contrast, over-reporting refers to attempts to exaggerate or claim negative traits or symptoms of psychopathology and minimize or deny positive traits; this response style is associated with potential and spurious elevated scores on clinical scales. The motivation to overreport, in contrast to underreporting, is typically intentional and engages the full awareness of the respondent, although there are some instances in which individuals may be unconsciously motivated to fabricate and exaggerate psychiatric symptoms (e.g., Factitious Disorder and Conversion Disorder). There are also a number of contexts in which overreporting may occur: Personal injury litigants or combat veterans may exaggerate the extent of psychological trauma they experience to maximize their chances of receiving financial compensation for disability claims; individuals genuinely experiencing psychopathology may exaggerate their symptoms as a cry for help; criminal litigants may claim the presence of psychopathological symptoms that they do not in fact possess in order to plead insanity as a way of avoiding criminal charges, prolonged imprisonment, and even the death penalty.

Irrelevant or inconsistent or random responding is another source of invalidation that can be assessed with validity scales. As noted by Rogers (1997a), irrelevant responding not only invalidates individuals' clinical profiles, but can also be associated with elevated scores on scales designed to detect overreporting biases. Consequently, irrelevant response biases can be easily mistaken for overreporting biases if there is no separate assessment of it (Rogers, 1997a).

Given that underreporting and overreporting response styles and irrelevant responding have the potential to invalidate MCMI protocols and that such responding likely occurs in a variety of important assessment contexts, the accurate detection of response biases is a critical aspect of MCMI interpretation. The purpose of the present chapter is to provide an overview of the modifying indices developed for use with the MCMI-I, MCMI-II, and MCMI-III and a review of the empirical literature addressing the validity of these indices.

DESCRIPTION AND SCALE OVERVIEW

The original MCMI contained two modifying indices related to response bias: the Validity Index and the Weight Factor Composite Score. When the MCMI-II was developed, the Weight Factor Composite Score was revised and renamed the Disclosure scale, and two additional modifying indices were added, the Desirability scale and the Debasement scale (Millon, 1987). The MCMI-III retained these three modifying indices in addition to the Validity Index (Millon, 1994), and we provide a brief description of these scales in their current form. Only those items from the MCMI-II versions of the modifying indices that were subsequently included in the MCMI-III were revised. These scales are described in detail next.

THE VALIDITY INDEX (V)

The current version of the V scale consists of three improbable statements designed to assess random responding or confusion (Craig, 1999). Responding true to two or more statements invalidates the test protocol. Responding true to only one statement indicates that a protocol has questionable validity and warrants caution in interpreting test scores.

THE WEIGHT FACTOR COMPOSITE SCORE

The Weight Factor Composite Score represented the deviation of the total raw score based on the eight basic personality scales from midrange. Positive scores greater than 8 were interpreted as suggesting a tendency to deliberately underreport; negative scores greater than −8 were interpreted as suggesting a deliberate tendency to overreport (Millon, 1983).

THE DISCLOSURE SCALE (X)

The X scale represents the degree of deviation from midrange with respect to an adjusted composite raw score derived from the 10 Clinical Personality Pattern scales (i.e., scales 1 through 8B). This scale represents a revision of the Weight Factor Composite Score originally developed for use with the MCMI-I. High scores indicate greater endorsement of psychopathology.

THE DESIRABILITY SCALE (Y)

The 23 items of the Y scale developed for the MCMI-II were selected if they were endorsed by at least 9 out of a sample of 12 clinical graduate students instructed to fake good, and had significantly higher endorsement frequencies in this sample than in a sample of 112 nonclinical respondents thought to be representative of the population (Millon, 1987). Instructions to fake good included exaggerating positive traits and denying faults (Millon, 1987). The MCMI-III version of the Y scale is a 21-item scale designed to detect defensive response styles, with high scores reflecting overreporting of virtues and the denial of psychological symptoms. Elevated scores do not invalidate a given profile; however, scoring adjustments for scales that correlate with the Y scale are made. Low scores are not interpreted.

THE DEBASEMENT SCALE (Z)

The 46 items of the Z scale developed for the MCMI-II were selected if they were endorsed by at least 9 out of a sample of 12 clinical graduate students instructed to fake bad, and had significantly higher endorsement frequencies in this sample than a general patient sample ($N = 400$; Millon, 1987). Instructions to fake bad included exaggerating negative traits and endorsing psychopathological symptoms. The MCMI-III version of the Z scale is a 33-item scale designed to detect response styles that reflect overreporting of psychopathology. Elevated scores do not invalidate a given profile; however, scoring adjustments for scales that correlate with the Z scale are made. Low scores are not interpreted. According to Craig (1999), high Z scale scores can also represent "acute emotional turmoil"; thus, scores on this scale may be confounded by genuine personality psychopathology.

EMPIRICAL REVIEW

Although the individual modifying indices were designed primarily to detect particular response styles, some studies have demonstrated that some of these scales are sensitive to other styles. For example, although the Z scale was designed to detect fake-bad responding, with high scores representing symptom exaggeration, lower scales on this scale have been used to detect fake-good responding. Following a recent meta-analysis by Baer and Miller (2002), we have provided a table describing the demographic and methodological characteristics of the various studies examining the MCMI modifying indices. Table 10.1 provides a summary of these studies, including instructional group, sample size, type of sample, mean age, level of education, number of female respondents, percentage of respondents of minority ethnocultural background, study design, and whether faking instructions were given for these studies.

DETECTION OF INCONSISTENT RESPONDING

Results from studies examining the utility of the V scale using the MCMI-II suggest that V scale scores can discriminate random profiles from protocols produced under standard instructions. Bagby, Gillis, and Rogers (1991) demonstrated that students instructed to respond randomly produced significantly higher V scale scores than did psychiatric inpatients who completed the MCMI-II under standard instructions. In addition, these authors found that the item endorsement frequency for individual V scale items in the inpatient sample was similar to that of the normative sample (Bagby et al., 1991). In contrast, the students instructed to respond randomly endorsed the V scale items at approximately chance levels (Bagby et al., 1991). Likewise, Retzlaff et al. (1991) reported that computer-generated random profiles were associated with significantly higher V scale scores than for students given standard instructions. In addition, computer-generated profiles created and based on a 95% true endorsement rule were associated with significantly higher V scale scores than computer-generated profiles based on a 95% false endorsement rule, those based on a 50% true endorsement rule, and the students responding to standard instructions; the mean

Table 10.1

Demographic and Methodological Summary of Studies Examining the Validity of the MCMI

Study	Group	N	Type	Age (Education) in Years	Education	Percent Female	Percent Min	Design	Fake Instruct
MCMI									
Langevin et al. (1988)	Std	247	SO	NR	NR	0	NR	BG	n/a
	Std	172	C	NR	NR	0	NR	BG	n/a
McNeil & Meyer (1990)	Std	144	F Inpts	NR	NR	0	20	DP	n/a
	Std	47	CI	31.3 (9.6)	10.9 (2.9)	0	11	BG sim	N
	FB	47	CI	30.4 (8.2)	11.4 (7.9)	0	—	BG sim	Y
Van Gorp & Meyer (1986)	Std	20	PI	39.4 (NR)	13.1 (NR)	2	NR	BG sim	N
	FG	13	PI	—	—	—	—	BG sim	Y
	RFP	15	PI	—	—	—	—	BG sim	Y
	FB	17	PI	—	—	—	—	BG sim	Y
	RFN	16	PI	—	—	—	—	BG sim	Y
	Neut	14	PI	—	—	—	—	BG sim	Y
	Std	17	GMI	53.4 (NR)	13.5 (NR)	2	NR	BG sim	N
	FG	13	GMI	—	—	—	—	BG sim	Y
	RFP	14	GMI	—	—	—	—	BG sim	Y
	FB	15	GMI	—	—	—	—	BG sim	Y
	RFN	17	GMI	—	—	—	—	BG sim	Y
	Neut	14	GMI	—	—	—	—	BG sim	Y
Wierzbicki (1993)	Std	44	Stu	NR	NR	57	NR	BG sim	N
	FB	45	Stu	NR	NR	60	NR	BG sim	Y

MCMI-II

Study / Group	N	Setting	M (SD)				Design	Valid
Bagby, Gillis, & Dickens (1990) 24.1 (10.4)								
FG	42	Stu	NR	NR	62	NR	BG sim	Y
FASL	36	Stu	NR	NR	64	NR	BG sim	Y
FDEP	38	Stu	NR	NR	74	NR	BG sim	Y
FADA	36	Stu	NR	NR	67	NR	BG sim	Y
Std	32	Stu	22.5 (6.6)	N	—	—	BG sim	Y
NR	67	NR	BG sim	—	—	—	BG sim	Y
Bagby et al. (1991)								
FG	28	Stu	—	—	37	9	BG sim	Y
FB	31	Stu	—	—	50	NR	BG sim	N
Std	129	PI	33.6 (9.7)	NR	73	NR	BG sim	n/a
Bagby et al. (1991)								
Rand	58	Stu	27.4 (9.5)	NR	—	NR	BG sim	Y
Std	50	Stu	25.8 (8.0)	NR	45	NR	BG sim	Y
FG	50	Stu	—	NR	—	NR	BG	n/a
FB	50	Stu	—	NR	—	4	BG	n/a
Blais, Benedict, & Norman (1995)								
Std	75	PI	35.9 (9.5)	NR	69	7	BG	n/a
Std	125	PI	39 (14.7)	NR	—	—	BG	n/a
Std	108	PI	—	—	0	NR	BG sim	n/a
Craig, Kuncel, & Olson (1994)								
Std	50	Inpts	38.6 (7.1)	12.5 (1.9)	0	NR	BG sim	Y
FG	51	Inpts	36.8 (7.3)	12.7 (1.4)	0	NR	BG sim	Y
FG	49	Inpts	37.8 (5.3)	12.6 (1.4)		NR	BG sim	Y

(continued)

233

Table 10.1 *Continued*

Study	Group	N	Type	Age (Education) in Years	Education	Percent Female	Percent Min	Design	Fake Instruct
Fals-Stewart (1995)	Std	62	SA	28.3 (6.6)	10.1 (1.9)	27	32	BG sim	N
	Std	62	SA	—	—	—	—	BG sim	Y
	FG	54	F	23.3 (4.8)	10.0 (2.3)	24	37	DP	n/a
Grossman & Craig (1995)	Std	131	Mar	38.8 (10.6)	NR	53	NR	n/a	n/a
Lees-Haley (1992)	Std	55	PTSD	38.9 (10.0)	NR	42	47	DP	n/a
	Std	64	Inj	39.1 (11.3)	NR	58	31	DP	n/a
Retzlaff, Sheehan, & Fiel (1991)	Std	50	Stu	NR	NR	66	NR	BG sim	N
	FG-ad	50	Stu	NR	NR	—	NR	BG sim	Y
	FG-cl	50	Stu	NR	NR	—	NR	BG sim	Y
	FB-ad	50	Stu	NR	NR	—	NR	BG sim	Y
	FB-cl	50	Stu	NR	NR	—	NR	BG sim	Y
	Rand 1	50	Cpu	n/a	n/a	n/a	n/a	BG sim	?
	Rand 2	50	Cpu	n/a	n/a	n/a	n/a	BG sim	?
	Rand 3	50	Cpu	n/a	n/a	n/a	n/a	BG sim	?
Retzlaff, Sheehan, & Lorr (1990)	Std	78	Stu	NR	NR	0	NR	BG	n/a
	Std	119	Stu	NR	NR	0	NR	BG	n/a
	Std	159	Stu	NR	NR	100	NR	BG	n/a
Streiner, Goldberg, & Miller (1993)	Std	134	PI	32.9 (9.8)	12.1 (1.3)	50	NR	n/a	n/a
Wetzler & Marlowe (1990)	Std	105	PI	37.1 (15.7)	NR	68	NR	n/a	n/a
Wierzbicki (1997)[a]	Std	NR	Stu	NR	NR	50	NR	BG sim	N
	FB	—	Stu	NR	NR	—	NR	BG sim	Y
	FG	—	Stu	NR	NR	—	NR	BG sim	Y

	FASL	—	Stu	NR	NR	—	NR	BG sim	Y
	FDEP	—	Stu	NR	NR	—	NR	BG sim	Y
	FADA	—	Stu	NR	NR	—	NR	BG sim	Y
MCMI-III									
Charter & Lopez (2002)[b]	Rand	40000	Cpu	n/a	n/a	n/a	n/a	BG sim	?
Daubert & Metzler (2000)	Std	160	PI	44.0 (NR)	NR	53	7	BG sim	N
	FG	80	PI	—	—	—	—	BG sim	Y
	FB	80	PI	—	—	—	—	BG sim	Y
Morgan, Schoenberg, Dorr, & Burke (2002)	Std	202	PI	33.4 (12.4)	12.5 (2.2)	55	13	WG	n/a
Schoenberg, Dorr, & Morgan (2003)	Std	111	Stu	NR	NR	NR	NR	BG sim	N
	FB	106	Stu	NR	NR	NR	NR	BG sim	Y
	Std	181	PI	33.9 (NR)	NR	55	NR	BG	n/a

[a] The total N for this study was 304. Sample size for individual subgroups was not reported.

[b] Specifically, this study used 8 eight subsets of computer-generated protocols based on the eight possible different combinations of gender, patient status (inpatient versus outpatient), and duration of Axis-I pathology (>4 weeks, <1 week, and 1 to 4 weeks).

Source: BG = Between-groups; C = Controls; CI = Correctional inmates; Cpu = Computer-generated; DP = Differential prevalence; F = Forensic chemical dependence evaluation clients; FADA = Fake alcohol/drug abuse; Fake instruct = Faking instructions given; FASL = Fake Antisocial Personality Disorder; FB = Fake bad; FB-ad = Fake bad, administrative context; FB-cl = Fake bad, clinical context; FDEP = Fake depression; FG = Fake good; FG-ad = Fake good, administrative context; FG-cl = Fake good, clinical context; F Inpts = Forensic inpatients; GMI = General, nonpsychiatric, medical inpatients; Inj = Non-PTSD personal injury claimants; Inpts = Nonpsychiatric inpatients; Mar = Marital therapy participants; % Min = Percentage of participants who were non-Caucasian; N = No; n/a = Not applicable; Neut = Role fake neutral; Outpts = Outpatients; PI = Psychiatric inpatients; PTSD = PTSD claimants; Rand = Randomly generated protocols; Rand 1 = Random protocol with 50% of items answered true; Rand 2 = Random protocol with 95% of items answered true; Rand 3 = Random protocol with 98% of items answered false; RFN = Role fake negative; RFP = Role fake positive; SA = Substance abuse treatment inpatients; sim = Simulation; SO = Sex offenders; Std = Standard instructions; Stu = Students; WG = Within-groups; Y = Yes; ? = Unclear for coding purposes.

V scale scores of the 95% false and 50% true computer-generated samples were also significantly higher than those of the students responding to standard instructions. There have been no attempts to replicate these findings using the revised 3-item MCMI-III V scale.

DETECTION OF UNDERREPORTING AND OVERREPORTING

Differences among the comparison groups used across various studies make it difficult to ascertain the stability of past results regarding the utility of the Y scale. The most replicated finding based on the MCMI-II version of the Y scale is that students instructed to fake good score higher on the MCMI-II Y scale than do those responding to standard instructions or instructions to fake bad (Bagby et al., 1990; Bagby, Gillis, Toner, & Goldberg, 1991; Retzlaff et al., 1991); there is also some evidence that the MCMI-II Y scale can make similar distinctions in clinical samples where inpatients have been instructed to fake good (Craig et al., 1994; Fals-Stewart, 1995). One study using the MCMI-III has replicated this result (Daubert & Metzler, 2000). Y scale scores may also be lower in comparisons of students instructed to fake bad versus either students or psychiatric inpatients given standard instructions, as well as among psychiatric outpatients responding to fake bad versus standard instructions (Schoenberg et al., 2003).

As with the Y scale, the Z scale appears to make appropriate group distinctions, although additional replication is needed to ascertain the reliability of past results and generalizability across assessment contexts. Nonetheless, several studies have demonstrated that students instructed to fake bad score higher on the MCMI-II Z scale compared with students responding to standard instructions or instructions to fake good (Bagby et al., 1990, 1991; Retzlaff et al., 1991), as well as psychiatric inpatients responding to standard instructions (Bagby et al., 1991). There is also some evidence that instruction to fake good is associated with significantly lower Z scale scores from analogue studies comparing students responding to fake good instructions versus students or psychiatric inpatients responding to standard instructions (Bagby et al., 1990, 1991; Retzlaff et al., 1991). Craig et al. (1994), as well as Fals-Stewart (1995), found that Z scale scores of inpatients being treated for substance abuse and/or dependence who were instructed to fake good did not differ from those who were given standard instructions. In addition, Fals-Stewart reported that Z scale scores of individuals being evaluated for substance dependence as part of a presentencing screening did not differ from those of substance abuse inpatients given standard instructions. However, there is preliminary evidence that Z scale scores were significantly lower among substance abuse and dependence inpatients instructed to fake good who were able to produce valid scores on the rel-evant clinical syndrome scales (i.e., Drug Dependence and Alcohol Dependence scores within the normal range) compared with those of similar inpatients responding to standard instructions. Lees-Haley (1992) also found that personal injury claimants classified as overre-porting versus those classified as responding honestly based on the MMPI-2 scored significantly higher on the Z scale. One study using the MCMI-III has replicated this result (Daubert & Metzler, 2000). Y scale scores may also be lower in comparisons of students instructed to fake bad versus either students or psychiatric inpatients given standard in-structions, as well as among psychiatric outpatients responding to fake bad versus standard instructions (Schoenberg et al., 2003).

Studies examining the Z scale of the MCMI-III indicate that these scores are significantly higher among students instructed to fake bad as compared with students or psychiatric inpatients responding to standard instructions (Schoenberg et al., 2003), as well as for psychiatric inpatients instructed to fake bad versus their responses when given standard instructions (Daubert & Metzler, 2000). In addition, there is preliminary evidence that psychiatric inpatients responding to fake good instructions are able to significantly lower scores on the Z scale compared with their own responses produced under standard instructions (Daubert & Metzler, 2000).

Studies using the MCMI-I reported that the Weight Factor Composite Score was positively correlated with the MMPI validity scales designed to assess overreporting but negatively correlated with the MMPI scales de-signed to assess underreporting (Langevin et al., 1988; McNeil & Meyer, 1990), suggesting that the Weight Factor Composite Score could provide an indication of the tendency to fake bad versus fake good.[2] However, subsequent investigations failed to support the ability of the Weight Fac-tor Composite Score to discriminate between protocols completed under standard instructions and those of respondents instructed to alter their

---

[2] Langevin et al. (1988) reported significant positive correlations between the MCMI-I Weight Factor Composite Score and the MMPI F scale ($r = .54$) and F through K index ($r = .68$), as well as significant negative correlations with the MMPI L ($r = -.20$) and K ($r = -.62$) scales in a mixed sample of sex offenders and sex offenders, police trainees, commu-nity volunteer controls, and nonviolent nonsex offenders. Separate correlations were not calculated for the individual samples. McNeil and Meyer (1990) provided partial replica-tion of these results in a sample of forensic inpatients classified as overreporting based on MMPI F scale scores; specifically, these authors reported that the Weight Factor Composite Score was significantly positively correlated with the MMPI F scale ($r = .72$) and significantly negatively correlated with the MMPI K scale ($r = -.57$) in this sample. McNeil and Meyer reverse-scored the Weight Factor Composite Score, thus the *r* values originally reported were $-.72$ for the correlation between the MMPI F scale and the Weight Factor Composite Score, and $.57$ for the correlation between the MMPI K scale and the Weight Factor Composite Score. For ease of comparison in this chapter, we re-versed the direction of the correlations.

responses (i.e., fake good or fake bad) or classified as either underreporting or bad based on external criteria. For example, Van Gorp and Meyer (1986) compared the MCMI Weight Factor Composite Scores of psychiatric inpatients and general medical inpatients asked to either respond honestly, fake good, or fake bad. These authors found that although respondents across both patient groups instructed to fake bad had higher Weight Factor Composite Scores than did those instructed to fake good, neither of these two conditions differed significantly from respondents instructed to complete the MCMI honestly (Van Gorp & Meyer, 1986). In contrast, Mc-Neil and Meyer (1990) reported that correctional inmates instructed to fake bad produced significantly higher Weight Factor Composite Scores than did those asked to respond honestly. Moreover, these authors found that forensic inpatients classified as overreporting based on MMPI F scale scores had significantly higher Weight Factor Composite Scores than did those with valid F scores, suggesting that the differences in Weight Factor Composite Scores could be generalized to a known group's sample.

The utility of the X scale, a revised version of the Weight Factor Composite Scores developed for the MCMI-II and retained for the MCMI-III, as a measure of overreporting is similarly unclear. Blais et al. (1995) reported significant negative correlations between X scores and MMPI-2 L ($r = -.34$), and K ($r = -.78$) in a psychiatric inpatient sample, consistent with previous results using the Weight Factor Composite Score and suggesting that the X scale may act as a measure of fake bad versus fake good response bias. In addition, however, these authors found that while scores on the X scale were significantly and positively correlated with scores on the MCMI-II Z scale ($r = .76$), which was specifically designed to assess overreporting, there was also a trend toward a positive correlation between X and Y scale scores ($r = .19$; Blais et al., 1995). In contrast, Grossman and Craig (1995) reported a significant positive correlation between the X scale and the Fake-Bad scale of the Sixteen Personality Factors Inventory ($r = .41$; 16PF; Cattell, Eber, & Tatsuoka, 1970, as cited in Grossman & Craig, 1995) and a significant negative correlation between the X scale and the 16- PF Fake-Good scale ($r = -.41$). Several studies have reported that scores on the X scale can discriminate students instructed to fake bad on the MCMI-II from those given either standard instructions or instructed to fake good (Bagby et al., 1990, 1991; Retzlaff et al., 1991); there is also preliminary evidence suggesting that X scale scores are lower among personal injury claimants classified as faking versus those classified as responding honestly based on the MMPI-2 (Lees-Haley, 1992). Yet, it is unclear whether this result can be generalized to other contexts. For example, Fals-Stewart (1995) reported that inpatients being treated for substance abuse who were instructed to fake good on the MCMI-II and individuals identified as underreporting who were being evaluated for substance dependence as part of a presentencing screening produced significantly lower scores on the X scale than did substance abuse inpatients given standard instructions. In contrast, Craig et al. (1994) found that X scale scores of inpatients being treated for substance abuse and/or dependence who were instructed to fake good did not differ from scores of those who were given standard instructions. However, a subsample of inpatients in the fake-good sample that produced valid scores on the relevant clinical syndrome scales (i.e., Drug Dependence and Alcohol Dependence scores within the normal range) were able to produce significantly lower X scale scores than did the inpatients responding to standard instructions.

A more recent study using the MCMI-III indicates that X scale scores are significantly higher among students instructed to fake bad as compared with either students or psychiatric inpatients responding to standard instructions (Schoenberg et al., 2003). Similar results have been reported for a within-group comparison of psychiatric inpatients responding to fake-bad versus standard instructions (Daubert & Metzler, 2000). In addition, there is preliminary evidence that psychiatric inpatients responding to fake good instructions are able to significantly lower scores on the X scale compared with their own responses produced under standard instructions (Daubert & Metzler, 2000).

There is mixed evidence that the V scale assesses overreporting in addition to irrelevant responding. Wierzbicki (1993) reported that both students instructed to respond honestly and those instructed to fake good produced significantly lower scores across 20 MCMI clinical scales and the V scale compared with students instructed to fake bad; however, no specific differences in V scale scores were published. Although this does not address whether the V scale does in fact assess confusion or lack of understanding of item content, it does suggest that higher scores may be associated with deliberate attempts to fake bad, thus presenting a potential confound for interpreting protocols in clinical contexts.

There is additional evidence based on studies using the MCMI-II that the deliberate instructions to fake bad result in significant elevations on the V scale. For example, Bagby et al. (1990) demonstrated that students instructed to fake bad produced significantly higher V scale scores than did students given standard instructions and students instructed to fake good. Similarly, Retzlaff et al. (1991) found that students faking bad produced significantly higher V scale scores than did students responding to standard instructions, although V scale scores of the students faking bad were still significantly lower than those from a sample of computer-generated profiles based on a 95% true endorsement rule. Interestingly,

Retzlaff et al. found that V scale scores of the students faking bad did not differ from those from a sample of computer-generated profiles based on a 95% false endorsement rule or those based on a 50% true endorsement rule. Unlike Bagby et al.'s results, V scale scores in the fake bad samples did not differ from those of students instructed to fake good. There have been no attempts to replicate these findings using the MCMI-III.

CLASSIFICATION ACCURACY

To date, the classification accuracy of the individual modifying indices in detecting irrelevant responding, overreporting, and underreporting remains uncertain due in part to the fact that few studies have examined this issue. Bagby et al. (1991) reported a mean overall correct classification (OCC) rate of 95.9% using an optimized cut-off score based on discriminant function analysis (DFA). This figure dropped slightly to 91% when adjusted for sample shrinkage. Although these results are promising, the stability of these figures is not established and additional research is needed.

In a study by Fals-Stewart (1995), the mean OCC rate was 58.9% using a cut-off score of Y scale > 75 on the MCMI-II for discriminating profiles produced by substance abuse patients instructed to fake good from substance abuse patients given standard instructions. The mean OCC rate in this study for discriminating forensic litigants identified as underreporting from the substance abuse patients given standard instructions was slightly higher, at 62.1%. Daubert and Metzler (2000) reported similar levels of accuracy using the MCMI-III to classify psychiatric outpatients instructed to fake good versus those given standard instructions; specifically, a cut-off score of Y scale > 85 was associated with an OCC rate of 64, while an optimal cut-off score of Y scale > 74 based on frequency distributions was associated with an improved OCC rate of 69.

The accuracy of the X and Z scales in detecting overreporting is variable. For example, Lees-Haley (1992) reported that the highest OCC rates possible for correctly classifying personal injury claimants determined to be overreporting versus those responding honestly based on the MMPI-2 were 73% using a cut-off score of X scale > 59 and 87% using a cut-off score of Z scale > 59. Using the MCMI-III, Daubert and Metzler (2000) found that a cut-off score of X scale > 84 correctly classified 71% of psychiatric outpatients instructed to fake bad versus those given standard instructions; the optimal cut-off score of X scale > 80 based on frequency distributions was associated with an OCC rate of 74%. For the same comparison, the standard cut-off score of Z scale > 85 was associated with an OCC rate of 64; the optimal cut-off score Z scale > 80 yielded an improved OCC rate of 71%. Finally, Schoenberg et al. (2003) reported an OCC rate of 63.4 for classifying students instructed to fake bad versus psychiatric inpatients using a cut-off score of Z scale > 62.

Several studies have examined classification accuracy using multiple modifying indices in combination. In general, this strategy is associated with greater accuracy than using individual scales. Using the MCMI-II, Bagby et al. (1990) used a stepwise DFA to assess the accuracy of the combination of V, X, Y, and Z scale scores for classifying students instructed to fake good, fake bad, or given standard instructions. A discriminant function composed of the V, Y, and Z scale scores correctly classified 84.4% of protocols in the initial classification phase and 66.7% of protocols when cross-validated; scores on the X scale did not enter into DFA. Wierzbicki (1997) reported that a discriminant function based on the same three modifying indices (V, Y, and Z scales) correctly classified 78.6% of protocols produced by students instructed to fake good versus those responding to standard instructions; OCC rates for classifying protocols produced by students instructed to fake bad ranged from 91.3% to 97.1% depending on specific instructions. A subsequent study by Bagby et al. (1991) found that a discriminant function composed of X, Y, and Z scale scores correctly classified 79.4% of protocols produced by students instructed to fake bad versus those responding to standard instructions in the initial phase and 70% in the cross-validation phase. A second discriminant function composed of X, Y, and Z scale scores correctly classified 74% of protocols produced by students instructed to fake good versus those responding to standard instructions in the initial phase and 72.6% in the cross-validation phase (Bagby et al., 1991). Finally, Daubert and Metzler (2000) found that using X, Y, and Z scale scores as multiple criteria for classifying protocols produced by adult psychiatric outpatients responding to fake good instructions versus those responding to standard instructions honestly was associated with OCC rates ranging from 70% to 74%; OCC rates associated with classifying protocols produced by adult psychiatric outpatients responding to fake good instructions versus those responding to standard instructions honestly using X, Y, and Z scale scores as multiple criteria ranged from 70% to 73%.

FUTURE DIRECTIONS

The most salient limitation of the literature regarding the MCMI modifying indices is the shortage of studies attempting to replicate or cross-validate previously published results. This precludes an evaluation of the utility of these scales for clinical purposes. As we argued earlier, response bias is a critical issue for clinical interpretation, and although most of the studies examined in this review have addressed the same research question, the methodological differences across these studies limit cross-study comparisons.

What can we conclude so far? The V scale appears to make clinically meaningful distinctions; however, there is also evidence that this scale is sensitive to deliberate attempts to overreport. The presence of this potential confound for interpretation warrants additional attention on the part of researchers. An expanded set of items may be needed to increase the construct validity of the V scale. Evidence supporting the utility of the X scale as a measure of overreporting is mixed, and convergent findings based on differential prevalence and known group designs is needed to determine the generalizability of previous results, which are based largely on analogue research designs. The Y scale is able to discriminate protocols produced by respondents deliberately instructed to underreport, yet classification accuracy in such settings is low. Likewise, the Z scale is able to discriminate protocols produced by respondents deliberately instructed to overreport, but stable classification accuracy rates have not been established. Future studies should continue to report group differences in scores on the modifying indices, but researchers should endeavor to use differential prevalence and known group designs with greater frequency. Moreover, effect sizes should be reported to facilitate cross-study comparisons. Additional information regarding the classification accuracy of the modifying indices is also recommended.

What is striking from this review is that the MCMI literature lags far behind that of other measures, most notably the MMPI-2 and PAI, in terms of capitalizing on methodological advances in response style and dissimulation research. Rogers (1997b) argued that to demonstrate the effectiveness of a specific scale, researchers must demonstrate convergent findings across several research designs, and that detection strategies underlying a given scale must be cross-validated across a variety of clinical samples. Although the MCMI literature examining the validity of the modifying indices has included several efforts to cross-validate results across different clinical comparison groups, researchers continue to rely almost exclusively on the analogue research design; thus, the effectiveness of the modifying indices has not yet been established. For example, only two studies (Daubert & Metzler, 2000; Schoenberg et al., 2003) examined the utility of the current MCMI-III modifying indices for discriminating feigned protocols from those completed under standard instructions, and both of these studies used between-groups, analogue research designs. Although this design has the advantage of convenience, there is evidence suggesting that different scales may not perform similarly across analogue and bona fide assessment contexts (Bagby & Marshall, 2004).To evaluate the utility of the modifying indices, MCMI researchers should therefore begin to make use of the differential prevalence design and the known group design. In the differential prevalence group design, a set of protocols from a group of respondents suspected of underreporting is compared to that of an honestly responding sample; in the known group design, scores on a measure or scale from a group of respondents who are independently identified as over- or underreporting (i.e., the known group) are analyzed for evidence of response dissimulation (Rogers, 1997b).

In addition to the use of nonanalogue designs, there are several other issues that should be addressed to bring the MCMI literature in line with current assessment literature based on alternative instruments. One such issue is the effect of coaching. Studies examining both underreporting (see, e.g., Butcher, Atlis, & Fang, 2000; Butcher, Morfitt, Rouse, & Holden, 1997; Cigrang & Staal, 2001) and overreporting (see, e.g., Bury & Bagby, 2002; Rogers, Bagby, & Chakraborty, 1993; Storm & Graham, 2000) suggest that the effectiveness of validity scales in detecting feigned protocols is substantially compromised when test takers are coached about the presence and operating characteristics of validity scales. Recent work using DFA suggests that scales designed to discriminate feigners from bona fide patients based on the overall validity scale profile may be less susceptible to the effects of coaching (Bacchiochi & Bagby, 2003, 2004; Rogers, Sewell, Morey, & Ustad, 1996). The development of scales for the MCMI-III that can accurately discriminate feigned protocols regardless of whether or not respondents are coached about the presence and operating characteristics of the modifying indices is necessary to advance the use of this instrument.

As noted by Rogers, Sewell, Martin, and Vitacco (2003), it also is important to examine the utility of overreporting validity scales based on different detection strategies. The MCMI-III V and Z scales both represent the rare symptoms strategy, with high scores indicating the endorsement of an unusually high number of rare symptoms; this strategy is based on the principle that individuals attempting to feign psychopathological symptoms are unable to distinguish rare symptoms from more common ones, the same principle underlying the MMPI-2 family of F scales (Rogers et al., 2003). Scales based on other detection strategies have also demonstrated utility in the detection of overreporting, and the development of supplementary scales for the MCMI-III based on other faking strategies is recommended. For example, scales based on the "erroneous stereotypes" detection strategy are designed to discriminate genuine patients from malingerers endorsing erroneous stereotypes regarding psychopathology (Rogers et al., 2003). Scales based on the "symptom severity" strategy are deigned to detect malingerers endorsing an unusually high number of disabling symptoms because they fail to account for symptom severity (Rogers et al., 2003). Finally, the strategy comparing "obvious and subtle symptoms" is based on the principle that feigners will tend to endorse more items that are obviously indicative of psychopathology as opposed to more subtle symptoms not recognized by laypersons (Rogers et al., 2003).

Regarding social desirability scales, results of several factor-analytic studies indicate that socially desirable responding consists of two response styles (e.g., Bagby & Marshall, 2004; Nichols & Greene, 1988, as cited in Nichols & Greene, 1997; Paulhus, 1984): self-deception and impression management. Self-deception has been broadly defined as a dispositional tendency to think of oneself in a favorable light; impression management refers to the deliberate attempt to distort one's responses to create a favorable impression on others. There is compelling evidence that the MMPI-2 underreporting validity scales have separate and unique associations with these two components; previous research regarding the MMPI-2 correlates of the Y scale are conflicted (Blais et al., 1995; cf. Morgan et al., 2002), suggesting that scores on the Y scale may reflect more than one of these forms of socially desirable responding. Future research examining the correlates of the Y scale with both the standard and supplementary scales of the MMPI-2 will be important for increasing our understanding of the operating characteristics of this scale.

Finally, classification rates for the MCMI-II and MCMI-III modifying indices have not been consistently reported across those studies that have examined this issue. For example, no studies have used the same cut-off scores when examining the classification accuracy of the individual modifying indices. Furthermore, the OCC rates are lower than those of the MMPI-2 scales, which are better validated than the MCMI modifying indices. Studies using multiple indices in combination have reported higher levels of classification accuracy, suggesting that this may be a more accurate method for identifying feigned protocols, although there have been insufficient studies examining this issue to justify the use of this method in clinical settings (see, e.g., Bagby et al., 1990, 1991).

CONCLUSIONS

Overall, the MCMI modifying indices appear somewhat effective in detecting underreporting, overreporting, and inconsistent response biases when respondents are deliberately instructed to feign. In spite of this, there is insufficient evidence regarding the generalizability of results based on analogue research designs to draw conclusions regarding the utility of the modifying indices in real-world settings; thus, research examining the utility of the modifying indices has only partially demonstrated the utility of these scales for identifying invalidating conditions. Given that the assessment of response bias is such a critical issue for clinicians involved in the assessment of personality psychopathology, further research addressing the utility of the MCMI modifying indices is imperative to justify the continued clinical use of this instrument.

REFERENCES

American Psychiatric Association. (1987). *Diagnostic and statistical manual of mental disorders* (3rd ed., rev.). Washington, DC: Author.

American Psychiatric Association. (1994). *Diagnostic and statistical manual of mental disorders* (4th ed.). Washington, DC: Author.

Bacchiochi, J. R., & Bagby, R. M. (2003, June). *Development of the malingering discriminant function index (M-DFI)*. Paper presented at the 38th annual Workshop and Symposium on the MMPI-2 and MMPI-A, Minneapolis, MN.

Bacchiochi, J. R., & Bagby, R. M. (2004, March). *Validation of the Malingering Discriminant Function (MDFI) for the MMPI-2*. Paper presented at the 2004 Midwinter Meeting of the Society for Personality Assessment, Miami, FL.

Baer, R. A., & Miller, J. (2002). Underreporting of psychopathology on the MMPI-2: A meta-analytic review. *Psychological Assessment, 14*, 16–26.

Bagby, R. M., Gillis, J. R., & Dickens, S. (1990). Detection of dissimulation with the new generation of objective personality measures. *Behavioral Sciences and the Law, 8*, 93–102.

Bagby, R. M., Gillis, J. R., & Rogers, R. (1991). Effectiveness of the Millon Clinical Multiaxial Inventory Validity Index in the detection of random responding. *Psychological Assessment, 3*, 285–287.

Bagby, R. M., Gillis, J. R., Toner, B. B., & Goldberg, J. (1991). Detecting fake-good and fake-bad responding on the Millon Clinical Multiaxial Personality Inventory-II. *Psychological Assessment, 3*, 496–498.

Bagby, R. M., & Marshall, M. B. (2004). Assessing underreporting response bias on the MMPI-2. *Assessment, 11*, 115–126.

Blais, M. A., Benedict, K. B., & Norman, D. K. (1995). Concurrent validity of the MCMI-II modifier indices. *Journal of Clinical Psychology, 51*, 783–789.

Bury, A. S., & Bagby, R. M. (2002). The detection of feigned uncoached and coached posttraumatic stress disorder with the MMPI-2 in a sample of workplace accident victims. *Psychological Assessment, 14*, 472–484.

Butcher, J. N., Atlis, M. M., & Fang, L. (2000). Effect of altered instructions on the MMPI-2 profiles of college students who are not motivated to distort their responses. *Journal of Personality Assessment, 75*, 492–501.

Butcher, J., Graham, J., Ben-Porath, Y. S., Tellegen, A., Dahlstrom, W., & Kaemmer, B. (2001). *Minnesota Multiphasic Personality Inventory-2 (MMPI-2): Manual for administration, scoring, and interpretation-Revised Edition*. Minneapolis, MN: University of Minnesota Press.

Butcher, J. N., Morfitt, R. C., Rouse, S. V., & Holden, R. R. (1997). Reducing MMPI-2 defensiveness: The effect of specialized instructions on retest validity in a job applicant sample. *Journal of Personality Assessment, 68,* 385–401.

Charter, R. A., & Lopez, M. N. (2002). Millon Clinical Multiaxial Inventory (MCMI-III): The inability of the validity conditions to detect random responding. *Journal of Clinical Psychology, 58,* 1615–1617.

Cigrang, J. A., & Staal, M. A. (2001). Readministration of the MMPI-2 following defensive invalidation in a military job applicant sample. *Journal of Personality Assessment, 76,* 472–481.

Craig, R. J. (1999). Essentials of MCMI-III assessment. In S. Strack (Ed.), *Essentials of Millon Inventories Assessment* (pp. 1–51). New York: Wiley.

Craig, R. J., Kuncel, R., & Olson, R. E. (1994). Ability of drug addicts to avoid detection of substance abuse on the MCMI-II. *Journal of Social Behavior and Personality, 9,* 95–106.

Daubert, S. D., & Metzler, A. E. (2000). The detection of fake-bad and fake-good responding on the Millon Clinical Multiaxial Inventory-III. *Psychological Assessment, 12,* 418–424.

Fals-Stewart, W. (1995). The effect of defensive responding by substance-abusing patients on the Millon Clinical Multiaxial Inventory. *Journal of Personality Assessment, 64,* 540–551.

Grossman, L. S., & Craig, R. J. (1995). Comparison of MCMI-II and 16 PF validity scales. *Journal of Personality Assessment, 64,* 384–389.

Langevin, R., Lang, R., Reynolds, R., Wright, P., Garrels, D., Marchese, V., et al. (1988). Personality and sexual anomalies: An examination of the Millon Clinical Multiaxial Inventory. *Annals of Sexual Research, 1,* 13–32.

Lees-Haley, P. R. (1992). Efficacy of MMPI-2 validity scales and MCMI-II modifier scales for detecting spurious PTSD claims: F, F-K, Faked Bad Scale, Ego Strength, Subtle-Obvious subscales, D. I. S., & DEB. *Journal of Clinical Psychology, 48,* 681–689.

McNeil, K., & Meyer, R. G. (1990). Detection of deception on the Millon Clinical Multiaxial Inventory (MCMI) *Journal of Clinical Psychology, 46,* 755–764.

Millon, T. (1983). *Millon Clinical Multiaxial Inventory manual.* Minneapolis, MN: National Computer Systems.

Millon, T. (1987). *Manual for the MCMI-II* (2nd ed.). Minneapolis, MN: National Computer Systems.

Millon, T. (1990). *Toward a new personology.* New York: Wiley.

Millon, T., & Davis, R. D. (1996). *Disorders of personality: DSM-IV and beyond* (2nd ed.). New York: Wiley.

Millon, T., Millon, C., & Davis, R. (1997). Manual for the Millon Clinical Multiaxial Inventory-III (MCMI-III) (2nd ed.). Minneapolis, MN: National Computer Systems.

Morey, L. C. (1991). *The Personality Assessment Inventory.* Lutz, FL: Psychological Assessment Resources.

Morgan, C. D., Schoenberg, M. R., Dorr, D., & Burke, M. J. (2002). Overreport on the MCMI-III: Concurrent validation with the MMPI-2 using a psychiatric inpatient sample. *Journal of Personality Assessment, 78,* 288–300.

Nichols, D. S., & Greene, R. L. (1997). Dimensions of deception in personality assessment: The example of the MMPI-2. *Journal of Personality Assessment, 68,* 251–266.

Paulhus, D. L. (1984). Two-component models of socially desirable responding. *Personality and Individual Differences, 46,* 598–609.

Retzlaff, P., Sheehan, E., & Fiel, A. (1991). MCMI-II report style and bias: Profile and validity scale analysis. *Journal of Personality Assessment, 56,* 466–477.

Retzlaff, P., Sheehan, E., & Lorr, M. (1990). MCMI-II scoring: Weighted and unweighted algorithms. *Journal of Personality Assessment, 55,* 219–223.

Rogers, R. (1997a). Current status of clinical methods. In R. Rogers (Ed.), *Clinical assessment of malingering and deception* (2nd ed., pp. 373–397). New York: Guilford Press.

Rogers, R. (1997b). Researching dissimulation. In R. Rogers (Ed.), *Clinical assessment of malingering and deception* (2nd ed., pp. 398–426). New York: Guilford Press.

Rogers, R., Bagby, R. M., & Chakraborty, D. (1993). Feigning schizophrenic disorder on the MMPI-2: Detection of coached simulators. *Journal of Personality Assessment, 60,* 215–226.

Rogers, R., Sewell, K. W., Martin, M. A., & Vitacco, M. J. (2003). Detection of feigned mental disorders: A meta-analysis of the MMPI-2 and malingering. *Assessment, 10,* 160–177.

Rogers, R., Sewell, K. W., Morey, L. C., & Ustad, K. L. (1996). Detection of feigned mental disorders on the Personality Assessment Inventory: A discriminant analysis. *Journal of Personality Assessment, 67,* 629–640.

Schoenberg, M. R., Dorr, D., & Morgan, C. D. (2003). The ability of the Millon Clinical Multiaxial Inventory-third edition to detect malingering. *Psychological Assessment, 15,* 198–204.

Storm, J., & Graham, J. R. (2000). Detection of coached general malingering on the MMPI-2. *Psychological Assessment, 12,* 158–165.

Streiner, D. L., Goldberg, J. O., & Miller, H. R. (1993). MCMI-II item weights: Their lack of effectiveness. *Journal of Personality Assessment, 60,* 471–476.

Van Gorp, W. G., & Meyer, R. G. (1986). The detection of faking on the Millon Clinical Multiaxial Inventory (MCMI). *Journal of Clinical Psychology, 42,* 742–747.

Wetzler, S., & Marlowe, D. (1990). "Faking bad" on MMPI, MMPI-2, and Millon-II. *Psychological Reports, 67,* 1117–1118.

Wierzbicki, M. (1993). Use of the MCMI subtle and obvious subscales to detect faking. *Journal of Clinical Psychology, 49,* 809–814.

Wierzbicki, M. (1997). Use of subtle and obvious scales to detect faking on the MCMI-II. *Journal of Clinical Psychology, 53,* 421–426.

CHAPTER 11

Validity of the MCMI-III™ in the Description and Diagnosis of Psychopathology

ANDREW G. RYDER AND SCOTT WETZLER

THE PUBLICATION of the third edition of the *Diagnostic and Statistical Manual for Mental Disorders* (*DSM-III*; American Psychiatric Association, 1980) introduced a formal separation between acute psychopathology on Axis I and personality disorders (PDs) on Axis II. Moreover, disorders on both axes were now described using formal operationalized criteria. These two innovations led to renewed research interest into the PDs (Livesley, 1998), an interest that was further encouraged by the publication of the original Millon Clinical Multiaxial Inventory (MCMI; Millon, 1983). By developing separate sets of scales for PDs and clinical syndromes and by keying the PD scales, in particular, to *DSM* constructs, the MCMI was well-situated to benefit clinicians and researchers who wanted to take advantage of the multiaxial approach. At the same time, the MCMI was developed based on Millon's biosocial model, thus providing test users with rich theoretical descriptions of PDs in contrast to the putatively atheoretical *DSM*.

Since this original publication, the MCMI-II (Millon, 1987) and MCMI-III (Millon, Millon, & Davis, 1994) have been released, keeping pace with successive editions of the *DSM*. Changing the instrument has ensured

This manuscript was prepared while the first author was a predoctoral intern in clinical psychology at Montefiore Medical Center, Bronx, NY.

that it remains linked to the diagnostic system and has provided the opportunity to improve the instrument in light of published research. On the other hand, the extensive nature of the revisions has called into question the extent to which research on older versions of the MCMI can be used to evaluate the most recent version, the MCMI-III. This latest edition, published in 1994, replaced over half of the items, changed the item-weighting system, significantly shortened the individual scales, and added two new scales (Rogers, Salekin, & Sewell, 1999). Moreover, the underlying theory has shifted from being primarily focused on behavioral principles (Millon, 1969) to a comprehensive system based on evolutionary theory (Millon & Davis, 1996). PDs are now ". . . seen as evolutionary constructs derived from the fundamental tasks that all organisms confront [that are] manifest across the entire matrix of the person, with expression throughout several clinical domains." (Millon & Meagher, 2004, p. 108) An evaluation of the MCMI-III, while it may use the conclusions from older research as a starting point, should be based as much as possible on research conducted using the latest edition. Such an evaluation, in the context of the instrument's validity and clinical utility in the assessment of psychopathology, is the major objective of this chapter.

OVERALL VALIDITY

Wetzler (1990) published a review of the original MCMI, evaluating several important domains of validity. This paper noted that both the content and the concurrent validity of the instrument appeared to be promising but suffered from a lack of research attention. Content validity, in particular, had not often been formally assessed, and concurrent validity had largely been limited to studies using self-report questionnaires. Factorial validity, meanwhile, was demonstrated by similar factor structures emerging in a variety of different samples. Finally, the MCMI was shown to be effective in detecting depression but considerably less so in the detection of mania and, especially, psychosis. The first part of this chapter reexamines Wetzler's conclusions for the MCMI-III, evaluating the content, concurrent, factorial, and diagnostic validity of this instrument using research published over the past ten years.

CONTENT VALIDITY

Wetzler (1990) reported findings suggesting that content validity had been established for the MCMI Paranoid, Dependent, and Avoidant scales using informal analysis. More formal content analysis by Widiger, Williams, Spitzer, and Francis (1985) demonstrated that the Antisocial scale was closer to the construct of psychopathy than the *DSM-III* disorder and that the Histrionic scale did not include features of shallowness, manipulativeness, and self-dramatization. Formal content analyses of the other scales have not been conducted.

In the second edition of the MCMI-III manual, Millon, Davis, and Millon (1997) describe the process leading to the development of the various versions of the MCMI, and we do not review this material here. Suffice it to say that the original MCMI was based on a clearly outlined model of personality and psychopathology. The research team selected from a pool of over 3,500 items to find sets matching each clinical construct, and these selections were then evaluated by a panel of eight mental health professionals. The combination of a clearly stated theory and careful procedures with empirical checks is strongly suggestive of good content validity. Unfortunately, the benefits of this approach do not extend to items new to the MCMI-III, where the research team adopted a considerably less stringent approach: "A substantial pool of new items for the MCMI-III was generated through the expert judgment of the senior author. These were then subjected to a rational scrutiny by research associates who worked on the revision project" (Millon et al., 1997, p. 26). Although we believe that it is reasonable to expect that the senior author would have an excellent grasp of his own theory, the lack of additional checks makes it more difficult to evaluate these new items (Rogers, Salekin, & Sewell, 2000). As a result, the content validity of the MCMI-III awaits a more careful evaluation.

CONSTRUCT VALIDITY

Wetzler's (1990) review of the original MCMI concluded that the various scales correlated with other self-report measures in expected ways, albeit with moderate correlations. It was argued that correlations with other assessment methods not based on self-report are more useful for the evaluation of concurrent validity. The Avoidant, Dependent, Dysthymia, Major Depression (at that time, Psychotic Depression), and Bipolar Mania (at that time, Hypomania) scales were found to exhibit adequate correlations with appropriate observer rating scales, but the Antisocial and Passive-Aggressive scales were considerably less impressive. The Avoidant scale, meanwhile, failed to show adequate discrimination. Unfortunately, there is still a lack of convergent validity studies in this area using different assessment methods, so the discussion of the MCMI-III that follows is based on self-report methods and does not avoid the problems of shared method variance. We therefore repeat the call for more research using a wider range of methodologies.

The MCMI-III manual evaluated construct validity by comparing the instrument with several collateral scales. However, the selected instruments are primarily relevant to Axis I psychopathology; no other measures of normal or abnormal personality were included. As no a priori theoretical expectations are provided, the approach taken is to simply go through the different collateral instruments and note the highly significant correlations obtained with specific MCMI-III scales. Unfortunately, although many of the high correlations make sense, many additional high correlations suggest a lack of discrimination. For example, the Hypomania subscale of the General Behavior Inventory has an expected correlation with MCMI-III Bipolar Mania, but has similar correlations with the Schizoid, Avoidant, Depressive, Negativistic, and Masochistic scales. Perhaps one could develop an explanation for why Hypomania is positively related to Schizoid PD and negatively with Histrionic PD, but such a theory would not follow from Millon's theory and in any event is not discussed in the text. This problem of poor discrimination is also addressed by Rogers and colleagues (1999), who argue that, in many cases, discriminant validity coefficients actually exceed convergent validity coefficients. The problem is attributable, in large part, to the high degree of intercorrelation between most of the MCMI-III scales; the clinician must keep this issue in mind when interpreting specific profiles.

Two studies have taken a different approach to assessing the convergent validity of the MCMI-III, with somewhat more promising results for the instrument. Craig and Olson (2001) found that most of the personality scales were moderately to highly correlated with self-descriptive adjectives that were expected to be related to the *DSM-IV* PDs. Only the Narcissistic and Compulsive scales showed problems, in both cases potentially attributable to the nonpathological aspects of these constructs. Locke (2000), meanwhile, compared the MCMI-III personality scales with scales measuring interpersonal features using the Circumplex Scales of Interpersonal Values. Only the Compulsive scale did not match predictions based on previous research, again because the scale appeared to be more prosocial than psychopathological. Both of these studies help to shed light on the constructs being measured by the various MCMI-III personality scales and suggest that caution should be used in interpreting the Compulsive scale.

FACTORIAL (STRUCTURAL) VALIDITY

A theory-driven instrument such as the MCMI-III should have an empirically observed structure corresponding to the structure predicted by the theory. Although Millon's complex model is not particularly amenable to standard factor-analytic techniques (Dyce, O'Connor, Parkins, & Janzin, 1997), some examples of theoretical constraints implied by this model are provided in the MCMI-III manual. In one case, Millon and colleagues (1997) note that the Narcissistic and Dependent scales should be related to one another, as both are passive patterns. Unfortunately, rather than testing these hypotheses, the manual simply presents a correlation matrix and states that the pattern is congruent with the evolutionary model; a look at the matrix reveals that the Narcissistic and Dependent scales are in fact correlated at −.55. Meanwhile, Histrionic PD is a low self, high other, active orientation, whereas Narcissistic PD is a high self, low other, passive orientation, yet these two prototypes are correlated at .70. The fit between the theory and the data leaves much to be desired.

Wetzler (1990) noted that factor analyses of the MCMI raw scale scores showed good stability over a range of patient populations, although it was noted that good stability in this case could be a product of high item overlap. A factor analysis by Strauman and Wetzler (1992) was found to be typical, with three dimensions being identified: depressive emotionality, paranoid and manic thinking, and schizoid thinking. Wetzler noted that these three factors correspond to the three pathological personality styles, Borderline, Paranoid, and Schizoid, respectively. The relation between these dimensions and the three DSM PD clusters was also explored and found to be less clear, although the validity of the cluster system itself has not been well established (Yang, Bagby, Ryder, & Costa, 2002).

Craig and Bivens (1998) also identified a three-factor solution for the MCMI-III and named these factors general maladjustment, paranoid behavior/thinking with emotional detachment, and antisocial acting-out. However, the pattern of loadings revealed a substantially different structure as compared with the analysis by Strauman and Wetzler (1992). Dyce and colleagues (1997) also found that the MCMI-III showed only modest correspondence with previous versions of the instrument, but added that this correspondence improves considerably when nonoverlapping versions of the scales are used. The authors also found excellent stability within versions of the MCMI. Again, one of the problems with comparing across versions appears to be the major changes in the extent of item overlap. More troubling for the general PD literature, the authors also note that the various MCMI PD correlation matrices are not strongly related to PD matrices using other assessment methods; as well, the various other methods are not strongly associated with each other.

Empirical efforts to confirm Millon's underlying theories have not been well supported in the literature. Dyce and colleagues (1997) tested numerous PD configurations and found a poor fit for models corresponding to the evolutionary model. Millon (1987) also proposed a circular organization of the PDs around two poles, representing affiliation and emotionality. Strack, Choca, and Gurtman (2001) tested this model statistically and found a moderate level of fit only when acquiescence bias was controlled, nonoverlapping scores were used, and two key assumptions of circumplex organization were relaxed. Even still, one of the two dimensions had to be changed to represent impulsivity versus compulsivity. These findings suggest, at best, that Millon's PD system could potentially be expressed as a circumplex if improvements were made both to the instrument and to the theory.

DIAGNOSTIC VALIDITY

Wetzler (1990) reported that, for the original MCMI, three studies comparing PD diagnoses with clinical judgment consistently found that the test diagnosed more PDs than did the practicing clinician. Notably, however, three additional studies found that the MCMI had good diagnostic efficiency in comparison with a structured interview, raising the possibility that the MCMI is in fact a better Axis II diagnostician than is the typical practitioner. For Axis I, the quality of the MCMI is dependent on the specific scale and disorder. Wetzler concluded that the Dysthymia scale showed moderately good diagnostic validity for Major Depression, but that the Hypomanic (now Mania), Psychotic Depression (now Major Depression), and Psychotic Thinking (now Thought Disorder) scales showed very poor diagnostic validity for Mania, Major Depression, and Schizophrenia, respectively. Millon and colleagues (1997) present sensitivity and positive predictive power for both the MCMI and MCMI-II, demonstrating a modest improvement, albeit with some individual scales showing a decline with the later version. On the MCMI, some of the weakest scales were for those constructs in which Millon's models differed most notably from *DSM*. On the MCMI-II, meanwhile, there was a notable drop on most scales measuring constructs with psychotic features, namely, the Schizoid scale and the three severe PDs.

When the MCMI-III was first published (Millon, 1994), only sensitivity and specificity were provided. Retzlaff (1996) calculated positive predictive power and negative predictive power using other data presented in the manual and found mean values of .22 (range = .00 to .58) and .89 (range = .30 to .99), respectively. These results for positive predictive power are, to say the least, problematic; on average, when a scale indicates a disorder is present, that disorder is actually present less than one quarter of the time. The second edition of the MCMI-III manual was published three years later and contained a new study of diagnostic validity using a smaller sample. The differences were dramatic, with positive predictive power now having a mean of .64 (range = .30 to .93). Hsu (2002) presented a range of additional diagnostic validity statistics, including the incremental improvement in positive predictive power that a test provides over chance, and found a mean increase from .11 to .61, a greater than fivefold improvement.

These wildly discrepant results deserve explanation, as the clinician's confidence in this instrument rises and falls dramatically depending on which study is referenced. Whereas the first study shows that even the Dysthymia scale is no longer a good indicator, the second study is resoundingly positive, showing particularly marked improvements for Major Depression, Mania, and Thought Disorder since the original MCMI. Retzlaff (1996) correctly notes that poor validity statistics do not necessarily indicate a poor test, and several authors have noted that the original study was indeed not well designed (Hsu, 2002; Millon et al., 1997; Retzlaff, 1996). Clinicians were asked to make diagnoses based on brand new *DSM-IV* criteria and at the same time had to include diagnoses for constructs that had been dropped from *DSM-IV* specifically because they were poorly established (Retzlaff, 1996). More problematic, patients were generally seen only once, and clinicians had an unknown degree of sophistication with PDs (Millon et al., 1997). In the 1997 study, by contrast, patients were seen a minimum of three times and clinicians were selected who had extensive previous experience with PDs in general and with Millon's model in particular.

In considering these striking differences, Hsu (2002) concurs with the view that the 1994 study underestimated diagnostic validity, but in addition argues that the 1997 study had design features that would lead to an overestimation. Most critical, the design of the latter study allowed for criterion contamination. Whereas in the original study, the clinician made the diagnostic ratings while the provisional MCMI-III was being completed by the patient, clinicians in the later study most often made diagnostic ratings long after the MCMI-III had been completed. Indeed, clinicians were told, "To ensure a sample of adequate size, we are encouraging the inclusion of patients whose MCMI-III results have already been obtained" (Millon et al., 1997, p. 89). Although clinicians were also warned not to include patients whose actual scores were clearly recalled, it is hard to imagine that their diagnostic conclusions were uninformed by the instrument (Rogers et al., 2000). The end result is that the diagnostic validity of the MCMI-III remains very much in question and awaits evaluation using, at a minimum, the kinds of studies that were conducted for the first two versions of the instrument.

PROFILE ANALYSIS

Traditional validity characteristics represent only one part of determining whether an instrument is useful for specific assessment situations that occur in clinical practice. It is, of course, important to be confident that scales measuring delusions and Thought Disorder, for example, are related to clinical syndromes such as Schizophrenia, but it is unlikely that a psychologist would be asked to administer an instrument such as the MCMI-III simply to determine whether or not Schizophrenia is present (Wetzler, Marlowe, & Sanderson, 1994). More frequently, the referral source is confident about the Axis I diagnosis and instead has other concerns, such as the clinical presentation, associated personality features, and implications for treatment (Wetzler, 1989). The second part of this chapter, therefore, focuses on specific assessment issues that arise in clinical practice and that afford the opportunity for the testing psychologist to make the greatest incremental contribution. We begin with a consideration of the state-trait issue and evaluate the extent to which the clinician can assume that the MCMI-III PD scales are measuring long-standing traits even in the context of acute distress. Then we evaluate the capacity of the MCMI-III to describe and differentiate patients with Unipolar Depression, Bipolar Disorder, and anxiety disorders, respectively. We conclude with an evaluation of two scales new to the MCMI-III, Depressive PD and PTSD. In each of these cases, we begin with a brief description of research findings based on previous versions of the MCMI and then evaluate whether these conclusions remain true for the MCMI-III.

THE STATE-TRAIT DISTINCTION

One feature of the MCMI-III that is potentially useful to clinicians is the distinction between the PD and Clinical Syndrome scales. The PD scales are designed to assess long-standing and stable aspects of character, whereas the Clinical Syndrome scales represent the acute symptomatic features of a current psychiatric illness; this distinction mirrors the separation between Axis I and Axis II. Ideally, the clinician is able to get a glimpse of underlying personality features that have persisted far longer than the immediate reason for seeking treatment, features that would be particularly resistant to change. The state-trait distinction thus has implications for treatment planning, the proper interpretation of scale elevations, and even for etiological hypotheses regarding the emergence of psychiatric illness from dysfunctional personality patterns.

Actually making this distinction, however, is difficult enough using a careful interview and becomes even more challenging when relying on a self-report inventory (Wetzler, 1990). Hirschfeld and colleagues (1983) have argued that changes in personality traits with acute syndrome change suggest that these putatively stable entities do not have a clinically significant independent existence. This perspective represents a serious attack on personality models such as Millon's, which propose that PDs may predispose individuals to acute Axis I syndromes. Bagby and Ryder (2000) note, however, that such a view overemphasizes the importance of absolute stability at the expense of relative stability. The latter property, assessed by test-retest correlations over the course of treatment, demonstrates the extent to which a personality trait remains a clinically meaningful entity in the context of acute change. Both forms of stability are important, and each has different implications for the proper interpretation of personality scales. Moreover, significant change in these scores should not be evaluated without consideration of the observed effect size; small but significant changes may not be clinically meaningful.

The original MCMI was used to estimate the prevalence and type of PDs associated with Axis I conditions (e.g., Reich & Troughton, 1988; Wetzler, Kahn, Cahn, Van Praag, & Asnis, 1990). Using BR $\geq$ 84, Wetzler (1990) noted that MCMI-based prevalence estimates of PDs were around 60% higher than estimates based on other methods and dropped by about 50% after recovery from the acute episode; such findings indicate a marked lack of absolute stability. Millon (1983) argued that because Clinical Syndrome scales are less stable than the PD scales over the course of treatment (average test-retest reliabilities of .67 and .80, respectively), the MCMI can make the state-trait distinction. A high test-retest coefficient certainly supports the relative stability of these scales, although whether a relatively small correlational difference should be interpreted as evidence of the state-trait distinction is unclear. More important, such an approach overlooks the potential weaknesses of individual scales. Piersma (1987), for example, found a low stability coefficient ($r = .27$) for the Borderline scale during a 5-week hospitalization. Such a result suggests that the MCMI-II Borderline scale should not be interpreted as evidence of long-standing personality pathology when assessed in the context of acute distress.

Following up on this work, Piersma and Boes (1997) conducted a treatment-outcome study using the MCMI-III. Setting a significance criteria of $p < .01$, they found that the Avoidant, Depressive, Aggressive, Passive-Aggressive, Borderline, and Paranoid personality scales decreased and the Histrionic, Narcissistic, and Compulsive scales increased 7 to 10 days following a psychiatric admission. The remaining personality scales showed nonsignificant decreases. Looking at Piersma and Boes's tabled data, we observe that the 11 decreasing scales change by an average of 6.5 BR score points and the 3 increasing scales change by an average of 4.7 BR score points. Taken together, the PD scales have a test-retest reliability of $r = .70$.

Only two of the scales have reliabilities of less than .60, namely, the Schizoid ($r = .52$) and Dependent ($r = .48$); the Borderline scale, meanwhile, has a markedly improved stability compared with the original MCMI ($r = .69$). The Clinical Syndrome scales decreased by an average of 10.1 BR score points and have an average test-retest reliability of $r = .63$.

The clinician may use the MCMI-III secure in the knowledge that none of the scales has disastrous relative stability coefficients like that found for the Borderline scale on the original MCMI. At the same time, the absolute stability for some scales remains problematic. For an instrument such as the MCMI-III, which uses BR scores to determine whether a diagnostic threshold has been passed, even small fluctuations can have implications for the classification of patients into clinical prototypes. Four PD scales showed a shift of at least 8 BR score points in the context of acute change: the Depressive (8.1), Avoidant (10.9), Passive-Aggressive (8.36), and Borderline (8.8). These changes occurred despite the MCMI-II's inclusion of corrective procedures designed to moderate PD scale scores when the Anxiety and/or Dysthymia scales are elevated. One should also keep in mind that this instability was found in a sample of patients hospitalized for their mood disorder, thus maximizing the distress and disorganization of these patients at intake.

Elevated PD scale scores in the context of acute psychopathology are far from invalid but need to be interpreted with caution. Scores higher than the upper cut-off of BR $\geq$ 85 can be safely interpreted but must be considered with increasing care as they approach the lower cut-off of BR $\geq$ 75. The MCMI-III PD scales contain both trait and state elements, as do previous versions of the instrument (Wetzler, 1990), and it is difficult to make a clear distinction between them as scores approach this lower cut-off. We concur with Choca and Van Denburg's (1997) argument that the personality scales are measuring the likelihood that a particular style is present, rather than necessarily indicating the presence of a PD. We would further contend that even when acute psychopathology is exaggerating PD scale scores, these elevations still provide the clinician with insight into the distressed patient's functioning. It would be risky to assume that a depressed patient with a Dependent score of BR = 78 has a long-standing dependent style, let alone a *DSM-IV* PD. We nonetheless do learn that this patient has, while depressed, a tendency to view himself or herself as a person who clings to others and is afraid of losing them. Such information, properly considered, remains clinically valuable.

The upward change in the Histrionic, Narcissistic, and Compulsive scales suggests that particular care must be used in their interpretation. This finding is of a piece with earlier descriptions of these scales as being negatively associated with the other MCMI-III scales, as well as being negatively associated with external measures of psychopathology. It appears that healthy functioning is associated with at least a moderate elevation on these scales, thus creating a risk of overpathologizing. Although MCMI-III scales are not designed to be interpreted when BR scores are below the cut-off, the clinician should consider the possibility of a poor self-concept when these scales are particularly low. At the same time, it is highly clinically significant when a mood disordered patient nonetheless produces an elevation on any of these scales. As with the other PD scales, these three scales can be used to generate reasonable hypotheses regardless of acute symptomatology, but conclusions about long-standing patterns should be tentative until stability following symptom resolution is observed.

MOOD DISORDERS

Wetzler and Marlowe (1993) found that patients diagnosed with Major Depressive Disorder had elevations on the Anxiety and Dysthymia Clinical Syndrome scales, as well as on the Avoidant, Dependent, and Borderline PD scales, compared with a heterogeneous patient comparison sample. The MCMI-II showed additional elevations on the Compulsive and Self-Defeating scales, indicating inwardly directed anger and rigid conformity. This study supported the diagnostic efficiency of the Dysthymia scale in the prediction of depression, but found poor results for the Psychotic Depression (now Major Depression) scale, in keeping with previous research. The authors also examined individuals in the manic state of a bipolar illness and found that scales designed specifically to assess for mania—MCMI Hypomania and MCMI-II Bipolar—were not sufficiently sensitive to detect mania in a consistent manner, replicating previous work. Although such a finding could be attributed to a social desirability bias during the manic phase, Wetzler, Khadivi, and Oppenheim (1995) reported that bipolar patients do not produce normal profiles while they are in the depressed phase. Neither the MCMI nor the MCMI-II scales were able to identify the presence of past manic episodes, and both groups of patients produced similar elevations on the Anxiety and Dysthymia scales. However, unipolar depressed patients also had PD scale elevations on the MCMI Dependent and Borderline scales and the MCMI-II Avoidant and Dependent scales; bipolar depressed patients, meanwhile, had elevations on the MCMI Passive-Aggressive and Borderline scales and the MCMI-II Dependent and Compulsive scales.

According to the second edition of the MCMI-III manual (Millon et al., 1997), and using a cut-off of BR = 85, the Major Depression scale was able to detect 65% of patients with this syndrome and 84% of patients for whom Major Depressive Disorder was the most prominent syndrome. An observed elevation on the Major Depression scale, meanwhile, resulted in a correct diagnosis 72% of the time. These figures show a marked improvement from previous versions of the scale. The Bipolar Manic scale was able to detect 44% of the patients with this syndrome and 64% of patients for whom Bipolar Disorder was the most prominent syndrome. An observed elevation on the Bipolar Manic scale, meanwhile, resulted in a correct diagnosis 57% of the time. These results are in the same range as those reported for the MCMI and MCMI-II and suggest, contra Goodwin and Jamison (1990), that patients with Bipolar Disorder can produce clinically meaningful test profiles. Surprisingly, the Dysthymia scale was less sensitive to Dysthymic Disorder than in previous versions, although interpretation of elevations on this scale was somewhat improved. The manual does not provide information on the diagnostic efficiency of the Dysthymia scale in the prediction of Major Depression. These results should be interpreted with caution given the continuing uncertainty about the potential for overestimation of diagnostic validity in the 1997 standardization study.

Until further research is conducted to clarify the situation, clinicians should interpret elevations on either the Major Depression or Dysthymia scale as potential evidence of a Major Depressive Episode. An elevation on Dysthymia alone may suggest a Major Depressive Episode as well, or may instead indicate the presence of Dysthymic Disorder. If a Major Depressive Episode has already been identified, an elevation on the Bipolar Manic scale suggests that Bipolar Disorder is present. The absence of such an elevation, in contrast, says little as to whether the depression being considered is unipolar or bipolar. Research based on previous versions of the MCMI suggested that a relatively high Narcissistic score may be associated with a bipolar illness. In the MCMI-III, the Narcissistic scale is negatively associated with most forms of psychopathology, including Major Depression, but lacks a significant correlation with MCMI-III Bipolar Mania, the Hypomania scale on the General Behavior Inventory, or Scale 9 of the MMPI-2. These findings are not sufficient to show that elevations on the Narcissistic scale necessarily indicate bipolar depression, but instead suggest that such an elevation provides a hypothesis that can be further tested using other methods, such as a clinical or structured interview. If, on the other hand, a diagnosis of Bipolar Disorder has already been established, elevations on the Narcissistic scale are more safely interpreted as part of the grandiosity that comes with mania and should not be seen as part of a long-standing personality pattern unless other data sources point in that direction.

ANXIETY DISORDERS

The Millon inventory does not contain scales keyed to the specific anxiety disorders, but instead has a single index of Anxiety. What research has been conducted in this area has tended to focus on the separation of anxiety and depression. Wetzler and colleagues (1990) compared patients with Panic Disorder, patients with Major Depressive Disorder, and normal controls. The only difference identified was that the depressed group had greater self-reported depression. No discrimination was provided by the MCMI Anxiety scale, which previous research has shown to be elevated in depressed patients. Better separation has been found using the MCMI-III in a study comparing patients with Major Depressive Disorder and Generalized Anxiety Disorder, two conditions that are difficult to differentiate in practice. Freeman, Kablinger, Rolland, and Brannon (1999) found that patients with Major Depressive Disorder had more frequent elevations (using a BR ≥ 75 cut-off) on the Dependent, Self-Defeating, Borderline, Dysthymia, and Major Depression scales, whereas those with Generalized Anxiety Disorder had more frequent elevations on the Compulsive and Anxiety scales. This increased differentiation may be attributable to sample selection, as the researchers excluded all patients who had clinically significant levels of both anxiety and depression.

According to the second edition of the MCMI-III manual (Millon et al., 1997), and using a cut-off of BR ≥ 85, the Anxiety scale was able to detect 57% of patients with an anxiety disorder and 64% of patients for whom an anxiety diagnosis was the most prominent syndrome. An observed elevation on the Anxiety scale, meanwhile, resulted in a correct diagnosis 80% of the time. This latter finding must be reconciled with previous work suggesting that the Anxiety scale is frequently elevated in cases of depression and may be due to high comorbidity with anxiety disorders in the depressed samples. Poor discriminant validity between the Anxiety and Dysthymia scales can be found on the various external validation criteria, with both scales correlating equally highly with a range of measures purporting to assess anxiety and depression. High scale intercorrelation becomes particularly problematic when trying to distinguish between conditions with high rates of comorbidity.

Whereas a high score on Anxiety alone is a good indicator that an anxiety disorder is present, a high Anxiety score in combination with elevations on Dysthymia and/or Major Depression is more problematic. An elevation on the Compulsive scale is also a good indicator of anxiety in such patients (Freeman et al., 1999), especially as the presence of depression is likely to exert a downward influence on this scale; for this reason, the absence of a Compulsive elevation does not speak to the absence of an anxiety disorder. Notably, the significant effect was generated by a minority of anxious patients having an elevation on this scale, in contrast to none of the depressed patients. Depressed patients are more likely than anxious patients to portray themselves as having a chaotic life with unstable and ambivalent relationships. Unfortunately, there is little information on the MCMI-III profiles characteristic of the different anxiety disorders. Sanderson, Wetzler, Beck, and Betz (1994) showed that these disorders differ in the overall and specific prevalence of *DSM-III-R* personality psychopathology using structured interview, but this question has not yet been examined using the MCMI-III.

PSYCHOSIS

The MCMI-III has two scales for the assessment of psychosis: Thought Disorder and Delusional Disorder. Thought Disorder is designed to measure the fragmented and bizarre thought processes found in Schizophrenia, and Delusional Disorder is designed to measure features of acute paranoia, including persecutory ideation, irrational jealousy, and grandiosity, seen in Schizophrenia and Delusional Disorder. Research using the older versions of the MCMI tends to show that these scales are not adequate for the identification of their target disorders. The study by Wetzler and Marlowe (1993) described earlier also included a sample of psychotic individuals and showed that neither scale, either alone or in combination, had good diagnostic efficiency for psychosis. They did find, however, that elevations were produced on the MCMI-II Dependent and Compulsive scales, reflecting the submissiveness, interpersonal fragility, and need for structure often seen in these patients. Surprisingly, PD scales associated with psychosis, such as the Paranoid, Schizoid, Schizotypal, and Borderline scales, did not show elevations.

According to the second edition of the MCMI-III manual (Millon et al., 1997), and using a cut-off of BR ≥ 85, the Thought Disorder and Delusional Disorder scales have positive predictive powers of .59 and .63 with sensitivities of .52 and .40, respectively. These findings represent a substantial improvement over previous versions of the instrument, improvement that might be attributed to the tendency of this second validation study to overestimate diagnostic validity. The Thought Disorder scale, in particular, can also be elevated by nonpsychotic patients with odd thinking patterns, as is sometimes observed in cases of Obsessive-Compulsive Disorder. This scale is best used as a general measure of chaotic and unusual thinking that may or may not be the result of an underlying psychotic process. The Delusional Disorder scale, meanwhile, is composed of two quite different sets of items, one set tapping paranoid suspiciousness and the other tapping grandiosity; the four prototypical items measure persecutory ideation. Although an elevation on this scale is not necessarily evidence of a frankly psychotic process, any elevation on this scale is sufficient cause for further clinical investigation, especially if one or more of the prototypical items are endorsed.

One missing ingredient in this discussion is the extent to which psychotic patients are actually able to produce valid profiles. Unfortunately, many of the studies in the literature, including those described by Millon and colleagues (1997), do not report the number of invalid profiles for specific clinical syndromes. What is clear is that many patients with psychotic disorders do in fact complete valid profiles, at least according to the criteria recommended in the test manual. In our clinical experience, patients with psychotic processes are often able to produce valid profiles containing useful information about personality styles, anxiety, and depression. However, as would be expected from the research described earlier, not all of these patients have prominent elevations on Thought Disorder and Delusional Disorder. Given the lack of empirical work in this area, the clinician should be especially careful to consider the MCMI-III findings for psychotic patients to be hypotheses in need of further confirmation rather than definitive statements about personality and psychopathology.

DEPRESSIVE PERSONALITY

The Depressive scale is new to the MCMI-III and is designed to capture the Depressive PD entity newly introduced in *DSM-IV*, a category reflecting what has traditionally been called "characterological depression" (Davis & Hays, 1997). Proponents of including this PD in future editions of *DSM* claim that the construct fills a hole in the current diagnostic system (e.g., Huprich, 2001; Phillips & Gunderson, 1999). Critics have argued, however, that the notion of depressive personality exhibits problematic overlap with depression and, especially, with Dysthymic Disorder (e.g., McLean & Woody, 1995; Ryder & Bagby, 1999; Ryder, Bagby, & Schuller, 2002). The inclusion of this new scale allows us to examine this issue in the context of Millon's model and the MCMI-III; it also provides a stringent test of the state-trait distinction by providing three separate scales for acute, chronic, and characterological depressive features.

The three scales are certainly highly intercorrelated, with the Depressive scale sharing its highest correlation with Dysthymia ($r = .79$). The Depressive and Major Depression scales, meanwhile, correlate at $r = .69$, and Dysthymia and Major Depression correlate at $r = .84$. Such associations are high, even in the context of an instrument that generally suffers from a high degree of scale intercorrelation. Piersma and Boes's (1997) treatment outcome study showed that the Depressive scale has some state-like quali- ties with a shift of 8.1 BR points during short-term hospital-based treatment for mood disorders. At the same time, greater shifts were demonstrated for Dysthymia (14.6) and especially for Major Depression (21.5). Davis and Hays (1997) studied a sample of psychiatric inpatients and found that 71% of patients with a BR ≥ 75 on the Depressive scale also had a BR score ≥ 75 on Major Depression. They also found that the Depres- sive scale makes a unique contribution to the prediction of state depression assessed by self-report. This latter result held even after controlling for the Avoidant, Dependent, and Negativistic scales, all measuring constructs thought to be theoretically related to depressive personality. The Depres- sive scale provides a measure of a depressive style that includes both state and trait components, but is more trait-like than other similar measures on the MCMI-III.

Unfortunately, there has not yet been any research on the comparative efficacy of the Depressive and Dysthymia scales. The relation between these constructs is at the center of the controversy regarding the proper status of Depressive PD. Ryder and colleagues (2002) noted that the cur- rent definition of these constructs allows many ways for one to meet cri- teria for Dysthymic Disorder and not Depressive PD, whereas the reverse relation is unlikely. This one-way overlap occurs because Dysthymia is much broader and less restrictive, including both medium- and long-term durations, early and late onset, and physical and psychological symp- toms. An inspection of the item content of the two scales shows that the same problem can be expected here. Although some of the items attempt to give some sense of the time frame involved, many others do not. As well, individuals who agree that they have had a depressive self-concept since childhood would likely endorse that they have felt poorly for several years. The biggest contribution to this conceptual and empirical overlap, however, is the neglect of somatic symptoms other than loss of energy on the Dysthymia scale, despite the fact that *DSM-IV* Dysthymic Disorder includes a number of different physical complaints. These complaints, moreover, are most likely to identify dysthymic individuals who do not in fact have Depressive PD (Bagby, Ryder, & Schuller, 2003; Ryder, Bagby, & Dion, 2001).

When interpreting these three scales, especially in assessment con- texts where a major mood disorder has already been established, the Major Depression scale should be interpreted first, followed by Dys- thymia, and then finally by the Depressive scale. An elevation on Major Depression supports the diagnosis of a Major Depressive Episode, which in turn colors interpretation of the other two scales. In this case, only a

strong elevation on these latter scales, at BR ≥ 85, should be taken as evidence of a long-standing condition; smaller elevations may have more
to do with a negative self-concept resulting from the acute condition. In
any event, an elevation on the Dysthymia scale may not have a clearly
different meaning from an elevation on the Depressive scale, and the clinician should not interpret the former as being evidence of the physical
symptomatology normally associated with Dysthymic Disorder.

TRAUMA AND PTSD

In the MCMI and MCMI-II, assessment of trauma and PTSD was
hampered by the lack of a specific scale measuring this symptom cluster. When a specific scale is lacking, users of broadband instruments
can turn to particular scale configurations associated with the disorder.
In a review of 10 studies, Craig (1997) found consistent support for the
Passive-Aggressive/Avoidant code type, sometimes with additional elevations on the Schizoid or Antisocial scale. Frequent elevations were
also observed on the Borderline, Anxiety, Dysthymia, Alcohol Abuse,
and Major Depression Clinical scales. Although it is unclear whether
this consistent personality profile contributes to the likelihood of developing PTSD or is a result of changes due to the onset of this disorder,
the picture of PTSD patients as angry yet passive, socially avoidant,
and withdrawn is in keeping with clinical descriptions (Craig &
Olson, 1997).

The MCMI-III provides a second and more direct means of assessing
PTSD by including a scale specific to its measurement. According to the
second edition of the MCMI-III manual (Millon et al., 1997), and using a
cut-off of BR ≥ 85, the PTSD scale was able to detect 53% of patients with
this syndrome and 88% of patients for whom PTSD was the most prominent syndrome. An observed elevation on the PTSD scale resulted in a
correct diagnosis 73% of the time. An independent study found somewhat lower figures, with the PTSD scale detecting 68% of patients with
this syndrome and a PTSD scale elevation accurately revealing the presence of PTSD only 43% of the time (Craig & Olson, 1997). In both studies,
the scale was very effective at ruling out PTSD. These figures could presumably be improved by conducting a separate assessment for the presence of a clinically significant trauma. Clinicians should certainly not
rely on a self-report measure to determine whether or not a trauma has
taken place and what its impact has been. Nonetheless, where trauma
has been determined by interview, the MCMI-III PTSD scale can be used
to determine whether clinically significant sequelae are present. This

information should be combined with other assessment data before a formal diagnosis is made.

Once a diagnosis of PTSD has been established, the PD scales can be used to elaborate on the overall clinical picture. Interestingly, the Craig and Olson (1997) study found a different code type in their admittedly small sample of substance abusers with PTSD, namely, a Schizoid/Antisocial pattern rather than a Passive-Aggressive/Avoidant pattern. This difference could be attributable to the prevalence of substance abuse in this sample; non-PTSD substance abusers in the same study had a predominantly Antisocial personality pattern. Allen, Coyne, and Huntoon (1998) found that women seeking inpatient treatment for complex PTSD following chronic trauma (Herman, 1992) were characterized by Depressive, Self-Defeating, and Dependent elevations. The authors note that this pattern is consistent with Herman's description of chronically abused patients as having disturbed interpersonal functioning with a tendency to repeat harmful patterns as a result of self-defeating behaviors. Allen, Huntoon, and Evans (1999) expanded this description of complex PTSD by using cluster analysis to classify these patients according to five different patterns observed on the MCMI-III PD scales. A decision tree allows for the classification of patients who have experienced prolonged trauma into one of these categories, each of which has its own clinical description and set of correlates.

Choca and Van Denburg (1997) argued that it is not appropriate to assume the presence of a trauma history on the basis of PD scale score elevations. We agree, and add that even a high PTSD scale score only adds one datum, and a potential hypothesis, to the clinical picture. Identifying a past event and evaluating whether it was sufficiently severe to cause trauma is challenging at best and should not be left to a self-report measure or indeed to any single data point. A better approach is to carefully establish the presence and extent of trauma history and then use the MCMI-III to evaluate the patient's subjective posttraumatic experience. Whether the trauma directly led to the personality disturbance or the disturbance was already in place is not a question that can be easily answered, and certainly not with the MCMI-III. Allen and colleagues (1998) further note that caution should be used when explaining MCMI-III PD scale results to traumatized patients; describing a long-standing pattern of self-defeating behaviors, for example, could easily be taken to mean blame and responsibility for the traumatic event. It is safer, and more productive, to focus on the PD scales as indicative of the current self-concept of the individual. Treatment can then include consideration of ongoing interpersonal patterns without being mired down in etiological questions.

CONCLUSION

The MCMI-III is the only major psychological assessment instrument that measures both major mental disorders and personality psychopathology, with the former tied to modern *DSM-IV* constructs and the latter based on a comprehensive theoretical system that also has an increasingly close correspondence to *DSM-IV.* One of the challenges in assessment is the separation of state and trait effects (Bagby & Ryder, 2000), and the MCMI-III is structured to appear ideally suited to this task. In reality, however, the instrument is only partially successful. The PD scales have both state and trait components, with some scales showing notable shifts even after brief treatment; interestingly, certain scale scores actually increase after treatment. Proper interpretation of the MCMI-III requires a knowledge of which scales are likely to change after a dysphoric state has been re-solved, and in which direction. Nonetheless, it is our contention that one can continue to interpret questionable elevations as representing the indi-vidual's current self-concept.

The MCMI-III, like previous editions of this instrument, is able to de-tect depressive states, although it is not particularly effective at making the fine-grained distinction between Major Depressive Disorder and Dysthymic Disorder. A new Depressive PD scale appears to add incre-mental prediction to the instrument in predicting mood disorders but is not clearly linked to a particular PD in such a way as to clearly separate this scale from Dysthymia. The MCMI-III is not as successful at detecting manic or psychotic episodes, although, according to Millon and col-leagues (1997), there have been considerable improvements over previous editions. Elevations that suggest the presence of a psychotic disorder, in particular, may actually represent unusual thinking more generally. Anxiety can be detected, although the instrument does not give informa-tion about specific anxiety disorders with the exception of PTSD. Finally, it should be noted that in general, the MCMI-III is very effective at ruling out psychopathology, with low elevations representing absence of disor-der the overwhelming majority of the time (Hsu, 2002). In short, the MCMI-III can be used to detect and differentiate broad categories of psychopathology but is considerably less effective at making finer diag-nostic distinctions.

Of course, as we noted in the introduction, the clinician rarely goes through an involved process to administer and interpret the MCMI-III sim-ply to make coarse diagnostic decisions. Assessment is also concerned—and may be primarily concerned—with identifying clinically meaningful differences between patients who belong in the same broad diagnostic cat-egory. Two patients might have Major Depression, but they will likely dif-fer in many other important ways. The MCMI-III has the capacity to detect some of these differences and to aid in their interpretation. We elaborate on this point by providing two clinical examples.

RF is a White American woman in her early 40s who has recently been diagnosed with a first episode of Major Depression. She has taken the MCMI-III and her diagnosis has been confirmed by a high elevation on Dysthymia (BR = 88); she also has a moderately high elevation on Anxiety (BR = 80), common in depressed individuals. Her PD scales show high elevations on Depressive PD (BR = 93) and Passive-Aggressive PD (BR = 86) and a moderately high elevation on Avoidant PD (BR = 77). Although both Depressive and Passive-Aggressive PDs are elevated by state dysphoria, the elevations are high enough to suggest that RF has these traits, if not necessarily these disorders. These elevations suggest that this patient has a tendency to see both herself and others in a negative light and to be accustomed to suffering as part of life. Her long-standing low self-esteem and tendency to express anger indirectly had often caused problems in relationships, and her current episode began shortly after her boyfriend raised the possibility of separation. The Avoidant PD elevation, in contrast, is best interpreted as current social avoidance secondary to depression and should not be seen as a long-standing or inflexible pattern in the absence of other evidence. RF reported being eager for therapy but at the same time brought an expectation that the therapeutic relationship would also be a difficult one. She was able to make a connection with the therapist but had a tendency toward passivity in session; she would then grow frustrated at her own self-perceived weakness and avoid sessions in order to "get back at" the therapist. Working on social avoidance created some positive events for RF, which in turn started to lift the depression, but she had a tendency to perceive herself as not deserving to be happy. Although the diagnosis of depression was evident and did not require confirmation by the MCMI-III, the test offered incremental information regarding associated personality traits relevant to her treatment.

BL is also a White American woman in her early 40s who has been diagnosed with a first episode of Major Depression. She has taken the MCMI-III and her diagnosis has been confirmed by high elevations on Dysthymia (BR = 90) and Major Depression (BR = 85). Her PD scales show a high elevation on Schizoid PD (BR = 95) and moderately high elevations on Self-Defeating PD (BR = 83) and Narcissistic PD (BR = 79). Like RF, BL has been keeping to herself, avoiding contact with others, but here this pattern appears to be a long-standing trait rather than a consequence of the depression. Also unlike RF, BL's social avoidance is based less on a fear of rejection by others and more on indifference or lack of interest in connecting with others. She states in therapy that she feels that other people are not good enough for her, reflected in her elevation on Narcissistic PD, an elevation that is particularly notable given the tendency of depression to suppress this scale. Indeed, it later emerged that the immediate trigger for her current episode was a narcissistic injury, in this case a setback at work. The elevation on Self-Defeating PD reflects a tendency while depressed to behave in such a way as to drive away those people who would be most likely to help her, whom she then dismisses as more evidence of their inferiority; this elevation may or may not represent long-standing traits. BL was resistant to the idea of therapy, often stating that she found it demeaning, but at the same time claimed that she was too proud to just give up. The constancy of the therapeutic relationship helped to provide a corrective experience to BL's self-defeating tendencies, but it was difficult to engage her emotionally beyond a certain point.

Although both cases describe women in their early 40s with first episodes of depression, the MCMI-III suggests different long-standing personality styles and different current self-concepts, with implications for the course of treatment. Psychiatric diagnoses are not homogeneous entities, and depression is no exception. Although depressed patients may bear a family resemblance to one another and the treatments may be fairly standard, the individual differences uncovered by the MCMI-III are of great interest and allow for increased individualization of treatment.

Unfortunately, the lack of research on the MCMI-III limits the level of confidence we may have in various clinical hypotheses. The largest immediate problem is the extent to which the two official validation studies contradict one another while violating accepted standards for establishing test validity. Although assessment is far more than simply establishing one-to-one links between scales and diagnoses, it is imperative that, as a first step, we increase our confidence that these scales are measuring what they are supposed to be measuring. The MCMI-III is in many ways the descendent of previous editions, but it deserves its own validation research. Interpretation is hampered by a lack of clarity regarding which scales can be read as intended, which scales should be ignored until they are improved, and which scales should be interpreted differently or cautiously.

Beyond general validity coefficients, there is a need for research specifically focused on particular assessment situations, for example, establishing the validity and interpretation of PD scales when the presence or absence of depression, mania, psychosis, and so on have already been determined. Common code types and their meanings within broad diagnostic categories should be studied and described, an effort that has begun in certain specific areas, such as complex PTSD. Finally, research is needed to evaluate the tenets of Millon's model, which is supposedly what is being measured by the MCMI-III PD scales. The model includes many testable hypotheses that await testing. Some of these hypotheses, especially those involving the underlying structure of the instrument, are very much in question. The past several years have seen the emergence of several competing dimensional models of personality psychopathology, models that tend to depart more radically from *DSM-IV* and that usually have less well developed underlying theories. They do have the advantage, however, of having clear and replicable structural properties. Some of these models, such as the Five-Factor Model of Personality (Costa & McCrae, 1985), also have the advantage of linking normal and abnormal personality. These dimensions can be interpreted along their entire length rather than being limited to high scores, as in the MCMI-III. More research is required to determine the role that can be played by Millon's model within this emerging discussion about dimensional PD models and the comparative validity and clinical utility of the MCMI-III with respect to alternative instruments.

REFERENCES

Allen, J. G., Coyne, L., & Huntoon, J. (1998). Complex posttraumatic stress disorder in women from a psychometric perspective. *Journal of Personality Assessment, 70,* 277–298.

Allen, J. G., Huntoon, J., & Evans, R. B. (1999). Complexities in complex posttraumatic stress disorder in inpatient women: Evidence from cluster analysis of MCMI-III personality disorder scales. *Journal of Personality Assessment, 73,* 449–471.

American Psychiatric Association. (1980). *Diagnostic and statistical manual of mental disorders* (4th ed.). Washington, DC: Author.

Bagby, R. M., & Ryder, A. G. (2000). Personality and the affective disorders: Past efforts, current models, and future directions. *Current Psychiatry Reports, 2,* 465–472.

Bagby, R. M., Ryder, A. G., & Schuller, D. R. (2003). Depressive personality disorder: A critical overview. *Current Psychiatry Reports, 5,* 16–22.

Choca, J. P., & Van Denburg, E. (1997). *Interpretive guide to the Millon Clinical Multiaxial Inventory* (2nd ed.). Washington, DC: American Psychological Association.

Costa, P. T., Jr., & McCrae, R. R. (1985). *The NEO Personality Inventory manual.* Odessa, FL: Psychological Assessment Resources.

Craig, R. J. (1997). A selected review of the MCMI empirical literautre. In T. Millon (Ed.), *The Millon inventories: Clinical and personality assessment* (pp. 303–326). New York: Guilford Press.

Craig, R. J., & Bivens, A. (1998). Factor structure of the MCMI-III. *Journal of Personality Assessment, 70,* 190–196.

Craig, R. J., & Olson, R. (1997). Assessing PTSD with the Millon Clinical Multiaxial Inventory-III. *Journal of Clinical Psychology, 53,* 943–952.

Craig, R. J., & Olson, R. E. (2001). Adjectival descriptions of personality disorders: A convergent validity study of the MCMI-III. *Journal of Personality Assessment, 77,* 259–271.

Davis, S. E., & Hays, L. W. (1997). An examination of the clinical validity of the MCMI-III Depressive Personality scale. *Journal of Clinical Psychology, 53,* 15–23.

Dyce, J. A., O'Connor, B. P., Parkins, S. Y., & Janzen, H. L. (1997). Correlational structure of the MCMI-III personality disorder scales and comparisons with other data sets. *Journal of Personality Disorders, 69,* 568–582.

Freeman, A. M., III, Kablinger, A. S., Rolland, P. D., & Brannon, G. E. (1999). Millon multiaxial personality patterns differentiate depressed and anxious outpatients. *Depression and Anxiety, 10*, 73–76.

Goodwin, F. K., & Jamison, K. R. (1990). *Manic-depressive illness*. New York: Oxford University Press.

Herman, J. L. (1992). Complex PTSD: A syndrome in survivors of prolonged and repeated trauma. *Journal of Traumatic Stress, 5*, 377–391.

Hirschfeld, R. M. A., Klerman, G. L., Clayton, P. J., Keller, M. B., McDonald-Scott, P., & Larkin, B. H. (1983). Assessing personality: Effects of the depressive state on trait measurement. *American Journal of Psychiatry, 140*, 695–699.

Hsu, L. M. (2002). Diagnostic validity statistics and the MCMI-III. *Psychological Assessment, 14*, 410–422.

Huprich, S. K. (2001). The overlap of depressive personality disorder and dysthymia, reconsidered. *Harvard Review of Psychiatry, 9*, 158–168.

Livesley, W. J. (1998). Suggestions for a framework for an empirically based classification of personality disorder. *Canadian Journal of Psychiatry, 43*, 137–147.

Locke, K. D. (2000). Circumplex scales of interpersonal values: Reliability, validity, and applicability to interpersonal problems and personality disorders. *Journal of Personality Assessment, 75*, 249–267.

McLean, P., & Woody, S. (1995). Commentary on depressive personality disorder: A false start. In W. J. Livesley (Ed.), *The DSM-IV personality disorders* (pp. 303–311). New York: Guilford Press.

Millon, T. (1969). *Modern psychopathology*. Philadelphia: Saunders.

Millon, T. (1983). *Millon Clinical Multiaxial Inventory manual* (3rd ed.). Minneapolis, MN: National Computer Systems.

Millon, T. (1987). *Manual for the MCMI-II*. Minneapolis, MN: National Computer Systems.

Millon, T. (1994). *MCMI-III Manual*. Minneapolis, MN: National Computer Systems.

Millon, T., & Davis, R. (1996). *Disorders of personality* (2nd ed.). New York: Guilford Press.

Millon, T., Davis, R., & Millon, C. (1997). *MCMI-III Manual* (2nd ed.). Minneapolis, MN: National Computer Systems.

Millon, T., & Meagher, S. E. (2004). The Millon Clinical Multiaxial Inventory-III (MCMI-III). In M. J. Hilsenroth & D. L. Segal (Eds.), *Comprehensive handbook of psychological assessment: Vol. 2. Personality assessment* (pp. 108–121). Hoboken, NJ: Wiley.

Millon, T., Millon, C., & Davis, R. (1994). *Millon Clinical Multiaxial Inventory-III manual*. Minneapolis, MN: National Computer Systems.

Phillips, K. A., & Gunderson, J. G. (1999). Depressive personality disorder: Fact or fiction? *Journal of Personality Disorders, 13*, 128–134.

Piersma, H. L. (1987). The MCMI as a measure of *DSM-III* Axis II diagnoses: An empirical comparison. *Journal of Clinical Psychology, 43*, 478–483.

Piersma, H. L., & Boes, J. L. (1997). MCMI-III as a treatment outcome measure for psychiatric inpatients. *Journal of Clinical Psychology, 53*, 825–831.

Reich, J. H., & Troughton, E. (1988). Comparison of *DSM-III* personality disorders in recovered depressed and panic disorder patients. *Journal of Nervous and Mental Diseases, 176*, 300–304.

Retzlaff, P. (1996). MCMI-III diagnostic validity: Bad test or bad validity study. *Journal of Personality Assessment, 65,* 431–437.

Rogers, R., Salekin, R. T., & Sewell, K. W. (1999). Validation of the Millon Clinical Multiaxial Inventory for Axis II disorders: Does it meet the Daubert standard. *Law and Human Behavior, 23,* 425–443.

Rogers, R., Salekin, R. T., & Sewell, K. W. (2000). The MCMI-III and the Daubert standard: Separating rhetoric from reality. *Law and Human Behavior, 24,* 501–506.

Ryder, A. G., & Bagby, R. M. (1999). Diagnostic viability of depressive personality disorder: Theoretical and conceptual issues. *Journal of Personality Disorders, 13,* 99–117.

Ryder, A. G., Bagby, R. M., & Dion, K. L. (2001). Chronic low-grade depression in a non-clinical sample: Depressive personality or dysthymia? *Journal of Personality Disorders, 15,* 84–93.

Ryder, A. G., & Bagby, R. M., & Schuller, D. R. (2002). The overlap of depressive personality disorder and dysthymic disorder: A categorical problem with a dimensional solution. *Harvard Psychiatry Review, 10,* 337–352.

Sanderson, W. C., Wetzler, S., Beck, A. T., & Betz, F. (1994). Prevalence of personality disorders among patients with anxiety disorders. *Psychiatry Research, 51,* 167–174.

Strack, S., Choca, J. P., & Gurtman, M. B. (2001). Circular structure of the MCMI-III personality disorder scales. *Journal of Personality Disorders, 15,* 263–274.

Strauman, T. J., & Wetzler, S. (1992). The factor structure of SCL-90 and MCMI scale scores: Within-measure and interbattery analyses. *Multivariate Behavioral Research, 27,* 1–20.

Wetzler, S. (1989). Parameters of psychological assessment. In S. Wetzler & M. M. Katz (Eds.), *Contemporary approaches to psychological assessment* (pp. 3–15). New York: Brunner/Mazel.

Wetzler, S. (1990). The Millon Clinical Multiaxial Inventory (MCMI): A review. *Journal of Personality Assessment, 55,* 445–464.

Wetzler, S., Kahn, R. S., Cahn, W., Van Praag, H. M., & Asnis, G. M. (1990). Psychological test characteristics of depressed and panic patients. *Psychiatry Research, 31,* 179–192.

Wetzler, S., Khadivi, A., & Oppenheim, S. (1995). The psychological assessment of depression: Unipolars versus bipolars. *Journal of Personality Assessment, 65,* 557–566.

Wetzler, S., & Marlowe, D. B. (1993). The diagnosis and assessment of depression, mania, and psychosis by self-report. *Journal of Personality Assessment, 60,* 1–31.

Wetzler, S., Marlowe, D. B., & Sanderson, W. C. (1994). Assessment of depression: Using the MMPI, Millon, and Millon-II. *Psychological Reports, 75,* 755–768.

Widiger, T. A., Williams, J. B., Spitzer, R. L., & Frances, A. (1985). The MCMI as a measure of *DSM-III. Journal of Personality Assessment, 49,* 366–378.

Yang, J., Bagby, R. M., Ryder, A. G., & Costa, P. T., Jr. (2002). Structure of personality disorder with a sample of Chinese psychiatric patients. *Journal of Personality Disorders, 16,* 317–331.

CHAPTER 12

The Diagnostic Efficiency of the MCMI-III™ in the Detection of Axis I Disorders

PAUL GIBEAU AND JAMES CHOCA

WE STUDIED the diagnostic accuracy of the Millon Clinical Multiaxial Inventory III (MCMI-III) under usual clinical conditions. MCMI-III-generated Axis I diagnoses from 371 clinical patients were compared to clinician-determined diagnoses, and the test's diagnostic operating characteristics were evaluated. The results indicated generally good specificity and negative predictive power, but a wide range of sensitivity levels and positive predictive power, suggesting that some scales may not be elevated when the disorder is present and some disorders may not be present when the scale is elevated (false positive). The Substance Abuse scales (B, T) and the Posttraumatic Stress Disorder scale (R) had particularly strong diagnostic efficiency statistics. The Thought Disorder (SS) and Delusional Disorder (PP) scales continue to experience problems in diagnosing thought disorder, a finding that was present in previous versions of the MCMI.

The MCMI (Millon, 1983) and its subsequent revisions (Millon, 1987, 1994, 1997a) has become a frequently used measure for personality disorders and clinical syndromes (Piotrowski, 1997; Watkins, Campbell, Nieberding, & Hallmark, 1995). Several books have been published on this test (Choca, 2003; Craig, 1993a, 1993b; Jankowski, 2002; McCann & Dyer, 1996; Millon, 1997b; Retzlaff, 1995; Strack, 1999), and it has been the subject of many scholarly reviews (Craig, 1999; Dana & Cantrell, 1988; Fleishauer, 1987; Greer, 1984; Haladyna, 1992; Hess, 1985, 1990; Lanyon, 1984; McCabe, 1984; Reynolds, 1992; Wetzler, 1990; Widiger, 1985).

The MCMI-III is a substantive revision of the MCMI-II. To improve its correspondence with *DSM-IV* (American Psychiatric Association, 1994) diagnostic criteria, 45 new items were added and two additional scales were introduced (Depressive Personality Disorder, Posttraumatic Stress Disorder), bringing the total of new items to 95; the item-weighting system was changed from a 3-point to a 2-point scale; other scales were reduced in length; and noteworthy items (i.e., critical items) pertaining to child abuse and eating disorders were added but not scored (Craig, 2001). It is uncertain how these changes will affect the test's utility, but one study found low congruence between MCMI-II and MCMI-III profiles among patients addicted to cocaine (Marlowe, Festinger, & Kirby, 1998).

Because Millon has raised the standard of measurement by introducing the base rate (BR) score, researchers had objective standards with which to compare a test's diagnoses with external criteria. Researchers have studied the test's convergent validity either by correlating the MCMI scales with similar measures or by reporting on the test's operating characteristics (Gibertini, Brandenberg, & Retzlaff, 1986) and its diagnostic power. The major operating characteristics of a test are its sensitivity, specificity, positive predictive power, negative predictive power, and overall diagnostic power. To study a test's diagnostic power, one needs to know the prevalence rate of a given disorder. *Prevalence* is the proportion of a population that have a particular disorder. It may be thought of as the "walk-in" probability that a patient has the disorder when the patient arrives for the diagnostic interview. *Sensitivity* is the percentage of patients known to have the disorder. *Specificity* is the percentage of patients known not to have the disorder. *Positive predictive power* (PPP) is the percentage of patients identified by the test as having the disorder and who actually do have the disorder. *Negative predictive power* (NPP) is the percentage of patients identified by the test as not having the disorder and who actually do not have the disorder. Finally, the *overall diagnostic power* (DP) of a test represents the global proportion of correct classifications.

There has been limited research on the MCMI-III in general and even less on its operating characteristics in particular. Moreover, the validity of this test has been the source of great controversy. Millon provided the prevalence, sensitivity, and specificity values obtained with the standardization data in the first edition of the MCMI-III test manual (Millon, 1994). Using these figures, Retzlaff (1996) calculated the PPP. Retzlaff noted that the PPP figures were uniformly poor, ranging from .00 to .32 for the Personality scales and from .15 to .58 for the Clinical Syndrome scales. Retzlaff proposed that the low PPP values were attributable to the poor quality of the external validity study. Others, however, questioned the value of the instrument given the poor validity scores (Rogers, Salekin, &

Sewell, 1999). The information was taken out of a second edition of the manual (Millon, 1997a), and data collected by Roger Davis (Davis, Wenger, & Guzman, 1997) were included instead.

For the personality disorders, the Davis, Wenger, and Guzman (1997) study showed scale sensitivities ranging from .44 (Negativistic) to .92 (Paranoid), with a median of .58; for the clinical disorders, scale sensitivity ranged from .67 (Bipolar: Manic) to .92 (Drug Dependence), with a median of .83. PPP values for the MCMI-III's Personality Disorders scales ranged from .30 (Self-Defeating) to .81 (Dependent), with a median of .67; for the Clinical scales, PPP ranged from .51 (Major Depression, Thought Disorder) to .70 (Anxiety), with a median of .58. Unfortunately, this study allowed the diagnostic formulation to be given by clinicians who had seen the test results and, therefore, compromised the integrity of the data (Choca, 2003; Rogers, Salekin, & Sewell, 2000). The fact that the values were so dramatically improved in comparison to the values of the first study was seen as further indictment of the data (Rogers et al., 2000).

In spite of literature in defense of the MCMI-III (Dyer & McCann, 2000), concerns continue to be expressed that the test's operating characteristics are problematic (Hsu, 2002). As a result, independent research is needed to learn how the test functions in a variety of contexts and with a variety of populations. Given that subsequent independent research often reported psychometric values lower than those in the test manuals (Craig, 1997a), it is also important for researchers to begin to study the MCMI-III's diagnostic properties. Although there is preliminary data on the PPP, NPP, and DP of the MCMI-III modifying indices in the detection of faking (Daubert & Metzler, 2000), there is a dearth of research on the test's other scales. Craig and Olson (1997) studied the utility of the MCMI-III PTSD scale among 228 substance abusers without PTSD compared to 32 with combat-related PTSD. They found that the PTSD scale (R) successfully differentiated between the PTSD and non-PTSD substance-abusing groups and was the best predictor of PTSD in a multiple regression equation, and the scale's sensitivity and specificity were even higher than those values reported in the test manual. The MCMI-III's Substance Abuse scales (B, T) were found to have higher sensitivity levels than reported for previous versions of the test but lower specificity levels in a sample of 164 inpatient substance abusers (Craig, 1997b). These were the only studies found to have researched the operating characteristics of the MCMI-III.

Although the MCMI-III has been used primarily as a measure of personality disorders, Millon's theory sees Axis I disorders as intimately related to Axis II disorders. His theory requires the clinician to understand the meaning of the clinical syndrome diagnosed by the MCMI in the light of the underlying personality structure, style, and/or disorder. Thus, a patient who scores in the diagnostic range on Major Depression and Narcissism may have experienced a narcissistic injury resulting in depression. A patient who scores in the diagnostic range on the Drug Abuse and Dependent scales may have initiated or escalated substance abuse in the face of perceived or actual loss of support, safety, and security. Thus, the operating characteristics of both the Personality Pattern scales and the Clinical Syndrome scales are critical in evaluating the test.

METHOD

Our study improves on previously published MCMI-III diagnostic power studies by (1) using a larger sample than those reported in earlier studies and (2) including a broad range of patients with a wider variety of psychiatric disorders. (Previously independent research has studied only substance abusers.) Furthermore, we were interested in learning how the test functions under more typical clinical conditions. This chapter reports our findings.

Participants

The patients for this study were in a variety of treatment settings in a Department of Veterans Affairs medical center in a large metropolitan area. A total of 371 patients composed the sample. There were 355 men and 16 women; 157 were Black, 174 were White, 23 were Hispanic, and 17 were from other races. A total of 287 were in outpatient psychiatric treatment, 47 were in inpatient substance abuse treatment, 25 were in inpatient medical and psychiatric treatment, and 12 were in a pain treatment program in general medicine.

Measure

The MCMI-III consists of 11 Clinical Personality Patterns scales (Schizoid, Avoidant, Depressive, Dependent, Histrionic, Narcissistic, Antisocial, Aggressive, Compulsive, Passive-Aggressive [Negativistic], Self-Defeating), three Severe Personality Pathology scales (Schizotypal, Borderline, Paranoid), and seven Clinical Syndromes scales (Anxiety, Somatization, Bipolar: Manic, Dysthymia, Alcohol, Drug, PTSD, Major Depression, Thought Disorder, and Delusional Disorder). It also has four modifier indices that serve as validity checks (Validity Index, Disclosure, Desirability, Debasement).

Procedure

A file search of the MCMI database in the medical center was conducted and resulted in more than 2,000 evaluations over a 4-year period. From this list we selected only those protocols that used the MCMI-III. Then we consulted their medical records and extracted their *DSM-IV* diagnoses. The diagnostic assignments were completed after a thorough interview in a multidisciplinary team setting, with typically more than one mental health professional having had contact with the patient. Although the MCMI-III is essentially a test for personality disorders and major clinical psychiatric syndromes, the existing database contained primarily Axis I disorders and only infrequently referenced a personality disorder. Because of this, we had to focus only on the diagnostic efficiency of the MCMI-III in relationship to the detection of clinical syndromes.

Many primary or secondary (i.e., comorbid) diagnoses included alcohol abuse, alcohol dependence, drug dependence, polydrug dependence, and so on; we collapsed these diagnoses into one entity as "substance abuse," especially because almost no patient had a single substance listed as his or her disorder. Similarly, the broad category of "depression" was selected because these scales have shown moderate overlap and redundancy in other research studies (Davis & Hays, 1997) and because the patient's medical record often included more than one depression-related diagnosis (i.e., Depression NOS, Major Depression, Dysthymia, and so on. Substance-Induced Mood Disorder was coded under both substance abuse and depression).

Expert licensed mental health clinicians in the VA medical center (psychiatrists, clinical psychologists, and clinical social workers) established all diagnoses before the MCMI-III was given. Thus, no diagnosis was based in part on psychological test findings. Although it would have been preferable to employ some type of standardized measure to establish the *DSM-IV* diagnosis (e.g., SCID-II; First, Spitzer, Williams, & Gibbon, 1997), we were interested in learning how the MCMI-III operates under usual clinical conditions. Except for rigorous studies, most clinical treatment settings rely on clinical diagnosis, where a brief contact for diagnostic purposes is all too often the norm. Thus, our interest was to determine how the MCMI-III operates under these real-world conditions.

Only valid MCMI-III profiles were used. Validity checks followed those prescribed in the manual (Validity Index < 2; Disclosure > 34 < 179). A total of eight profiles were discarded because of validity problems, leaving the total sample at 371.

RESULTS

The full range of operating characteristics, including sensitivity, specificity, PPP, NPP, and DP, were calculated for all Axis I disorders using BR scores of both >74 and > 84. Both values are reported because both

Table 12.1

Operating Characteristics of MCMI-III Clinical Syndrome Scales

Scale	Dx	Prevalence	Sensitivity	Specificity	PPP	NPP	DP
Anxiety	BR > 74	.42	.73	.35	.13	.91	.39
	BR > 84	.42	.55	.58	.14	.90	.57
Somatoform	BR > 74	.03	.50	.81	.03	.98	.80
	BR > 84	.03	.08	.89	.08	.97	.87
Bipolar: Mania	BR > 74	.10	.19	.92	.22	.91	.85
	BR>84	.10	.05	.98	.29	.90	.89
Dysthymia	BR > 74	.42	.73	.58	.56	.75	.65
	BR > 84	.42	.32	.86	.62	.63	.63
Alcohol/Drug	BR > 74	.48	.64	.90	.85	.72	.77
	BR > 84	.48	.37	.97	.92	.62	.68
PTSD	BR > 74	.11	.83	.79	.34	.97	.80
	BR > 84	.11	.41	.92	.39	.92	.86
Major Depression	BR > 74	.42	.45	.79	.60	.67	.65
	BR > 84	.42	.26	.90	.67	.63	.63
Thought Disorder	BR > 74	.05	.09	.86	.05	.94	.82
	BR > 84	.05	.04	.96	.07	.94	.91
Delusional Disorder	BR > 74	.12	.23	.93	.31	.89	.85
	BR > 84	.12	.09	.96	.24	.89	.86

DP = Diagnostic power; Dx = Diagnostic cut-off score; NPP = Negative predictive power; PPP = Positive predictive power.

MCMI-I and MCMI-II literature varied on the criteria used to establish an MCMI personality disorder or clinical syndrome. Some researchers used BR > 74, reflecting the presence of traits associated with the disorder, and/or a BR > 84, reflecting the presence of the disorder at the diagnostic level. Understandably, the operating characteristics of these scales will differ, not only based on sample size and prevalence rates of the disorder, but also based on the external criterion. Other researchers have also used other diagnostic tests and clinical diagnosis for the external criterion. Table 12.1 displays our findings.

One way to measure the validity of a test is to look at its incremental validity. Here we are interested in whether or not the test findings are greater than the base rate of the disorder. If predicting the base rate of occurrence of the disorder within a population is less accurate than test findings, then the test would be considered an improvement in diagnostic efficiency. The results here indicate that the sensitivity levels of all MCMI-III Clinical Syndrome scales were higher than the prevalence rate of the disorder when the diagnostic cut-off was BR > 74. When the cut-off score was increased to BR > 84, the scales of Anxiety, Somatoform, and PTSD exceeded prevalence statistics, whereas the scales of Bipolar: Mania, Dysthymia, Substance Abuse, Major Depression, Thought Disorder, and Delusional Disorder had sensitivity levels lower than the base rate occurrence of those disorders in this population. On the other hand, except for the Anxiety and Dysthymia scales, the MCMI-III specificity levels were quite good, with values ranging in the .80s and .90s. As would be expected from raising the diagnostic threshold for the presence of a disorder, specificity levels were higher at BR > 84 than at BR > 74 across all scales, and sensitivity levels were lower.

Sensitivity levels are useful for group data, but the clinician needs to know whether or not the test can detect the disorder if the individual patient has the disorder. PPP provides this data. At BR > 74, PPP ranged from .03 (Somatoform) to .85 (Substance Abuse), with a median of .21; at BR > 84, PPP ranged from .14 (Anxiety) to .92 (Substance Abuse), with a median of .31.

DISCUSSION

We found generally acceptable DP of the MCMI-III Clinical Syndrome scales with a good proportion of correct classifications. With the exception of Anxiety, the test had high specificity levels, indicating that scores were not likely to be elevated when the disorder is absent. Similarly, the test's NPP, or the probability that the disorder is absent when the scale is not elevated, was generally quite good. However, the wide range of sensitivity levels and the PPP were of concern. This suggests that some scales may not be elevated when the disorder is present (sensitivity) and that some disorders may not be present when the scale is elevated (PPP). This latter situation is generally referred to as false positives.

It is important to look at the operating characteristics of individual scales. For example, even though the PPP of the PTSD scale was .34 at BR > 74 and .39 at BR > 84, this was still 3 times better than chance, or the prevalence rate of the disorder, which was .11. In this population, the prevalence of mania was 10%, so the probability of not having this disorder was 90%. The NPP of the Bipolar: Mania scale was 91%; thus, the incremental validity of a negative test finding on this scale was only 1%.

The strong performance of the PTSD scale (R) corroborates the only other study published to date on this scale's operating characteristics. In a large sample of substance-abusing patients with and without PTSD, Craig and Olson (1997) reported a sensitivity level of scale R at .68, specificity at .83, PPP at .43, NPP at .93, and DP at .80 when the prevalence was .16. In our study with a prevalence of .11, scale R's sensitivity was .83, specificity was .79, PPP was .34, NPP was .97, and DP was .80 using the same BR value (> 74) as reported in the Craig and Olson study. Thus, in both studies, scale R showed substantial incremental validity and good diagnostic power. This scale has correlated well with other PTSD self-report measures and was able to differentiate between PTSD treatment and non-PTSD treatment groups (Hyer, Boyd, Stanger, Davis, & Walters, 1997).

These results continue to demonstrate problems with the MCMI-III in diagnosing psychotic disorders. The sensitivity and PPP for Bipolar: Mania and Major Depression (both of which could occur with or without psychotic manifestations) and for Thought Disorder and Delusional Disorder (both of which were designed to detect psychotic conditions) were generally poor. However, for Mania, the PPP was twice the base rate of the disorder, therefore showing incremental validity, even though it was accurate between 22% and 29% of the time, depending on the diagnostic cut-off score. The PPP for Major Depression was about 1.5 times better than the prevalence rate, but sensitivity levels were modest at best. However, the two scales designed to detect psychotic conditions showed variable performance. The Thought Disorder Scale (SS) had both low sensitivity levels and PPP, and the Delusional Disorder scale (PP) had low sensitivity levels and mediocre PPP, but this still was an improvement over the prevalence rate of the disorder. These results are consistent with the problems with these scales previously identified by Jackson, Greenblatt, Davis, Murphy, and Trimakas (1991), who found the MCMI-I insensitive in the detection of Schizophrenia. Other research also found previous versions of the MCMI to be insensitive to Thought Disorder related to Schizophrenia (Bonato, Cyr, Kalpin, Predergast, & Sanhueza, 1988; Patrick, 1988; Wetzler & Marlowe, 1993).

The Substance Abuse scales (B and T), as a combined entity, showed good PPP, with a prevalence rate of .48; this finding is consistent with previous research which reported on the diagnostic efficiency of these two scales. With a prevalence of 100%, the sensitivity of Drug Abuse (T) was .82 and the PPP was 1.00; with a prevalence of 80%, the sensitivity of Alcohol (B) was .80 and the PPP was .59 (Craig, 1997b). In our study, with a prevalence rate of 48%, the sensitivity was .64 and the PPP was .85.

In reflecting on the sensitivity levels and PPP obtained here and also those of similar studies, it is important to remember that there is no gold standard for Axis I disorders. It is impossible to determine whether the problem with low diagnostic efficiency on some scales lies with the test, the method used to establish the diagnosis, or both. However, it may be argued that MCMI-III scales Alcohol, Drug, and PTSD appear to perform well, while others perform poorly in a clinical setting with a population similar to that used here and where the clinical diagnosis is made by an unstructured clinical interview. It is also possible that clinicians simply missed the diagnoses of Anxiety and Thought Disorder, which would not be the fault of the test. Also, when prevalence rates are extremely low, reflecting a low rate of occurrence, as evidenced by a prevalence rate of .03 in somatoform disorders, any diagnostic method would have difficulty capturing this diagnosis.

Our study does have several factors that limit its findings. First, the sample was mostly male veterans who were socially disadvantaged and impoverished; hence, these results may not generalize to other populations. Second, the diagnoses, though based on *DSM-IV* criteria and typically benefiting from the input of several mental health professionals, were not examined for accuracy or reliability. A more rigorous research methodology might have required at least a subsample of judges to study interjudge reliability, but this was not feasible under this research design. This is certainly a limitation from a methodological point of view, but it also reflects ecological validity in a clinical sense, in that most psychiatric diagnoses at mental health centers are made by a single clinician. Our stated purpose was to evaluate how the MCMI-III operates under real-world conditions. More objective diagnostic specifications would be required for studies that sought to determine how a test operates under ideal conditions, whereas we sought to study how the test functions in situations more often encountered by clinicians. We believe that there is a place for this kind of methodology in research, as there is no objective standard or biological marker for the presence of Axis I disorders and because clinician diagnosis is most often used in many research publications and in actual practice.

REFERENCES

American Psychiatric Association. (1994). *Diagnostic and statistical manual of mental disorders* (4th ed.). Washington, DC: Author.

Bonato, D., Cyr, J., Kalpin, R., Predergast, P., & Sanhueza, P. (1988). The utility of the MCMI as a *DSM-III* Axis I diagnostic tool. *Journal of Clinical Psychology, 44,* 867–875.

Choca, J. P. (2003). *Interpretive guide to the Millon Clinical Multiaxial Inventory* (3rd ed.). Washington, DC: American Psychological Association.

Craig, R. J. (Ed.). (1993a). *The Millon Clinical Multiaxial Inventory: A clinical and research information synthesis.* Hillsdale, NJ: Erlbaum.

Craig, R. J. (1993b). *Psychological assessment with the Millon Clinical Multiaxial Inventory (II): An interpretive guide.* Odessa, FL: Psychological Assessment Resources.

Craig, R. J. (1997a). A selected review of the MCMI empirical literature. In T. Millon (Ed.), *The Millon inventories: Clinical and personality assessment* (pp. 303–326). New York: Guilford Press.

Craig, R. J. (1997b). Sensitivity of MCMI-III scales T (Drugs) and B (Alcohol) in detecting substance abuse. *Substance Use and Misuse, 32,* 1385–1393.

Craig, R. J. (1999). Overview and current status of the Millon Clinical Multiaxial Inventory. *Journal of Personality Assessment, 72,* 390–406.

Craig, R. J. (2001). Essentials of MCMI-III assessment. In S. Strack (Ed.), *Essentials of Millon inventories assessment.* New York: Wiley.

Craig, R. J., & Olson, R. (1997). Assessing PTSD with the Millon Clinical Multiaxial Inventory-III. *Journal of Clinical Psychology, 53,* 943–952.

Dana, R., & Cantrell, J. (1988). An update on the Millon Clinical Multiaxial Inventory (MCMI). *Journal of Clinical Psychology, 44,* 760–763.

Daubert, S. D., & Metzler, A. E. (2000). The detection of fake-bad and fake-good responding on the Millon Clinical Multiaxial Inventory III. *Psychological Assessment, 12,* 418–424.

Davis, R. D., Wenger, A., & Guzman, A. (1997). Validation of the MCMI-III. In T. Millon (Ed.) *The Millon inventories: Clinical and personality assessment* (pp. 327–362). New York: Guilford Press.

Davis, S. E., & Hays, L. W. (1997). An examination of the clinical validity of the MCMI-III Depressive Personality disorder. *Journal of Clinical Psychology, 46,* 770–774.

Dyer, F. J., & McCann, J. T. (2000). The Millon Clinical Inventories, research critical of their forensic application, and Daubert criteria. *Law and Human Behavior, 24,* 487–497.

First, M. B., Spitzer, R. L., Williams, J. B., & Gibbon, M. (1997). *Structured Clinical Interview for Disorders (SCID).* Washington, DC: American Psychiatric Association.

Fleishauer, A. (1987). The MCMI-II: A reflection of current knowledge. *Noteworthy Response, 3,* 7.

Gibertini, M., Brandenberg, N., & Retzlaff, P. (1986). The operating characteristics of the Millon Clinical Multiaxial Inventory. *Journal of Personality Assessment, 50,* 554–567.

Greer, S. (1984). Testing the test: A review of the Millon Multiaxial Inventory. *Journal of Counseling and Development, 63,* 262–263.

Haladyna, T. M. (1992). Review of the Millon Clinical Multiaxial Inventory-II. In J. J. Kramer & J. C. Conoley (Eds.), *Eleventh mental measurement yearbook* (pp. 532–533). Lincoln: University of Nebraska Press.

Hess, A. K. (1985). Review of Millon Clinical Multiaxial Inventory. In J. Mitchell, Jr. (Ed.), *Ninth mental measurements yearbook* (Vol. l, pp. 984–986). Lincoln: University of Nebraska Press.

Hess, A. K. (1990). Review of the Millon Clinical Multiaxial Inventory-III. In J. Mitchell, Jr. (Ed.), *Mental measurements yearbook.* Lincoln: University of Nebraska Press.

Hsu, L. M. (2002). Diagnostic validity statistics and the MCMI-III. *Psychological Assessment, 14,* 410–422.

Hyer, L., Boyd, S., Stanger, E., Davis, H., & Walters, P. (1997). Validation of the MCMI-III PYTSD scale among combat veterans. *Psychological Reports, 80,* 720–722.

Jackson, J. L., Greenblatt, R. L., Davis, W. E., Murphy, T. T., & Trimakas, K. (1991). Assessment of schizophrenic inpatients with the MCMI. *Journal of Personality Assessment, 51,* 243–253.

Jankowski, D. (2002). *A beginner's guide to the MCMI-III.* Washington, DC: American Psychological Association.

Lanyon, R. (1984). Personality assessment. *Annual Review of Psychology, 35,* 667–701.

Marlowe, D. B., Festinger, D. S., & Kirby, K. C. (1998). Congruence of the MCMI-II and MCMI-III in cocaine dependence. *Journal of Personality Assessment, 71,* 15–28.

McCabe, S. (1984). Millon Clinical Multiaxial Inventory. In D. Keyser & R. Sweetland (Eds.), *Test critiques* (Vol. I, pp. 455–456). Kansas City, MO: Westport.

McCann, J., & Dyer, F. J. (1996). *Forensic assessment with the Millon inventories.* New York: Guilford Press.

Millon, T. (1983). *Millon Clinical Multiaxial Inventory Manual* (3rd ed.). New York: Holt, Rinehart and Winston.

Millon, T. (1987). *Millon Clinical Multiaxial Inventory-II: Manual for the MCMI-II.* Minneapolis, MN: Pearson Assessments.

Millon, T. (1994). *Millon Clinical Multiaxial Inventory-III: Manual.* Minneapolis, MN: Pearson Assessments.

Millon, T. (1997a). *Millon Clinical Multiaxial Inventory-III: Manual* (2nd ed.). Minneapolis, MN: Pearson Assessments.

Millon, T. (Ed.). (1997b). *The Millon inventories: Clinical and personality assessment.* New York: Guilford Press.

Patrick, J. (1988). Concordance of the MCMI and the MMPI in the diagnosis of three *DSM-III* Axis I disorders. *Journal of Clinical Psychology, 44,* 186–190.

Piotrowski, C. (1997). Use of the Millon Clinical Multiaxial Inventory in clinical practice. *Perceptual and Motor Skills, 84,* 1185–1186.

Retzlaff, P. (Ed.). (1995). *Tactical psychotherapy of the personality disorders: An MCMI-III-based approach.* Needham Heights, MA: Allyn & Bacon.

Retzlaff, P. (1996). MCMI-III validity: Bad test to bad validity study. *Journal of Personality Assessment, 66,* 431–437.

Reynolds, C. R. (1992). Review of the Millon Clinical Multi-axial Inventory-II. In J. J. Kramer & J. C. Conoley (Eds.), *Eleventh mental measurement yearbook* (pp. 533–535). Lincoln: University of Nebraska Press.

Rogers, R., Salekin, R. T., & Sewell, K. W. (1999). Validation of the Millon Clinical Multiaxial Inventory for Axis II disorders: Does it meet the Daubert standard? *Law and Human Behavior, 23,* 525–443.

Rogers, R., Selekin, R. T., & Sewell, K. W. (2000). The MCMI and the Daubert standard: Separating rhetoric from reality. *Law and Human Behavior, 24,* 501–506.

Strack, S. (1999). *Essentials of Millon inventories assessment.* New York: Wiley.

Watkins, C. E., Campbell, V. L., Nieberding, R., & Hallmark, R. (1995). Contemporary practice of psychological assessment by clinical psychologists. *Professional Psychology: Research and Practice, 26,* 54–60.

Wetzler, S. (1990). The Millon Clinical Multiaxial Inventory: A review. *Journal of Personality Assessment, 55,* 445–464.

Wetzler, S., & Marlowe, D. B. (1993). The diagnosis and assessment of depression, mania, and psychosis by self-report. *Journal of Personality Assessment, 60,* 1–31.

Widiger, T. A. (1985). Review of the Millon Clinical Multiaxial Inventory. In J. Mitchell, Jr. (Ed.), *Ninth mental measurements yearbook* (Vol. I, pp. 986–988). Lincoln: University of Nebraska Press.

CHAPTER 13

On the Decline of MCMI-Based Research

ROBERT J. CRAIG AND RONALD E. OLSON

BASED ON a review of all published studies from 1984 through 2001, we found a statistically significant decline of MCMI-based research studies, peaking in 1990 and showing a consistent decline thereafter. In this chapter, we offer possible reasons for this decline and implications for the training of psychologists.

The Millon Clinical Multiaxial Inventory (MCMI), as revised (Millon, 1983, 1987, 1994), has become a popular instrument in the assessment of personality disorders and major clinical syndromes (Piotrowski, 1997; Watkins, Campbell, Nieberding, & Hallmark, 1995). It has a substantial literature and research base (Butcher & Rouse, 1996; Craig, 1993a, 1997), published interpretive manuals (Choca, 2004; Craig, 1993b), commercially available computer interpretive services (Craig, 1994), and several specialty books (McCann & Dyer, 1996; Millon, 1997; Retzlaff, 1995). Despite this impressive array of scholarly work, we had the impression that there has been a diminution of MCMI-based research over the past several years. To verify if such a trend existed, we decided to review and tally the total number of MCMI studies published each year.

METHOD

Studies published from 1984 through 2001 on all three versions of the MCMI were tallied. The initial MCMI appeared in 1983, though Millon researchers had been well aware of this instrument's development and had access to it for research purposes prior to its actual publication. Two studies were published on the precursor to the MCMI, the Millon Illinois

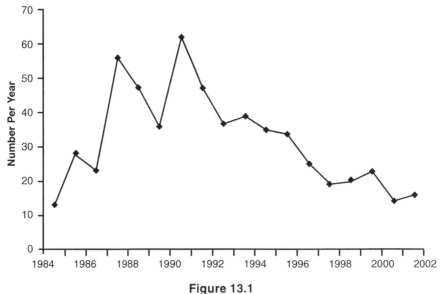

Figure 13.1
MCMI published research studies.

Self-Report Inventory (MISRI), in 1980, and studies on the MCMI also appeared in 1981 (3), 1982 (1), and 1983 (3), but it seemed reasonable to begin the count one year after the test's actual publication date.

A computer search was generated using the keyword "MCMI" (abbreviated and spelled out) and subject headings of "personality tests" of all MCMI studies from 1981 to 2001 in English-speaking journals, using the search engines Psychological Abstracts and MEDLINE. This ensured that the database was constant across all the years included in this review. These searches were done independently, twice, at different locations, and using different personnel to improve the accuracy of the final count. We individually inspected these references and eliminated those that only mentioned the test. Dissertations and book chapters were excluded. We included only reports that used the MCMI for research.

RESULTS

The results are graphically displayed in Figure 13.1. The data visually demonstrate a recent decline in published MCMI-based research studies, peaking in 1990 and then showing a consistent decline through 2001.[1] To determine if this decline was statistically significant, we used two approaches. First, the data were divided into two curves, one from 1984 to

---

[1] There were 27 research reports in 2002 and 14 in 2003.

1990, when the number of published studies was rising, and another from 1991 to 2001, when the number of published studies was on the decline. A linear regression was applied to these data; the slope of the line was 5.21 and was statistically significantly, positive at $p = -.31$. The data from 1991 to 2001 have a significantly negative slope of -3.09, $p < .0005$. This means that there was a significant rise in MCMI publications up to 1990 and a significant decline thereafter. Next the data were divided into two 9-year segments, and independent T-tests were conducted. The average number of MCMI publications from 1984 to 1992 was 38.78, $SD = 15.86$. From 1993 to 2001, the average number of MCMI publications was 25, $SD = 8.97$. There were significantly fewer publications in the latter years ($t = 2.27$, $df = 16$, $p = .037$).

DISCUSSION

Why has there been a decline in MCMI-based research? The data point to no conclusions, so any suggestions remain speculative. One leading hypothesis that might account for this decline is related to the effects of HMO reimbursement practices. Many psychologists may have used the MCMI for clinical assessment of patients and then conducted retrospective analysis of data in their private practice files. With reduced reimbursement for routine psychological assessment, such data may not be as frequently available for analysis as they once were. This hypothesis is consistent with a similar trend in the MMPI research literature, where there has been a decrease in the use of the MMPI-2 in the assessment of substance abusers (Craig, 2002). To test this hypothesis, we considered reviewing all institutional affiliations cited in the MCMI research studies to determine if there was a decline in studies emanating from practice or from university settings. However, this proved to be too cumbersome and unreliable. For example, there are psychologists who may cite their university affiliations but who referenced their data collection from clinics and other practice settings. Hence, an institutional citation might not be a reliable indicator of the true source of the data. However, this hypothesis remains a viable but disturbing possibility.

Another possibility pertains to the source of funding for research institutions. Much research funding derives from a few psychiatrically oriented branches of the National Institute of Mental Health and from the National Science Foundation. Most of this money is devoted to studies of the major Axis I disorders, especially Schizophrenia and Bipolar Disorders. There seems to have been a reduced interest in the study of Axis II disorders from these funding sources. To the extent that dissertations, and their subsequent publications, emanate from projects under the direction of an advisor whose funding is derived from NIMH/NSF, where the focus is on treatment of severe disorders, this could be another reason for the decline in MCMI-based research.

Another possibility is that the trend documented here is part of a larger overall decline in published research on many other personality assessment instruments, perhaps for similar reasons. One way to test this hypothesis is to conduct a similar review of another major personality instrument. Testing this hypothesis is beyond the scope of this review, but it is worth exploring.

A final possibility is that psychologists have lost interest in the MCMI as an assessment tool and have turned to instruments that have greater clinical utility. This does not seem likely in view of the continued (and even increasing) popularity of the test among practitioners, as cited in previous test usage reviews (Piotrowski, 1997; Watkins et al., 1995).

Perhaps the MCMI will experience the same fate as the Thematic Apperception Test (TAT). Kaiser and Prather (1990) documented a decline in the number of published studies on the TAT, yet the test remains in the top 10 of commonly used psychological tests.

Research on the MCMI clearly needs to continue if the science of assessment with this instrument is to advance. Basic studies on the test's reliability and validity, which were prolific with the MCMI-I and MCMI-II (Craig, 1997), are comparatively absent for the MCMI-III. Hopefully, psychologists will find a way to continue to research this instrument.

IMPLICATIONS FOR TRAINING

The results reported here have serious consequences for the field of assessment and training. As a result of our assessments, clients can gain or lose employment opportunities, custody, personal freedoms, remedial help, and financial damages. If the validating research associated with those decisions lose empirical support, what might this mean for assessment psychology? Should we train students in our assessment courses on instruments that may be falling into disuse among researchers (but apparently not among clinicians)? Should we teach instruments that have a declining literature base and thus lack incremental empirical validity, especially for use in forensic areas where both the adequacy of the instrument as well as the skill of the clinician are imperative in rendering expert opinion (*Daubert v. Merrell Dow Pharmaceuticals,* 1993; Heilbrun, 1992)? These questions are not easily answered but need to be debated.

What is clear is the need to investigate whether or not this evident decline in MCMI-based research is also true of other popular assessment instruments. If that trend is replicated across several instruments, this has implications not just for assessment psychology but for psychology as a profession.

Psychological tests have validity coefficients that are similar to, and even indistinguishable from, those of many medical tests (Meyer et al., 2001). We need to improve our advocacy of well-validated instruments among those we train who will use those instruments in their career and among those who influence public policy. Only then will succeeding generations receive the full benefit from our competence.

REFERENCES

Butcher, J. N., & Rouse, S. V. (1996). Personality: Individual differences and clinical assessment. *Annual Review of Psychology, 47,* 87–111.

Choca, J. P. (2004). *Interpretive Guide to the Millon Clinical Multiaxial Inventory* (3rd Ed.). Washington, DC: American Psychological Association.

Craig, R. J. (Ed.). (1993a). *The Millon Clinical Multiaxial Inventory: A clinical research information synthesis.* Hillsdale, NJ: Erlbaum.

Craig, R. J. (1993b). *Psychological assessment with the Millon Clinical Multiaxial Inventory (II): An interpretive guide.* Odessa, FL: Psychological Assessment Resources.

Craig, R. J. (1994). *MCMI-II/III interpretive system.* Odessa, FL: Psychological Assessment Resources.

Craig, R. J. (1997). A selected review of the MCMI empirical literature. In T. Millon (Ed.), *The Millon inventories* (pp. 303–326). New York: Guilford Press.

Craig, R. J. (2002). *Assessment of contemporary substance abusers with the MMPI/MMPI-2: A review of code types.* Manuscript submitted for editorial consideration.

Daubert v. Merrell Dow Pharmaceuticals, Inc., 113 S. Ct. 2786 (1993).

Kaiser, R. E., & Prather, E. N. (1990). What is the TAT? A review of ten years of research. *Journal of Personality Assessment, 55,* 800–803.

Heilbrun, K. (1992). The role of psychological testing in forensic assessment. *Law and Human Behavior, 16,* 257–272.

McCann, J. T., & Dyer, F. J. (1996). *Forensic assessment with the Millon inventories.* New York: Guilford Press.

Meyer, G. J., Finn, S. E., Eyde, L. D., Kay, G. G., Moreland, K. L., Dies, R. R., et al. (2001). Psychological testing and psychological assessment: A review of evidence and issues. *American Psychologist, 56,* 128–165.

Millon, T. (1983). *Millon Clinical Multiaxial Inventory manual.* New York: Holt, Rinehart and Winston.

Millon, T. (1987). *Millon Clinical Multiaxial Inventory-II: Manual for the MCMI-II.* Minneapolis, MN: National Computer Systems.

Millon, T. (1994). *Millon Clinical Multiaxial Inventory-III* Minneapolis, MN: National Computer Systems.

Millon, T. (1997). *Millon Clinical Multiaxial Inventory-III manual* (2nd ed.). Minneapolis, MN: Pearson Assessments.

Piotrowski, C. (1997). Use of the Millon Clinical Multiaxial Inventory in clinical practice. *Perceptual and Motor Skills, 84*, 1185–1186.

Retzlaff, P. (1995). *Tactical psychotherapy for the personality disorders: An MCMI-III-based approach.* Boston: Allyn & Bacon.

Watkins, C. E., Campbell, V. L., Nieberding, R., & Hallmark, R. (1995). Contemporary practice of psychological assessment by clinical psychologists. *Professional Psychology: Research and Practice, 26*, 54 60.

CHAPTER 14

Using Critiques of the MCMI to Improve MCMI Research and Interpretations

Louis Hsu

THIS CHAPTER provides information relevant to the critical interpretation of MCMI scales and scale scores and to the design and data analysis of future MCMI studies. For each of the major criticisms of the MCMI, an attempt is made to (1) indicate why this criticism is important, (2) discuss its implications for the analysis and interpretation of scale scores, (3) assess the extent to which it applies to the most recent version of the MCMI, and (4) suggest its implications for future research.

THE PATHOLOGY BIAS OF MCMI SCALES

Dana and Cantrell (1988), who examined 10 reviews of the original version of the MCMI, drew attention to the consistency of reviewers' criticisms of the pathology bias of MCMI scales. In particular, they noted that the MCMI tends to classify too many normals as disordered (see also Cantrell & Dana, 1987; Hess, 1998; Widiger, 2001). Similarly, Keller, Butcher, and Slutske (1990) stated that there are "broad concerns about its [the MCMI's] tendency to overpathologize compared to clinicians' judgments" (p. 348).

Empirical evidence to support these views may be illustrated with a study of the utility of the MCMI-I as a screening instrument in a university setting. Holliman and Guthrie (1989), who administered the MCMI-I

I would like to thank Gretchen Gibbs for very helpful advice (which I followed) concerning organization of topics in this chapter.

to 241 college freshmen, found that 92% would have been classified as having a psychiatric disorder, using one or more scales at or above BR 75 as the criterion for the presence of Axis I or Axis II disorders. Using the higher BR 85 criterion, 70% would still have been classified as distressed. These classifications greatly exceed all other estimates of the prevalence of psychiatric disturbances in an unselected college sample.

In fairness to Millon, it should be noted that the MCMI manuals admonish against using the MCMI scales with normal populations. For example, Millon (1987) states, "The MCMI-II should be administered, scored, and interpreted only with individuals who are involved in mental health services stemming from genuine emotional, social, or interpersonal difficulties" (p. 107). Furthermore, Millon, Davis, and Millon (1997) note:

> The MCMI-III is not a general personality instrument to be used with normal populations or for the purpose other than diagnostic screening or clinical assessment. . . . Normative data and transformation scores of the MCMI-III are based entirely on clinical samples and are applicable only to individuals who evidence problematic emotional and interpersonal symptoms or who are undergoing professional psychotherapy or a psychodiagnostic evaluation. (p. 6)

The intended objective of the MCMI is clearly to discriminate among disorders rather than to differentiate between normal and disordered individuals (see Millon, 2003, p. 957).

Nevertheless Millon et al. (1997) indicate that it is appropriate to use the MCMI in child custody evaluations to address "the chief referral question [which] is whether a parent is able to discharge parental responsibilities adequately" (p. 144), in criminal trials to interpret criminal confessions, in neuropsychological settings to provide "a valid measure of emotional and personality functioning" (p. 144), in the diagnosis of Posttraumatic Stress Disorder (PTSD), in correctional settings to provide information relevant to criminal relapse, and in marital counseling to guide decisions about whether or not individuals should seek therapeutic interventions. It would appear that in all of these applications, the pathology bias of the MCMI and the ability of the MCMI-III to differentiate between normal and disordered individuals in the specific context in which the test is used should be considered important.

FUTURE RESEARCH ON THE PATHOLOGY BIAS OF THE MCMI-III

Widiger (2001) notes that "clinicians working within . . . settings in which substantial clinical symptomatology is not commonplace (e.g., college counseling or divorce mediation center) might find that the MCMI-III overestimates the extent of psychopathology" (pp. 768–769). This view is consistent with the findings of Holliman and Guthrie (1989) and with Hess's (1998) statement that "it seems [that virtually] no one taking the MCMI can appear normal" (p. 666).

Given the known pathology bias of earlier versions of the MCMI, and given the potential serious consequences of false positive MCMI diagnoses, it would be very desirable to conduct studies on the extent to which the MCMI-III scales tend to overestimate levels of pathology in each context in which the MCMI-III has been recommended or used, especially in those contexts in which MCMI-III "red flag diagnostic terms" (Hess, 1998, p. 666) could be used to justify important real-world decisions concerning the test taker (decisions concerning child custody, parole, treatment, competency to stand trial, competency in relation to wills, hirings, and firings). For example, in child custody evaluations, it would be desirable to obtain empirical information about the risk that MCMI-III labeling could result in an incorrect decision concerning a parent's ability to "discharge parental responsibilities adequately" (Millon et al., 1997, p. 144).

Studies aimed at testing explanatory hypotheses concerning the psychopathology bias of the MCMI-III are also needed. For example, one explanation of this pathology bias in normals may involve the susceptibility of MCMI-III scales to the acquiescence response set (see LaVoie, 1991). The vast majority of MCMI-III items are keyed True (see following for details); therefore, persons who tend to acquiesce (a tendency that increases with increase in ambiguities of item content; see Guilford, 1954; Jackson & Messick, 1958) also tend to respond in the pathological direction. Possibly, factors related to respondents' predisposition and ability to detect ambiguities in item content could affect their tendency to acquiesce, which would in turn affect their estimated levels of pathology as determined by MCMI-III scales. To the extent that normal persons detect ambiguities in MCMI-III item content, they are likely to acquiesce and also to appear disordered. Differences in predisposition and ability to detect ambiguities between normals and disordered persons would result in differences in the extent of pathology biases of MCMI-III scales for normal versus disordered persons.

Research that addresses the validity of potential explanations of the bias might involve reversing (when semantically possible) the phrasing of True-keyed items (rewriting items so that the negative responses would generally be indicative of presence of the disorder) and determining if the pathology bias decreased in the reverse-keyed scales (see Messick, 1991). The sizes of these effects could be compared (within groups) to measures of predispositions and abilities of respondents to detect ambiguities in item content, or could be compared (across groups) with group predispositions and abilities to detect ambiguities in item content.

A second, tentative explanation of the pathology bias might focus on the possible existence of differences in meanings of a given response (say,

True) when this response comes from normal versus disordered individuals (see Craig & Olson, 2001; Widiger, 2001; Widiger & Sanderson, 1995). For many MCMI items, a True response appears to have pathological meaning only if given by someone who fits Millon's description of a disorder. As noted by Widiger (2001), "Persons with the respective personality disorders might endorse the item in the [keyed] direction, but it is also evident that persons who do not have maladaptive personality traits would have to endorse these items in the same direction" (p. 768). For example, item 80, "It is very easy for me to make many friends," or item 57, "I think I am a very sociable and outgoing person," or item 88, "I never sit on the sidelines when I'm at a party," all of which are keyed True on scales 4 and 5 (i.e., a True response is viewed as pathological), might well indicate normalcy when answered True by a normal person, but pathology when answered True by a person who fit Millon's description of scale 4 (Histrionic) or 5 (Narcissistic) disorders (e.g., "[Histrionics engage in] facile and enterprising manipulation of events, through which they maximize the attention and favors they receive and avoid the indifference and disapproval of others. . . . Tribute and affection must be constantly replenished and are sought from every interpersonal source and in every social context"; Millon et al., 1997, p. 17).

Contrasts of proportions of True responses of normal versus disordered criterion groups to each of the 175 MCMI-III items would provide much-needed information relevant to the validity of this potential explanation of the pathology bias of MCMI scales. It is important to realize that, to the extent that this explanation is correct, items and scales of the MCMI-III lack validity with respect to discrimination of normal versus disordered individuals. For example, if the same (or if a larger) proportion of normals as of histrionics or narcissistics answered the above three questions True, then these items (as keyed in the MCMI-III manual) could not be considered valid in relation to discriminating normals from histrionics or narcissistics. In general, the fact that persons who have a disorder tend to respond in a certain way to an item does not necessarily imply that this response is indicative of the presence of the disorder, because normals who do not have the disorder may be at least as likely to respond in this way to this item. Scales composed of items of this type would, of course, not be valid.

The current dearth of research on these topics suggests that Reynolds's (1992) caveat concerning use of the MCMI-II with nonclinical populations is also relevant to the MCMI-III:

> Clinicians must be extremely careful in using the MCMI-II with nonclinical populations such as in child custody evaluations, foster-parent studies, employment testing in all settings but especially in police agencies, security,

and nuclear energy settings where one might be strongly tempted to use the MCMI-II, and in criminal forensic work where one is presumed innocent and mentally healthy—the latter not being the assumption of the MCMI-II. (p. 534)

ITEM OVERLAP ISSUES

Virtually all authors who have evaluated the MCMI-I, MCMI-II, and MCMI-III have drawn attention to both positive and negative implications of item overlap (item sharing across scales). On the positive side, item sharing allows the generation, for each test taker, of a 20+ scale clinical profile from information gathered in a very short testing session. (It generally takes less than 30 minutes for a patient to respond to between 171 [MCMI-II] and 175 [MCMI-I and MCMI-III] items.) Also on the positive side, item overlap reflects and is generally consistent with Millon's bioevolutionary theory of personality development and psychopathology, a theory that has frequently been praised, even by some of the MCMI's most severe critics; for example, Widiger (1999) considers this theory to be "tremendously rich and grand in its coverage" (p. 388). On the negative side, item overlap has many drawbacks that, in the view of most reviewers of the MCMI, should not be ignored. In fact, Wetzler (1990), who reviewed the MCMI-II, described item overlap among scales as "the most limiting psychometric feature of the MCMI" (p. 447).

Among major problems associated with item overlap are the following:

1. Item sharing causes unacceptably high correlations of MCMI-I and MCMI-II scales intended to measure different traits (nonconvergent correlations). Several of these correlations exceed the average of the convergent correlations (correlations of MCMI-I and MCMI-II scales with identical names; LaVoie, 1991).
2. Item overlap across scales may inhibit differential diagnoses of similar disorders (LaVoie, 1991; Millon, 1987; Wetzler, 1990), as well as "interpretations of MCMI profiles" (Wetzler, 1990, p. 447).
3. Results of principal components analyses of scales with and without item overlap "diverge to a remarkable degree with regard to factor size, factor loadings, and factor priority (as judged by percentage of variance accounted for)" (LaVoie, 1991, p. 460).
4. The MCMI-II cannot be used to study covariation among personality disorders because of the extensive degree of item overlap (Wetzler, 1990): The "interrelationships among scales appear to be artifactual rather than a function of intrinsic conceptual relationship among dimensions" (p. 447).

5. The factor structure (obtained in factor analyses and principal components analyses) is built in by item overlap among the scales (Farley & Cohen, 1974; Retzlaff & Gibertini, 1987; Wetzler, 1990).

6. The built-in structure prevents "disconfirming [Millon's] theory of psychopathology" (LaVoie, 1991, p. 464); as noted by Widiger (1985), "Covariations suggested by Millon's theory . . . are built into the tests through the item overlap among scales" (p. 987).

7. Similarities among MCMI factor structures obtained with different groups can be largely attributed to item overlap (Gibertini & Retzlaff, 1988; Retzlaff & Gibertini, 1990).

8. Lack of independence of measurement errors causes spurious scale correlations (Bashaw & Anderson, 1967; Budescu & Rogers, 1981; Hsu, 1992).

EXTENT OF ITEM OVERLAP IN THE MCMI-III

Problems associated with item overlap will be present whenever scales share items, but of course, the seriousness of these problems can be expected to depend on the extent of the item overlap. According to LaVoie (1991), item overlap was worse in the MCMI-II than in the MCMI-I; he noted that the ratio of the average number of items per scale to number of items in the inventory actually increased from $37/175 = 0.21$ in the MCMI-I to $40/171 = 0.23$ in the MCMI-II. However, using the same index, it is apparent that item overlap is much less of a problem in the MCMI-III than in the two earlier versions. The ratio of the average number of items per scale to total number of items in the inventory for the MCMI-III is only $16/175 = 0.09$.

Table 14.1 was generated to (1) provide more detailed information about the extent of item overlap in the MCMI-II and MCMI-III and (2) allow for scale-by-scale comparison of the extent of overlap in these two versions. The entries were calculated from the scale composition information provided in the MCMI-II and MCMI-III manuals (Millon, 1987; Millon et al., 1997). The first two columns show the MCMI-II and MCMI-III percentages of items in each scale that appear on at least one other scale. For example, 97.1% of scale 1 items in the MCMI-II appear on at least one other scale, whereas only 81.2% of scale 1 MCMI-III items appear on at least one other scale. The last two columns indicate, for each scale, how many other scales share its items (one average). Thus, for example, the typical item in scale 1 is shared by 3.75 MCMI-III scales and by 6.37 MCMI-II scales. Table 14.1 entries show that the item-overlap has been greatly reduced in the MCMI-III relative to the MCMI-II but that nonnegligible item overlap is still present in the MCMI-III.

Table 14.1

Comparison of Item Overlap in MCMI-II and MCMI-III Scales

Scale	Percentage of Overlapping (Shared) Items in This Scale		Typical (Mean) Number of Scales Sharing Items with This Scale	
	MCMI-II	MCMI-III	MCMI-II	MCMI-III
1	97.1	81.2	6.37	3.75
2	100.0		6.42	
2A		93.7		4.31
2B		93.3		4.80
3	100.0	75.0	6.86	3.06
4	100.0	94.1	7.38	3.41
5	100.0	79.2	7.0	3.21
6A	100.0	100.0	6.62	4.12
6B	100.0	80.0	6.87	2.95
7	100.0	82.4	6.82	3.59
8A	100.0	87.5	7.29	3.62
8B	100.0	86.7	6.80	3.53
S	97.7	93.7	5.82	4.25
C	100.0	100.0	6.77	4.69
P	100.0	100.0	5.89	2.53
A	100.0	92.9	6.48	2.71
H	100.0	91.7	6.26	3.67
N	91.9	69.2	6.30	3.62
D	100.0	100.0	6.19	5.07
B	95.7	66.7	5.96	3.20
T	100.0	78.6	6.53	3.43
R		81.2		4.31
SS	97.0	82.4	5.76	4.29
CC	100.0	100.0	6.26	3.88
PP	100.0	76.9	5.41	2.31
Y	100.0	100.0	6.39	4.29
Z	100.0	100.0	6.28	3.79

IMPLICATIONS OF ITEM OVERLAP FOR INTERPRETATIONS OF
MCMIs IN RESEARCH AND IN CLINICAL PRACTICE

Millon (1987) justified the extensive item overlap among MCMI scales by noting that sharing of items was guided by his theory of psychopathology: "Scale overlap with the MCMI-I and MCMI-II was both anticipated and guided by the polythetic structural model and the dynamic features of its underlying theory" (p. 37). He argued that this model and its underlying theory implied that "many items should overlap . . . scales" (p. 36). Nevertheless, in response to Wiggins's (1982) critique of built-in correlations caused by item overlap in the MCMI-I, Millon adopted item weights (1, 2, 3) specifically for the purpose of reducing item-overlap-caused interscale correlations: "A major goal that prompted the development of differential item weights was the reduction of high levels of scale [correlations] that was built into the MCMI-I" (p. 131).

What should be noted, in relation to Millon's (1987) defense of item overlap and of his revision of the MCMI to address the problem of built-in correlations, is that critics of item overlap have not objected to the high correlations among MCMI scales per se, but to the possibility that the sizes of correlations among scales might be artifacts of item sharing (see, in particular, Wiggins, 1982, p. 211). "Differential item weighting" (the "overlap"-reducing strategy adopted in the construction of the MCMI-II) will affect interscale correlations, but it need not eliminate or even reduce spurious effects of item sharing. It simply complicates these spurious effects.

An extreme (and admittedly unrealistic) example may be used to illustrate how item overlap can cause the eight problems that were noted earlier (see also Hsu & Maruish, 1992). Consider that scales X and Y are constructed to measure levels of disorders X and Y. A test constructor who develops these scales believes in theory 1, which postulates that the levels of disorders X and Y are manifested in the same symptoms. The two scales are therefore made up of identical true-false (symptom) items, each of which is unit-weighted and keyed in the same direction (on scale X as on scale Y). Given that (as is the case with the MCMI) each subject responds to each item in the inventory exactly once, it is apparent that the correlation of scale X and Y total scores will be exactly 1.00, irrespective of (1) the size or composition of the patient group, (2) the contents of the items, and (3) how the patients responded to the items (patients could even have chosen their responses by tossing a coin or a die). Such a correlation of 1.00 would, of course, be entirely consistent with theory 1, but clearly, this correlation could hardly be interpreted as empirical support for theory 1. It would simply reflect how disorders X and Y were defined in theory 1.

If theory 2 postulated that each symptom of one disorder never co-occurred in the same patient with the presence of the other disorder, items in scales X and Y would be keyed in the opposite direction, and the correlation of X and Y would be −1.00 for any set of patients, irrespective of item contents and of how these patients responded to the items. The correlation would be −1.00 even if patients responded at random to all items. Once more, the numerical value of the correlation provides no empirical support for the theory (theory 2) but only reflects how the disorders were defined in the theory.

Item overlap among MCMI scales is, of course, never as extensive as in this example, but what is apparent is that, to the extent that overlap is present, correlations of scales as well as statistical analyses involving these correlations (e.g., exploratory principal components and factor analyses, confirmatory factor analyses, MANOVAs, MANCOVAs, discriminant function analyses, multiple regression analyses) and relations of elevations of scale scores in a patient's profile (differential diagnoses, discriminant validity) can be expected to reflect how the theory that led to the construction of the MCMI scales defined its constructs rather than whether or not the theory is valid.

Item overlap issues are, of course, not limited to scales that share items within an inventory (which I will call case A), but are also present when items are shared across scales that are not in the same inventory (case B), or when item contents are matched to external criteria (case C). The principal differences between effects of item overlap in A and B are implied by the fact that a single response determines each shared item's score on all scales in which this item appears in the same inventory (case A), whereas K responses determine the shared item's scores in the K inventories (case B). In the extreme example of theory 1, the correlation of scales X and Y, given case A, has to be 1.00 even if the only factor that affects item scores is measurement error (e.g., patients choose their responses using some random process, e.g., coin tosses). More generally, to the extent that scales within an inventory share items, correlations of these scales can be spuriously affected by lack of independence of measurement errors of overlapping items. Furthermore, in case A, similarities of factor structures across samples could be largely or completely determined by item overlap. (For a detailed explanation of how case A experimental dependence of responses of subjects to overlapping items can control factor structures of scales, and for methods of adjusting correlations of personality scales for spurious effects of case A overlap with unit-weighted items, see Bashaw & Anderson, 1967; Budescu & Rodgers, 1981; Hsu, 1992.)

In case B, the correlation of the same scale (for the extreme example of theory 1) included in two different inventories is expected to be less than 1.00 because each patient need not respond to each overlapping item in the same way in the two inventories. In this example, the observed correlation could be viewed as a reliability coefficient (and its value would, unlike in case A, actually be .00 with random responding). More generally, to the extent that case B scales share items (that are keyed in the same direction), the correlations of these scales should be viewed as measures of reliability (rather than measures of concurrent validity).

When contents of items in MCMI scales are matched to external criteria (case C), correlations of item or scale scores with criteria will be reduced not just by experimental independence of measurement errors, but also by the extent to which item contents differ from the criteria. Widiger (1999) provides illustrations of such differences. For example, "the second DSM-IV schizoid criterion is 'almost always chooses solitary activities.' The comparable test item (Item 27) is 'When I have a choice, I prefer to do things alone'" (p. 378). The extent of this type of "overlap" in the MCMI-III is not negligible: Daubert and Metzler (2000) found that "there is a strong degree of concordance between MCMI-III items and specific diagnostic criteria. Fully 84% (105) of the 125 relevant diagnostic criteria statements in the *Diagnostic and Statistical Manual of Mental Disorders* (4th ed., rev., *DSM-IV*; American Psychiatric Association) have a directly corresponding item on the MCMI-III" (p. 418). The extent to which correlations of (or diagnostic efficiency statistics for) MCMI-III items and scales with *DSM-IV* diagnostic criteria provide evidence of validity of the MCMI can perhaps be considered to depend on the extent to which the *DSM-IV* criteria are considered valid.

The extensive differences between the MCMI-II and MCMI-III (e.g., the MCMI-III includes 95 items that were not included in the MCMI-II) seem to reflect a shift from item overlap among MCMI scales motivated by Millon's theory (in the MCMI-I and MCMI-II) to overlap between MCMI-III item contents and *DSM-IV* criteria motivated by the need to improve concordance between MCMI diagnoses and *DSM-IV* diagnoses. Widiger (1999) noted:

> Many (if not most) of the MCMI-III items were . . . written or re-written to represent the *DSM-IV* diagnostic criteria rather than the self-other, pleasure-pain, and active-passive . . . constructs [of Millon's theory]. In the section [of the 1997 manual] . . . that is concerned with item development, examples of items for each of the scales are provided. All of the examples refer to *DSM-IV* diagnostic criteria. No mention is made in the presentation of examples of the theoretical construct from which the scales were purportedly derived. (p. 378)

The problem associated with these changes is that "most of the diagnostic criteria for the *DSM-IV* personality disorders were not [in spite of Millon's membership in the committee that developed the *DSM-IV*] based on Millon's . . . theoretical model" (p. 378).

Obtaining empirical evidence of validity of Millon's theory using the MCMI-I or MCMI-II has been hampered primarily by the extensive experimental dependence associated with item sharing of scales within each of the earlier versions of the MCMI (see, in particular, LaVoie, 1991). Obtaining empirical evidence of validity of Millon's theory using the MCMI-III has been hampered not by item overlap (which, as noted earlier, has been considerably reduced relative to earlier MCMI versions) but by the lack of clear, explicit, and testable specification of how MCMI-III scales are linked to Millon's theory (see Widiger, 1999). However, researchers who are not interested in the validity of Millon's theory but in assessing validity of the MCMI-III in relation to the *DSM-IV* may view overlap of item contents with *DSM-IV* criteria (case C overlap) as desirable (assuming they consider *DSM-IV* criteria valid), in the sense that it is this type of overlap that is likely to increase agreement of classifications based on MCMI-III scales and classifications based on the *DSM-IV*.

FUTURE RESEARCH ON ITEM OVERLAP

Future research related to item overlap might focus on different issues for cases A, B, and C. In case A, existing methods that adjust correlations of scales within an inventory for spurious effects of experimental dependence (see Bashaw & Anderson, 1967; Budescu & Rodgers, 1981; Hsu, 1992) could be generalized to inventories (such as the MCMI-II and MCMI-III) that include multiple weighting of items. Alternatively, Monte Carlo studies could be carried out to provide empirical estimates of scale and interscale parameters, as well as of the factor structure parameters, when patients respond at random or when they respond in some other manner (response styles) that ignores item contents or that takes content into account to create a desired impression. Note that with case A item overlap, nonzero correlations will be caused by the item overlap in all of these situations. These nonzero correlations will, in turn, cause spurious factor structures to emerge in principal components analyses, as well as in both exploratory and confirmatory factor analyses. More specifically, Monte Carlo studies could simply involve generation of N sets of random responses (one set per simulated respondent) to the 175 MCMI-III items, scoring (weighted raw scores and/or BR scores) of these items to obtain the 24 MCMI-III scale scores, correlations of these scale scores, and determination of factor structures. These correlations and factor structures would reflect spurious case A item overlap effects and could then be used as baselines against which to evaluate and interpret correlations and factor structures obtained from real patient groups. Similarly, Monte Carlo studies could be used to estimate response set or response style effects on MCMI-III scale, interscale, and factor structure parameters.

According to Gynther and Green (1982), case B item overlap is a "widespread problem" that results in "spuriously high validity coefficients" (p. 372). However, future case B item overlap studies could also be considered to provide empirical information about (a) consistency of responding to the same items and item sets across inventories and

(b) context effects. These studies would also yield useful information about the extent to which scales that supposedly measure different constructs in different inventories, and whose correlations are generally interpreted as nonconvergent correlations, correlate because of the item sharing.

Future case C overlap studies could include, but not be limited to, diagnostic validity (efficiency) studies of the MCMI-III (see the section on Biases in Diagnostic Efficiency Statistics). However, to address possible low values of these indices, investigations might focus on assessing how well items in a scale designed to measure a *DSM-IV* disorder adequately sample the "domain of the targeted construct" (Haynes, Nelson, & Blaine, 1999, p. 142). For example, researchers might attempt to determine the extent to which the 16 items of the new PTSD scale of the MCMI-III are "proportionally distributed across the three major symptom clusters of PTSD outlined by the DSM-IV" (Haynes et al., 1999, p. 142). To the extent that these 16 items achieve this goal of proportional sampling, the MCMI-III PTSD scale could be expected to be a valid indicator of *DSM-IV* PTSD. Because the names of the MCMI-III scales actually match names of *DSM-IV* categories, this type of study could be used to assess the extent to which items in each of the MCMI-III scales represent the symptom clusters of the corresponding *DSM-IV* category.

BASE RATE SCORES VERSUS RAW SCORES: INTERPRETATION AND DATA ANALYSIS ISSUES

Users of the MCMI-III can choose between two types of MCMI scale scores: weighted raw scores (often simply called raw scores) and base rate (BR) scores that are transformations of the weighted raw scores. In general, BR scores have received positive evaluations from critics and have been chosen over raw scores by both clinical practitioners and researchers. However, weighted raw scores have been recommended over BR scores (see Millon, 1987) to researchers who carry out statistical analyses of MCMI data (see also Holmes, 1987). Closer examination of the definitions of raw and BR scores is necessary for a critical assessment of the major implications of the choice of raw versus BR scores by both researchers and practitioners.

Weighted Raw Scores

The weighted raw score for each MCMI-III scale is defined as the sum of weighted item scores of the items that compose this scale. For each prototypal item (a prototypal item is an item considered "central . . . to the definition of [the] construct" measured by the scale; Millon et al., 1997, p. 2) that a patient answers in the keyed direction, 2 points are added to his or her total score for that scale. For each nonprototypal item answered in the keyed direction, 1 point is added to his or her raw score for that scale.

RELATIONS OF RAW SCORES TO BASE RATE SCORES

The MCMI-III BR scores are nonlinear transformations of the weighted raw scores. According to the revised MCMI-III manual (Millon et al., 1997), the transformation of raw scores to BR scores, though nonlinear, is "monotonic" (p. 62), which, according to the authors, means that "higher raw scores *always* [italics added] mean higher base rate scores (before secondary adjustments are made)" (p. 62). However, after an examination of the MCMI-III manual's BR transformation tables (Millon et al., 1997, Appendix C), it becomes apparent that the manual's description of the relation of raw to BR scores needs to be revised, and that the revision has important implications for data analysis and interpretation. For many of the 24 scales (specifically, 9 out of 24 scales for males and 11 out of 24 scales for females), the statement "higher raw scores always mean higher base rate scores (before secondary adjustments are made)" is not accurate. For example, for the Narcissism scale, an increase of 7 points at the upper end of the raw score range is associated (for females) with an increase of 0 points on the BR scale (see Figure 14.1). In contrast, an increase of 7 raw score points at the lower end of the raw score range corresponds to an increase of 38 points on the Narcissistic BR scale (see Millon et al., 1997, p. 174). Thirty-eight points on the BR scale is not negligible because it is 33% of the BR score range (viz., 0 to 115). Thus, depending on the location of the BR score change, the same increase in raw scores can correspond to absolutely no change in the BR score or to a BR increase that is one-third of the entire range of BR scores.

DATA ANALYSIS IMPLICATIONS OF RAW-TO-BR SCORE
TRANSFORMATION RULES

A nonlinear transformation of an interval scale is inadmissible because it results in loss of equality of units in the transformed scale (see Stevens, 1951). One implication of the fact that BR scores are nonlinear (and in fact, not even strictly monotonic) transformations of raw scores is that if raw scores of an MCMI-III scale can be considered interval measurements of a

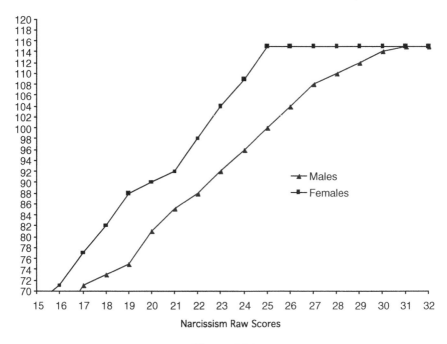

Figure 14.1

Relation of MCMI-III Narcissism raw and BR scores for males and females.

construct (as suggested by Millon, 1987, p. 183), then the BR scores for that scale cannot be interval measurements of the same construct (see also Holmes, 1987). Similarly, if BR scores are interval measurements, of a construct then raw scores cannot be interval measurements of the same construct. Thus, if parametric tests of significance (which require at least interval-level measurements when researchers are interested in answering nontrivial real-world questions) are defensible for one type of measurement (say, raw scores) because this type of measurement has interval-scale properties, then these tests would be indefensible for the other type of measurement (say, BR scores).

According to the MCMI-II manual (Millon, 1987), "Raw scores are more appropriate than base rate scores when the statistical analysis to be performed on MCMI-II results require[s] the use of interval level measurement" (p. 183). However, in the majority of published research on the MCMI-I, MCMI-II, and MCMI-III, statistical analyses (which require interval-level measurements) were explicitly carried out on MCMI BR scores. In several additional studies that have analyzed MCMI-III data using parametric statistical methods, authors did not indicate whether the methods were applied to raw scores or to BR scores. Perhaps the fact that correlations of raw and BR scores reported in the manuals are generally high (e.g., in the 1997 MCMI-III manual, they are all greater than .82) has led researchers to believe that the choice of type of score to analyze is unimportant with respect to conclusions drawn from the significance tests. However, such a belief would not be justified. This will first be demonstrated when the same transformation rule is applied to all raw scores collected in a study, that is, when all persons who receive the same raw score are assigned the same BR score, and then when different transformation rules are applied to different persons (males and females with the same raw score are assigned different BR scores).

CONFLICTS IN RESULTS WHEN A SINGLE TRANSFORMATION RULE IS USED

Consider that the efficacy of a treatment is investigated in a single-group pretest-treatment-posttest design involving 22 female patients. Suppose the pre- and posttreatment raw Narcissism scores of these patients are as follows (the entire data set is provided so that the reader can verify the surprising conclusions drawn below): (24,25), (31,30), (30,29), (29,28), (28,27), (27,26), (26,25), (24,25), (24,25), (31,30), (24,25), (31,30), (30,29), (29,28), (28,27), (27,26), (26,25), (24,25), (24,25), (31,30), (28,27), (27,26).

A correlated t test of the difference between the pre- and posttreatment means of raw scores yields evidence of a statistically *significant reduction in Narcissism raw scores* for this group of 22 patients ($t = -2.34$, $p < .03$, two-tailed test). However, after transforming these raw scores into BR scores (using the Narcissism Raw to BR Score Transformation Table for females; Millon et al., 1997, p. 174), the correlated t test applied to the BR scores yields evidence of a statistically *significant increase in Narcissism BR scores* for this group of patients ($t = 2.81$, $p < .01$, two-tailed test). This example shows that the choice of type of score (raw versus BR) to be analyzed via parametric significance tests can lead to either a conclusion of *significant beneficial effects* of the treatment or to a completely contradictory conclusion of *significant harmful effects* of the treatment, even when the same transformation table is used to convert raw scores to BR scores for all patients in the study.

CONFLICTS WHEN TRANSFORMATION RULES DIFFER FOR
DIFFERENT GROUPS

It should be noted that the raw-to-BR score transformation rules differ across gender groups. Thus, raw and BR scores are not interchangeable in relation to data analyses, not only because of nonlinearity of

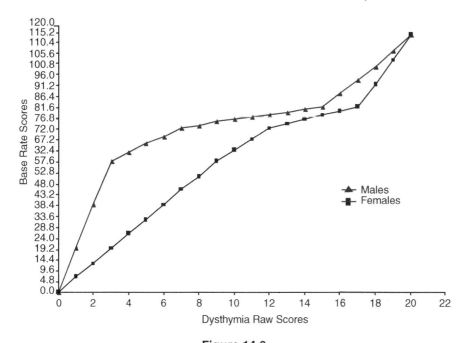

Figure 14.2
Relation of MCMI-III Dysthymia raw and BR scores for males and females.

transformations within gender groups, but also because of the differences in transformation rules across gender groups. This is apparent in Figure 14.2, which shows the relation of Dysthymia BR scores to Dysthymia raw scores of males and females.

Given the MCMI-III manual's (Millon et al., 1997) raw-to-BR score transformation rules for males and females, the BR score of males who obtain a raw score of 3 on the Dysthymia scale is 60, whereas the BR scores of females who obtain the same raw score of 3 is 20. Thus, males and females who have identical raw scores on the Dysthymia scale can differ by 40 (i.e., 60 − 20 = 40) points on the Dysthymia BR scale. A 40-point difference on the BR scale is not negligible because the within-group standard deviation of these scores is generally reported to be somewhere between 20 and 25: With a standard deviation of 20, a 40-point difference is a two standard deviation difference. In terms of Cohen's effect size d, this corresponds to an effect size of 2.0, which is 2.5 times larger than what Cohen has described as a "large" effect size. When *t* or *F* tests are used to test contrasts of means of males and females, it would of course be easy to demonstrate that, even with very small samples, males and females could differ significantly on the Dysthymia BR scale, despite the fact that they obtained identical Dysthymia raw score means. Once more, it is clear that conclusions drawn from parametric hypothesis testing could very well be determined by the choice of type of score to be analyzed.

Another implication is that imbalance in gender composition of contrasted groups in comparative efficacy studies could markedly affect results of significance tests. For example, if most subjects in a group exposed to treatment A were males, and most subjects in a group exposed to treatment B were females, it would be possible for two groups that had identical raw score means to have significantly different BR score means. Clearly, the choice of types of score to analyze could determine conclusions about relative efficacy of two treatments. Effect size (and other parameter) estimates would, of course, also be affected by this choice.

Future Research Related to Raw-to-BR Score Transformation Rules

Several issues related to Raw-to-BR score transformation rules need to be addressed in future investigations. Millon (1987) recommended the use of raw scores in statistical analyses, but the majority of MCMI researchers have used BR scores in their statistical analyses. Because conflicting conclusions could be drawn when the same parametric tests are applied to raw versus BR scores, this is not a trivial issue. One approach to this problem for investigators who have access to the data is to perform data analyses on both types of scores to assess whether conflicting conclusions would result. Alternatively, investigations might focus on identifying the contexts and questions for which raw scores can be demonstrated to approximate interval measurements of the targeted construct more closely than BR scores obtained from a single, or from more than one, raw-to-BR score transformation table(s) (and vice versa). For example, issues related to the justification of gender differences in transformation rules could be addressed. As demonstrated earlier, the same raw score can correspond to very different BR scores for males versus females. This suggests that the same raw score should have very different real-world meanings for males versus females. To what extent are differences in BR scores of males and females who obtain the same raw score (see, e.g., Figure 14.2) justifiable in terms of differences between males and females on meaningful external criteria? Questions of interest might be: are females who have much lower BR scores than males (but the same raw scores) on a specific scale less likely to attempt suicide—after controlling (empirically or statistically) for performances on the other scales in the inventory? Are males and females who have the same BR score profiles equally likely to attempt suicide? Alternatively, are males and females who have equal raw (rather that BR) scores equally likely to attempt suicide? Clearly, studies of this type would be relevant to (1) the choice of type of score to use when parametric statistical methods are used to address specific questions, (2) the choice of type of score to use in clinical settings, and (3) the debate concerning the relevance of research to clinical practice. The choice of type of score to analyze might also be made on purely pragmatic grounds. For example, in a study whose objective is to develop MCMI-based models for predicting some outcome (e.g., suicide attempts) researchers might fit logistic regression models to both raw scores and BR scores and determine (from cross-validation results) which type of score vector (vector of raw scores, or vector of BR scores) leads to more accurate predictions.

RESPONSE SETS

As noted by Messick (1991), "It has been presumed that the score a person attains on a ... psychological test is determined by relevant responses to the specific content of the stimulus items" (p. 161). However, he adds that the

> respondent may characteristically bring to tests of certain formats (such as true-false ...) various test taking attitudes and habits (such as the tendency to agree when in doubt) that produce a cumulative effect on his or her scores. Aspects of item and test form, then, may differentially influence an individual's mode of item response and permit or even facilitate the operation of preferred or habitual styles of response. ... A test presumed to measure one characteristic may thus also inadvertently be measuring another characteristic (response set). (pp. 161–162)

As noted by Aiken (1989), there are two types of response sets that are of particular concern in inventories such as the MCMI: acquiescence and social desirability. Due to space limitations, only problems associated with the acquiescence response set are discussed in this chapter.

The MCMI-I has been criticized (LaVoie, 1991) for having too many True-keyed items: The proportion of True-keyed items in this version of the MCMI was .83. In his critique of the second version of the MCMI, LaVoie noted that the situation had not improved: In the MCMI-II, "less than 100 [items] are negatively keyed [out of 880]" (p. 460). Instead of reducing the proportion of positively keyed items, the MCMI-II actually increased that proportion, from .83 to .89 (i.e., $(880 - 100)/880 = .886$). In the MCMI-III, the situation has also not improved: Out of 416 keyed items, 380 are positively keyed (True-keyed). Thus, in the MCMI-III, the proportion of positively keyed items has increased to .91.

More detailed information relevant to a comparison of the extent of the acquiescence response set problem in the MCMI-II and MCMI-III is provided in Table 14.2, which lists the percentage of True-keyed items on each scale. (These percentages were calculated from MCMI manual information about item composition and keying in MCMI-II and MCMI-III scales.) Most noteworthy is the fact that the number of scales consisting entirely of True-keyed items (i.e., 100% True-keyed) in the MCMI-III is more than double that of the MCMI-II (i.e., the MCMI-III has 17 scales in which all items are True-keyed, whereas the MCMI-II has 8 such scales). This is important because the impact of the acquiescence response set is maximum when the percentage of True-keyed items deviates maximally from 50%. In fact, two scales composed entirely of unit-weighted True-keyed items would be expected to have a correlation close to 1.00 if variability in subjects' responses was determined entirely by the variability in their tendencies to acquiesce. In the MCMI-II, there are 28 pairings of 100% True-keyed scales (i.e., $_8C_2 = 28$). But in the MCMI-III, this number is almost 5 *times* larger (viz., $_{17}C_2 = 136$). To the extent that acquiescence response set is present in contexts in which the MCMI is administered, it is likely to spuriously increase correlations of all pairs of 100% True-keyed scales, and because the number of pairs of these scales is nearly 5 times larger in the MCMI-III than in the MCMI-II, this problem is potentially much more serious in the MCMI-III than it was in the MCMI-II. It would appear that conditions conducive to acquiescence response set problems have become progressively worse with each revision of the MCMI. This could be due, at least in part, to the internal consistency criteria used in item selection; that is, False-keyed items in scales composed mostly of True-keyed items may very well have had low internal consistency statistics. Thus, because one criterion for deletion of items in revisions of the MCMI was low internal consistency statistics (see Millon et al., 1997), False-keyed items may well have been systematically discarded in each successive revision of the MCMI. This conjecture could easily be confirmed or refuted by those who have access to the relevant item internal consistency statistics.

FUTURE RESEARCH ON ACQUIESCENCE

Responses to MCMI items are, of course, not completely determined by the acquiescence response set. However, at this time, there is little information about the extent to which variabilities in respondents' tendencies to acquiesce spuriously affect elevations of their MCMI scale scores, the intercorrelation of MCMI scales, differential diagnoses, or the factor structures of scales in the MCMI inventories. In fact, there is no discussion of these topics in the MCMI manuals. More research in this area

Table 14.2

Acquiescence-Set–Relevant Statistics
for MCMI-II and MCMI-III Scales

| Scale | Percentage of True-Keyed Items | |
	MCMI-II	MCMI-III
1	71.4	87.5
2	87.8	
2A		87.5
2B		100.0
3	59.5	93.8
4	80.0	41.2
5	81.6	58.3
6A	88.9	94.1
6B	84.4	100.0
7	55.3	47.1
8A	92.7	100.0
8B	97.5	100.0
S	90.9	100.0
C	100.0	100.0
P	100.0	100.0
A	96.0	100.0
H	96.8	100.0
N	89.2	100.0
D	91.7	100.0
B	93.5	93.3
R		100.0
T	98.3	100.0
SS	100.0	100.0
CC	100.0	100.0
PP	100.0	100.0
Y	100.0	47.6
Z	100.0	100.0

would be particularly welcome for the MCMI-III in view of the fact that spurious effects of the acquiescence response set are likely to be much more serious in the MCMI-III than in earlier MCMI versions.

Empirical approaches to the detection and control of acquiescence response set effects have been described in Messick (1991), and Strack, Lorr, Campbell, and Lamnin (1992), among others. Messick noted that "if the same content is tapped in true-keyed and false-keyed forms and consistently higher trait scores are obtained with one form than with the other, then an agreement response set may be a contaminating influence" (p. 162). Revising most items would involve little more than making a minor modification so that the False-keyed item describes a behavior that is the complement of that described in the True-keyed item. For example, the item "It is very easy for me to make many friends" might be modified to "It is NOT very easy for me to make many friends"; the item "People usually think of me as a reserved and serious-minded person" could be changed to "People DO NOT usually think of me as a reserved and serious-minded person." To the extent that acquiescence response set is negligible, respondents should give opposite responses to corresponding items on the two forms. A study that would involve revising all (or most) of the 175 MCMI items and administering of the original and revised forms to the same pool of subjects (with a suitable time interval between forms to control for memory effects, and counterbalancing to decrease carryover effects) should provide useful information about the extent to which acquiescence response set affects (1) individual scores on MCMI-III scales, (2) intercorrelation of MCMI-III scales, and (3) factor structures of these scales.

The most popular method of attempting to control (or at least clarify or assess) for the acquiescence response set effects consists of constructing "balanced" scales (Meier, 1994). A balanced scale has half of its items keyed True and the other half keyed False. After rekeying enough of the MCMI-III items to obtain 24 balanced scales, researchers could compare results obtained with these scales to results obtained with the unaltered MCMI scales. Absence of differences in elevations and shapes of the 24-scale profiles of test takers would provide support for the view that acquiescence response set effects were negligible.

Researchers might also consider developing an Acquiescence scale constructed from MCMI items and modeled after the TRIN scale of the MMPI-2. The TRIN scale consists of pairs of items that have been matched (within-pairs) for opposite meaning. Thus, a patient who endorsed (answered True to) both items in a pair would add 1 point to his or her Acquiescence score. The construction of such a scale would not require adding items to the MCMI but identifying pairs of contradictory items that could then be scored as in the MMPI-2 TRIN scale.

BIASES IN DIAGNOSTIC EFFICIENCY STATISTICS

According to the current MCMI-III publishers (Pearson Assessments), the MCMI-III was designed to detect "Axis I and Axis II disorders based on the new *DSM-IV* classification system, [and identify] the personality disorders that underlie a patient's presenting symptoms" (http:www.pearsonassessments.com/tests/mcmi_3.htm#norms). Similarly, Widiger (1999) noted that "a major purpose of the MCMI-III is to provide a valid assessment of the DSM-IV personality disorders. . . . Its success as a clinical instrument is dependent primarily on its validity as a measure of the DSM-IV personality disorders" (p. 379).

The extent to which the MCMI-III provides valid assessment of *DSM-IV* personality disorders has been measured primarily with diagnostic efficiency statistics (also called diagnostic validity statistics), the most popular of which are sensitivity (SE), specificity (SP), positive predictive power (PPP), and negative predictive power (NPP). According to Millon et al. (1997), "The use of diagnostic efficiency statistics as evidence of external validity [constitutes] . . . a unique aspect of the MCMI-III" (p. 144). They note:

> The advantages of using these operating statistics are numerous. In essence, they make validity results accessible to lay jurors by answering a series of probability questions. Such questions include (a) what are the chances that someone who has X disorder will be identified by the test as having this disorder [SE], (b) what are the chances that someone who does not have X disorder will be correctly classified by the test as not having it [SP], and (c) what are the chances that someone who is found by the test to have X disorder actually does have it [PPP]? (p. 144)

SEs, SPs, and PPPs were reported for the MCMI-III in two separate studies (Millon, 1994; Millon et al., 1997).

Several important issues are relevant to the interpretation of diagnostic efficiency statistics and to the assessment of diagnostic validities of MCMI-III scales. These issues concern implications of (1) the choice of diagnostic validity statistics on the assessment of validities of scales, (2) prior knowledge and backgrounds of clinicians involved in studies that yield diagnostic validity indices on biases of these indices, (3) effects of base rates of disorders across diagnostic settings on generalizability of diagnostic validity statistics, and (4) effects of differences in demographics of the patients across diagnostic settings on generalizability of the diagnostic validity statistics.

Choosing Diagnostic Validity Statistics

To avoid possible biased assessments of diagnostic validities of MCMI-III scales, future diagnostic validity studies of the MCMI-III should report more than SEs, PPPs, and hit rates (these were the only diagnostic validity statistics reported in the 1997 MCMI-III manual). Several problems with studies that report only these statistics should be noted. First, it is possible for a scale that has no discriminating ability whatsoever to yield an SE = 1.00. This can be achieved by simply adopting a diagnostic cut-off score low enough to classify all patients as having the disorder. Then 100% of those who have the disorder will be correctly diagnosed by the scale as having the disorder, and so the SE will be 1.00. Of course, adopting such a cut-off score would necessarily result in an SP = .00. Reporting the SP whenever the SE is reported would provide the reader information about exactly what the costs are, in terms of specificity, of high sensitivities (or vice versa). In the case of most MCMI-III scales, high SPs were attained by using high diagnostic cut-off scores, which in turn resulted in relatively low SEs. Thus, focusing exclusively on the reported SEs could result in unnecessarily pessimistic evaluations of these scales.

Second, it is often possible to attain a very high PPP for a scale that has very little discriminating ability by choosing a sufficiently high diagnostic cut-off score. But this cut-off score may well cause a very low NPP. Therefore, when PPPs are reported, it is suggested that NPPs also be reported to inform the reader about the costs in terms of lowered NPPs of high PPPs (or vice versa).

Third, the PPP, which is generally considered the most important of the diagnostic efficiency statistics (see, e.g., Millon, 1994; Retzlaff, 1996), carries little information about values of other diagnostic validity statistics. The coefficients of determination (i.e., the squared correlations) of PPPs of the 24 MCMI-III scales with 5 other diagnostic validity statistics of the 1994 MCMI study extended from .0018 to .0164 (Hsu, 2002). These low coefficients of determination indicate that a scale that has a high PPP could perform very poorly when validity is assessed by any or all of the other measures of diagnostic efficiency; hence, there is a need to report more than PPPs. In particular, Hsu noted that in the 1994 validity study, the MCMI-III Anxiety scale, which had the highest PPP of the 24 scales, had the lowest value (out of 24) of each of five other diagnostic efficiency statistics. Reporting only PPPs of scales could clearly be misleading.

Fourth, none of the most popular diagnostic validity statistics (SE, SP, PPP, and NPP) adjusts for chance agreement between scale-based diagnoses and *DSM-IV* diagnoses. This is a problem because of the fact that a scale that appears to have high diagnostic validity as determined by these statistics may actually be performing worse than chance. In fact, Hsu (2002) showed that, in the 1994 study, the scale that had the highest PPP of the 24 MCMI-III scales consistently performed worse than chance, as determined by five chance-corrected diagnostic validity indices. This suggests the need to report chance-adjusted diagnostic validity statistics in future diagnostic validity studies of the MCMI-III. Cut-off score– and base rate–independent diagnostic validity statistics (see Hsu, 2002) should also be reported.

EXPERIMENTAL DESIGN CHARACTERISTICS RELEVANT TO THE INTERPRETATION OF DIAGNOSTIC VALIDITY STATISTICS

Diagnostic efficiency statistics are not only useful as measures of the diagnostic validities that can be understood by "lay jurors" (Millon et al., 1997, p. 144) and clinicians in their evaluations and interpretations of MCMI scales and scale scores, but also as measures that can be used by researchers to compare diagnostic validities of different versions of the same MCMI scales. Because the MCMI has undergone two extensive, time-consuming, and costly revisions, the major goal of which was to improve the diagnostic efficiency of the scales, it would seem reasonable to ask whether the most recent version of the MCMI is in fact superior to its predecessors in this respect.

To address this question, Millon et al. (1997) compared the SEs and PPPs of corresponding scales of the MCMI-I, MCMI-II, and MCMI-III (see Millon et al., 1997, tables 4.4 and 4.5). In relation to the MCMI-II and MCMI-III, the conclusions drawn by Millon et al. with respect to Axis I scales were that "although sensitivity statistics are mixed relative to the MCMI-II, positive predictive power statistics are generally higher, and in some cases much higher than for the MCMI-II . . . the diagnostic criterion validity of the MCMI-III is comparable and, for some Axis I scales, marginally superior to that of the MCMI-II" (pp. 100–101). Concerning Axis II MCMI scales, Millon et al. concluded that "the shift in Axis II diagnostic efficiency statistics from the MCMI to the MCMI-II and MCMI-III shows a modest but generally upward trend in the instrument's sensitivity and positive predictive power" (p. 102).

The upward trend in the MCMI's diagnostic validity statistics has been questioned by Hess (1998), Choca (2001), Widiger (2001), and more recently by Hsu (2002). To understand the problems associated with estimation of the diagnostic validities of MCMI-III scales, it should first be noted that the two diagnostic validity studies carried out by Millon (in 1994 and in 1997) yielded very different estimates of diagnostic validities of the scales, and that the 1997 diagnostic efficiency statistics were consistently much higher than the corresponding 1994 statistics (see Table 14.3).

After drawing attention to some very disappointing diagnostic efficiency statistics reported in the 1994 MCMI-III manual, Hess (1998) wrote:

> Reviewers of the first two editions of the MCMI were appropriately critical but quite hopeful and even enthusiastic for the MCMI [but that] the third

Table 14.3

Comparison of Average Diagnostic Validity Statistics of the
MCMI-III 1994 and 1997 External Validity Studies

Diagnostic Validity Statistic	1997	1994	Difference	Ratio
Sensitivity	0.670	0.275	0.394	2.431
Specificity	0.968	0.860	0.107	1.125
Positive Predictive Power	0.640	0.223	0.417	2.871
Negative Predictive Power	0.964	0.887	0.078	1.088
Quality of IPPP	0.608	0.109	0.499	5.560
Quality of INPP	0.637	0.156	0.481	4.081
Cohen's Kappa	0.610	0.128	0.482	4.766
Cohen's Effect Size	2.362	0.588	1.774	4.015
Area under ROC Curve	0.937	0.653	0.285	1.436

Note: Each entry is the mean of 24 values (14 from MCMI-III Personality Disorder scales; 10 from MCMI-III Axis I Disorder scales) of a diagnostic validity index. IPPP = Incremental validity of a positive test score; INPP = Incremental validity of a negative test score.

This table originally appeared in Hsu, L. M. (2002). Diagnostic validity statistics and the MCMI-III. *Psychological Assessment, 14,* 410–422 as is used with permission of the American Psychological Association.

edition (i.e., the MCMI-III) represents a regression; the MCMI's promissory notes are past due. The user of the MCMI-III does so at his or her own risk. (p. 667)

Choca (2001) made similar but somewhat less critical comments concerning the diagnostic validity statistics reported in the 1994 MCMI-III manual: "The operating characteristics [i.e., diagnostic validity statistics] of the first two editions [i.e., the MCMI-I and MCMI-II] spoke well for those instruments. In contrast, the operating characteristics for the MCMI-III left something to be desired" (p. 766). Similarly, Widiger (2001) described the low values of the diagnostic validity statistics reported in Millon (1994) for the MCMI-III as "remarkably poor results [even though] they were based on the test authors' own validation data" (p. 768). Widiger, who, unlike Hess (1998) and Choca (2001), had access to diagnostic validity statistics reported in the 1997 MCMI-III manual (Millon et al., 1997), noted that there were impressive increases in these statistics from 1994 to 1997. However, he also drew attention to the fact that little information was provided in the 1997 manual to explain this "substantial improvement" (p. 768).

Hsu (2002) provided detailed information about the marked improvements in the 1997 diagnostic validities of MCMI-III scales (see Table 14.3

for a summary). Millon et al. (1997) and Retzlaff (1996) accounted for these improvements primarily in terms of limitations of the 1994 study that led to underestimation of validities of the MCMI-III scales. The principal flaws of the 1994 study—which apparently were not recognized as such at the time the study was designed—were identified as lack of familiarity of therapists with their patients, and with the "theoretical and clinical grounding of personality constructs" (Millon et al., 1997, p. 102). It was primarily these flaws that motivated the diagnostic validity study whose results were reported in the 1997 MCMI-III manual. In the 1997 validity study, "some 75 clinicians who were well acquainted with the MCMI and with Millon's (1990) evolutionary theory and who had participated in earlier MCMI research projects were invited to participate" (Millon et al., 1997, p. 88). A characteristic shared by all clinicians who took part in the 1997 study was that of "having substantial direct contact with the patients they were to evaluate" (p. 88): The minimum contact time was 3 hours and the maximum was 60 hours.

The 1997 diagnostic validity study overcame some of the major flaws of the 1994 study, and undoubtedly the correction of these flaws accounted for some of the increases in the 1997 diagnostic validity statistics. However, a criterion contamination problem (which was acknowledged but not considered important by Millon et al., 1997) was noted in Choca's (2001) otherwise very positive evaluation of the MCMI-III: Choca described the MCMI-III as "one of the greatest contributions made to the field during his professional life" (p. 766), but also indicated that, unfortunately, "the research design [used in the 1997 validity study] allowed clinicians who had seen the MCMI-III results to assign the diagnoses, obviously contaminating the data" (p. 766). Hsu (2002) provided more information concerning criterion contamination as well as the possibility of confirmatory bias and availability heuristics biases in the 1997 study.

Given the problems of criterion contamination, confirmatory bias, and availability heuristics, it would be very desirable to demonstrate in future studies that diagnostic validity statistics as high as the ones reported in the 1997 MCMI-III manual (Millon et al., 1997) can actually be obtained when (1) clinicians who are asked to classify patients according to the *DSM-IV* (American Psychiatric Association) do so prior rather than after seeing their patients' MCMI-III scores, and (2) clinicians who participate in the study are not required to fill out both the ratings that determine each patient's *DSM-IV* diagnoses and the patient's MCMI-III scores on a single form (MCMI-III scale names are identical to those of the *DSM-IV* categories and are listed in the same order on the form as the *DSM-IV* categories; see Hsu, 2002). The MCMI-III manual (Millon et al., 1997) is exemplary in allowing public scrutiny of important procedural details of the 1997 study by providing readers a copy of the form distributed to clinicians who participated in this study.

Also, given the criteria used in the selection of clinicians who were invited to take part in the 1997 study (in particular (1) participation in earlier MCMI research projects prior to the 1997 study and (2) familiarity with Millon's evolutionary theory), it would be desirable to assess the extent to which the high values of the diagnostic validity statistics reported in the 1997 study are limited to clinicians who meet these criteria.

BASE RATES OF DISORDERS AND GENERALIZABILITY

Craig (1999) recommended that "clinicians who use the MCMI as part of their testimony are expected to have a working knowledge of diagnostic efficiency statistics in areas being evaluated as well as the latest research in this area" (p. 297). Because Millon et al. (1997) have suggested that the MCMI-III can be used in a wide variety of settings (e.g., child custody cases, prisons), this working knowledge should include awareness of the major factors that limit generalizability of diagnostic efficiency statistics across settings.

Three major requirements for diagnostic validity statistics to generalize across diagnostic settings are as follows: (1) The same disorders must be present across the two settings; (2) patients in a disorder category in one setting must be comparable (e.g., in severity and type) to patients in the same disorder category in the second setting; and (3) the base rates of these disorders in one setting must match those of the other setting. If requirement 1 is not met, then the diagnostic efficiency statistics obtained in one setting are irrelevant to the second setting. For example, there is little reason to believe that the population of parents involved in child custody cases is identical or even closely similar in terms of disorder and clinical syndrome categories to the exclusively clinical population used to generate the diagnostic validity statistics of the 1997 MCMI-III study. If requirement 2 is not met, then the SEs and SPs obtained in one setting will be irrelevant to the second setting. For example, although the same disorders might be present in both settings, the severities or types of these disorders might differ radically across settings. As a consequence, the SE of an MCMI-III scale (the probability that a person who has the disorder will exceed the diagnostic cut-off score) used to detect this disorder could be radically different across settings (see Kraemer, 1992).

Some of the most popular diagnostic efficiency statistics (e.g., PPP and NPP) are base rate–specific (Gibertini, Brandenburg, & Retzlaff, 1986). Thus, even if exactly the same set of disorders and syndromes occur in two diagnostic settings (say, a community mental health center and a mental hospital), the values of these diagnostic efficiency statistics obtained in one setting would differ in the second setting if the base rates of these conditions differed across settings. For example, the fact that the Schizoid scale has a PPP = .83 in a setting with BR of .20 does not imply that the same PPP would be obtained in another setting with a different BR. In fact, Gibertini et al. estimated that if the BR was .01, the PPP would not be .83 but .10, which is clearly not a trivial difference. Methods exist for estimating PPPs and NPPs across settings that differ in base rate (see, e.g., Gibertini et al., 1986; Hsu, 2002), but these methods assume that requirements 1 and 2 are tenable.

Diagnostic efficiency statistics may be considered biased if they provide misleading information about the diagnostic validity of MCMI-III scales. This section drew attention to several sources of this type of bias:

1. Limiting diagnostic efficiency statistics to those that are not adjusted for chance can suggest that scales have high diagnostic validity when these scales are performing at or below chance levels. In particular, very high PPPs (or very high NPPs, SEs, or SPs) can occur with scales that perform at or below chance levels.
2. Limiting attention to SEs and PPPs ignores the negative relations of these indices (caused by changes in diagnostic cut-off scores) with SPs and NPPs and could suggest unnecessarily optimistic or pessimistic evaluations of scales.
3. Lack of familiarity of clinicians with their patients and with theories of psychopathology can result in poor criterion measures and lead to underestimation of diagnostic validities of scales in external validity studies used to generate diagnostic efficiency statistics.
4. Criterion contamination, confirmatory bias, and availability heuristics can cause overestimation of diagnostic validities of scales.
5. Changes across diagnostic settings in disorder categories, severities and subtypes of disorders, and base rates can decrease generalizability of diagnostic efficiency statistics reported in MCMI-III manuals.

REFERENCES

Aiken, L. W. (1989). *Assessment of personality.* Needham Heights, MA: Allyn & Bacon.

Bashaw, W. L., & Anderson, H. E. (1967). A correction for replicated error in correlation coefficients. *Psychometrika, 32,* 435–441.

Budescu, D. V., & Rodgers, J. L. (1981). Corrections for spurious influences on correlations between MMPI scales. *Multivariate Behavioral Research, 16,* 483–497.

Cantrell, J. D., & Dana, R. H. (1987). Use of the Millon Multiaxial Clinical Inventory (MCMI) as a screening instrument at a community mental health center. *Journal of Clinical Psychology, 43,* 366–375.

Choca, J. (2001). Review of the Millon Clinical Multiaxial Inventory-III Manual (2nd ed.). In J. C. Impara & B. S. Plake (Eds.), *Fourteenth mental measurements yearbook* (pp. 765–767). Lincoln, NE: Buros Institute of Mental Measurements.

Craig, R. J. (1999). Testimony based on the Millon Clinical Multiaxial Inventory: Review, commentary and guidelines. *Journal of Personality Assessment, 73,* 290–304.

Craig, R. J., & Olson, R. E. (2001). Adjectival descriptions of personality disorders: A convergent validity study of the MCMI-III. *Journal of Personality Assessment, 77,* 259–271.

Dana, R. H., & Cantrell, J. D. (1988). An update on the Millon Clinical Multiaxial Inventory (MCMI). *Journal of Clinical Psychology, 44,* 760–764.

Daubert, S. D., & Metzler, A. E. (2000). The detection of fake-bad and fake-good responding on the Millon Clinical Multiaxial Inventory. *Psychological Assessment, 12,* 418–424.

Farley, F. H., & Cohen, A. (1974). Scale interdependency effects and the smallest space analysis of structure. *Psychological Bulletin, 81,* 766–772.

Gibertini, M., Brandenburg, N., & Retzlaff, P. (1986). The operating characteristics of the Millon Clinical Multiaxial Inventory. *Journal of Personality Assessment, 50,* 554–567.

Gibertini, M., & Retzlaff, P. D. (1988). Factor invariance of the Millon Clinical Multiaxial Inventory. *Psychopathology and Behavior Assessment, 10,* 65–74.

Guilford, J. P. (1954). *Psychometric methods.* New York: McGraw-Hill.

Gynther, M. D., & Green, S. B. (1982). Methodological problems in research with self-report inventories. In P. C. Kendall & J. N. Butcher (Eds.), *Handbook of research methods in clinical psychology.* New York: Wiley.

Haynes, S. N., Nelson, K., & Blaine, D. D. (1999). Psychometric issues in assessment research. In P. Kendall, J. N. Butcher, & G. N. Holmbeck (Eds.), *Handbook of research methods in clinical psychology.* New York: Wiley.

Hess, A. K. (1985). Millon Clinical Multiaxial Inventory. In J. V. Mitchell, Jr. (Ed.), *The ninth mental measurement yearbook* (Vol. 1, pp. 984–986). Lincoln: University of Nebraska Press.

Hess, A. K. (1998). Review of the Millon Clinical Multiaxial Inventory-III. In J. C. Impara & B. S. Plake (Eds.), *Thirteenth mental measurements yearbook.* Lincoln, NE: Buros Institute of Mental Measurements.

Holliman, N. B., & Guthrie, P. C. (1989). A comparison of the Millon Clinical Multiaxial Inventory and the California Psychological Inventory in assessment of a nonclinical population. *Journal of Clinical Psychology, 45,* 373–382.

Holmes, N. R. (1987). [Letter to the editor]. *Military Medicine, 153,* 330.

Hsu, L. M. (1992). Correcting correlations of personality scales for spurious effects of shared items. *Multivariate Behavioral Research, 27,* 31–41.

Hsu, L. M. (1994). Item overlap correlations: Definitions, interpretations, and implications. *Multivariate Behavioral Research, 29,* 127–140.

Hsu, L. M. (2002). Diagnostic validity statistics and the MCMI-III. *Psychological Assessment, 14,* 410–422.

Hsu, L. M. (2004). Biases of success rate differences shown in Rosenthal and Rubin's Binomial Effect Size Displays. *Psychological Methods, 9*, 183–197.

Hsu, L. M., & Maruish, M. E. (1992). *Conducting publishable research with the MCMI-II: Psychometric and statistical issues.* Minneapolis: National Computer Systems.

Jackson, D. N., & Messick, S. (1958). Content and style in personality assessment. *Psychological Bulletin, 55*, 243–252.

Keller, L. S., Butcher, J. N., & Slutske, W. S. (1990). Objective personality assessment. In G. Goldstein & M. Hersen (Eds.), *Handbook of psychological assessment* (2nd ed., pp. 345–386). New York: Pergamon Press.

Kraemer, H. C. (1992). *Evaluating medical tests.* Newbury Park, CA: Sage.

LaVoie, A. L. (1991). Millon Clinical Multiaxial Inventory-II. In D. J. Keyser & R. C. Sweetland (Eds.), *Test critiques* (Vol. VIII, pp. 457–470). Austin, TX: ProEd Publishing.

Meier, S. T. (1994). *The crisis in psychological measurement and assessment: A historical survey.* New York: Academic Press.

Messick, S. (1991). Psychology and methodology of response styles. In R. E. Snow & D. E. Wiley (Eds.), *Improving inquiry in social science* (pp. 161–200). Hillsdale, NJ: Erlbaum.

Millon, T. (1987). *Manual for the MCMI-II.* Minneapolis: National Computer Systems.

Millon, T. (1990). *Toward a new personology.* New York: Wiley.

Millon, T. (1994). *MCMI-III Manual.* Minneapolis, MN: National Computer Systems.

Millon, T. (2003). It's time to rework the blueprint: Building a science for clinical psychology. *American Psychologist, 58*, 949–961.

Millon, T., Davis, R., & Millon, C. (1997). *MCMI-III Manual.* (2nd ed.). Minneapolis, MN: National Computer Systems.

Retzlaff, P. D. (1996). MCMI-III diagnostic validity: Bad test or bad validity study. *Journal of Personality Assessment, 66*, 431–437.

Retzlaff, P. D., & Gibertini, M. (1987). Factor structure of the MCMI basic personality scales and common-item artifact. *Journal of Personality Assessment, 51*, 588–594.

Retzlaff, P. D., & Gibertini, M. (1990). Factor-based special scales for the MCMI. *Journal of Clinical Psychology, 46*, 47–52.

Reynolds, C. R. (1992). Review of the Millon Clinical Multiaxial Inventory-II. In J. J. Kramer & J. C. Connoley (Eds.), *The eleventh mental measurements yearbook* (pp. 533–535). Lincoln, NE: Buros Institute of Mental Measurements.

Stevens, S. S. (1951). Mathematics, measurement and psychophysics. In S. S. Stevens (Ed.), *Handbook of experimental psychology* (pp. 1–41). New York: Wiley.

Strack, S., Lorr, M., Campbell, L., & Lamnin, A. (1992). Personality disorder and clinical syndrome factors of MCMI-II scales. *Journal of Personality Disorders, 6*, 40–52.

Wetzler, S. (1990). The Millon Clinical Multiaxial Inventory (MCMI): A review. *Journal of Personality Assessment, 55*, 445–464.

Widiger, T. A. (1985). The Millon Clinical Multiaxial Inventory. In J. V. Mitchell, Jr. (Ed.), *The ninth mental measurements yearbook* (Vol. 1, pp. 986–988). Lincoln: University of Nebraska Press.

Widiger, T. A. (1999). Millon's dimensional polarities. *Journal of Personality Assessment, 72,* 365–389.

Widiger, T. A. (2001). Review of the Millon Clinical Multiaxial Inventory-III. *Fourteenth mental measurements yearbook* (pp. 767–769). Lincoln: Buros Institute of Mental Measurements.

Widiger, T. A., & Sanderson, C. J. (1995). Assessing personality disorders. In J. Butcher (Ed.), *Clinical personality assessment: Practical approaches* (pp. 380–394). New York: Oxford University Press.

Wiggins, J. S. (1982). Circumplex models of interpersonal behavior in clinical psychology. In P. Kendall & J. N. Butcher (Eds.), *Handbook of research methods in clinical psychology* (pp. 183–222). New York: Wiley.

APPENDIX A

Diagnoses Associated with MCMI Codes Types

LISTED IN Appendix A are MCMI modal code types that have been reported in the empirical literature. An individual patient may or may not have the same diagnosis or problems associated with that code type. To the extent that certain code types are commonly associated with a particular problem or diagnosis across several samples, the probability that an individual patient with this same code type would also have that same problem or diagnosis would increase. In any case, the individual clinician bears the final responsibility for the use of any of this material.

Appendix A presents the code types along with the source, sample size, and diagnosis or problem. A "Within Normal Limits" code type is defined as one where the base rate scores are <75. An asterisk (*) before the personality disorder scale indicates that the scales were >60 and <75. The clinical code types listed here were based on the highest two or three basic personality disorder scales, provided that the base rate scores were >74. Following the year of publication is a designation of whether the group was tested with the MCMI-II or MCMI-III. If there is no designation, it can be assumed that the group was tested with the MCMI-I. Occasionally, the designation "Type" followed by a number is listed in the diagnosis column. Here, the author conducted a cluster analysis and reported this code type as one of the typological analyses. The references listed are in the References at the end of the book.

The second listing (pp. 345–356) allows the reader to look up an MCMI code type according to a patient's diagnosis or problem area. The format remains the same as in the first listing.

This is a greatly expanded version of an article originally published in the *Journal of Clinical Psychology*, 1995, 51, 352–360. This material is used by permission of John Wiley & Sons, Inc.

Within Normal Limits (WNL)	Sample Size	Diagnosis
Tuokko et al. (1991)	79	Head-injured patients
Divac-Jovanovic et al. (1993)	67	Outpatients w/o personality disorders
Dagan et al. (1996)	47	Sleep Disorder patients
Craig, Bivens, & Olson (1997) – III	45	Type IV heroin/cocaine addicts
McMahon, Malow, et al. (1998) – II	40	Type III inpatient substance abusers
King (1998) – II	312	College students
Allen, Huntoon, & Evans (1999) – III	23	Women with PTSD
Nadeau et al. (1999)	173	Sexual dysfunction patients
Sugihara & Warner (1999) – III	60	Mexican American male batterers
Gunsalus & Kelly (2000) – III	132	College students
Boyle & Le Dean (2000) – III	36	Community sample
	36	Psychiatric outpatients
Petrocelli, Glaser, et al. (2001) – II	58	Psychiatric outpatients
	39	Mildly depressed patients
Kristensen & Torgersen (2001) – II	99	Mothers of Selective Autism children
	87	Fathers of Selective Autism children
Petrocelli, Glaser, Calhoun, et al. (2001) – II	40	Type I psychiatric outpatients
McCann et al. (2001) – III	130	Female child custody seekers
	127	Male child custody seekers
Piersma et al. (2002) – III	50	College counselees
Wise (2002) – II	84	Convicted offenders
Cohen et al. (2002)	24	Community controls
Espelage et al. (2002) – II	31	Type I Eating Disorder patients
Schwartz et al. (2004) – III	366	Male prison inmates
*1		
Joffe et al. (1988)	23	Depressed patients
*2A		
Joffe et al. (1988)	23	Obsessive-Compulsive PD patients
Garner et al. (1990)	19	Bulimics with poor treatment outcome, pretest code
Norman et al. (1993)	17	Anorexics
Wetzler et al. (1995)	158	Bipolar PD patients
Nadeau et al. (1999)	34	Rapists

Within Normal Limits (WNL)	Sample Size	Diagnosis
*238A		
Choca et al. (1990)	471	White psychotic inpatients
Chick et al. (1993)	107	Psychiatric inpatients
*28A		
Millon (1987) – II	184	Dysthymic Disorder patients
*28B		
Millon (1987) – II	133	Dysthymic Disorder patients
*3		
Barnett & McCormack (1988)	147	Child molesters
Kennedy et al. (1990)	44	Eating Disorder patients
McMahon & Tyson (1990)	15	Female alcoholics with transient depression, admission code
Libb, Stankovic, Sokol, et al. (1990)	28	Major Depression patients, discharge code
Bryer et al. (1990)	359	General psychiatric patients
McNeil & Meyer (1990)	11	Forensic inpatients
Ahrens, Evans, & Barnette (1990)	1757	Prison inmates
Davis & Greenblatt (1990)	27	Young, White schizophrenics
	17	Young, Black nonparanoid schizophrenics
Jackson et al. (1991)	X	White schizophrenics, symptom nonreporters
Greenblatt & Davis (1992)	263	White nonangry, nonpsychotic inpatients
Fals-Stewart (1992)	43	Type IV drug addicts in therapeutic community
Wetzler & Marlowe (1993)	75	Psychiatric inpatients, not depressed
Chick et al. (1994)	245	Psychiatric inpatients
McCann, Flynn, & Gersh (1992) – II	42	Psychiatric inpatients
Wetzler & Marlowe (1993) – II	65	Depressed psychiatric inpatients
	95	Psychiatric inpatients, not depressed
	81	Nonpsychotic psychiatric inpatients

(continued)

Within Normal Limits (WNL)	Sample Size	Diagnosis
	29	Psychotic psychiatric inpatients
	24	Type V polydrug-abusing inpatients
Donat (1994) – II	24	Type V polydrug-abusing inpatients
Chantry & Craig (1994a) – II	202	Child molesters
	195	Adult rapists
Chantry & Craig (1994b) – II	115	Type I child molesters
McKee & Klohn (1994)	135	Pretrial defendants
Wetzler et al. (1995) – II	26	Bipolar PD patients
Lecic-Tosevski et al. (2002) – I	19	Civilians air-attacked (Cluster II)
*32		
Piersma (1989a)	98	Major Depression patients, at discharge
*328A		
Choca et al. (1990)	235	Black psychiatric inpatients
*37		
Jay et al. (1987)	25	Headache patients
Joffe & Regan (1991)	20	Depressed, family history, code in remission
Craig & Olson (1995) – II	23	Type IV marital therapy patients
*38A		
Cantrell & Dana (1987)	72	Mental health outpatients
Craig et al. (1985)	106	Alcoholics
May & Bos (2000) – III	25	ADHD patients with comorbidity
*4		
Garber et al. (1990)	17	Bulimics with good treatment outcome, pre- & postcode
Tisdale et al. (1990)	32	Female outpatients in therapy
Yeager et al. (1992)	1000	General psychiatric outpatients
Wetzler & Marlowe (1993)	50	Nondepressed psychiatric inpatients
Matano et al. (1994)	116	Male alcoholics
	84	Female alcoholics
Terpylak & Schuerger (1994)	32	Undergraduate college students

Within Normal Limits (WNL)	Sample Size	Diagnosis
Barrett & Etheridge (1994)	28	College students
Richman & Nelson-Gray (1994)	197	College student panickers
	350	College student nonpanickers
Hastings & Hamberger (1994)	23	Nonviolent community, poor premorbid history
	20	Violent community violent, good premorbid history
Baggi et al. (1995)	42	TMJ patients
	42	Community controls
Parry, Ehlers, et al. (1996)	X	Late Luteal Phase Dysphoric Disorder females; both follicular and luteal phase had same code type
Sugihara & Warner (2000) – III	45	Mexican American male non-batterers
May & Bos (2000) – III	26	ADHD patients
Sinha & Watson (2001) – II	99	College males
*45		
Wall et al. (1990)	18	Normals with high alpha on EEG
Donat (1994) – II	62	Type I polydrug inpatients
Lecic-Tosevski et al. (2002)	19	Civilians air-attacked (Cluster III)
*5		
Mannis et al. (1987)	52	Keratoconus patients (eye disorder)
Retzlaff & Gibertini (1990a)	124	Air Force alcoholics
Jackson et al. (1991)	X	Black schizophrenics, symptom nonreporters
Barrett & Etheridge (1994)	18	College students
Retzlaff, Sheehan, & Fiel (1991) – II	50	University students
Chantry & Craig (1994a) – II	205	Aggressive felons (nonsexual crimes)
Hastings & Hamberger (1994)	33	Batterers with good premorbid history
Murphy et al. (1993) – II	24	Happily married men

(continued)

Within Normal Limits (WNL)	Sample Size	Diagnosis
*53		
Ownby et al. (1991)	800	Offenders, presentencing
*54		
Butters et al. (1986)	52	Air Force trainees, returned to duty
Retzlaff & Gibertini (1987a)	350	Air Force pilot trainees
Holliman & Guthrie (1989)	85	Nondistressed students
Yeager et al. (1992)	144	Drug addicts in residential treatment
Matano et al. (1994)		Male alcoholics (Cluster I)
Lecic-Tosevski et al. (2002)	71	Civilians air-attacked (Cluster I)
*56A		
Robert et al. (1985)	25	Misc. psychiatric patients
Craig (1984)	71	Opiate addicts, program completers
Craig (1985)	100	Opiate addicts
Marsh et al. (1988)	163	Opiate addicts
McMahon & Davidson (1986a)	74	Alcohlics, not depressed
Craig & Olson (1990)	86	Heroin addicts
Lorr & Strack (1990) – II	28	Type IV misc. psychiatric patients
Calsyn, Wells, et al. (2000)	141	Methadone patients (light drug (users), pretreatment
*58A		
Craig (1984)	29	Opiate addicts, program dropouts
*6A		
Hastings & Hamberger (1994)	66	Batterers with poor premorbid history
*6A5		
Bartsch Hoffman (1985)	17	Type IV alcoholics
Calsyn, Wells, et al. (2000)	141	Methadone patients (heavy drug users), pretreatment
	89	Methadone patients (light drug users), pre- & posttreatment
	141	Methadone patients (heavy drug users), posttreatment

Within Normal Limits (WNL)	Sample Size	Diagnosis
*6B		
Millon (1987) – II	35	Passive-Aggressive PD patients
Craig & Olson (1995) – II	70	Males in marital therapy
Murphy et al. (1993) – II	24	Nonviolent males in discordant relationships
*6B7		
Millon (1987) – II	42	Obsessive-Compulsive PD patients
*6B8A		
Fals-Stewart & Lucente (1994) – II	191	Non-cognitively impaired substance abusers
*7		
Donat (1988)	23	Alcoholics
Mayer & Scott (1988)	21	Type III alcoholics
Herron et al. (1986)	129	Laminectomy patients
	92	Good response to treatment
	37	Poor response to treatment
Hamberger & Hastings (1986)	12	Type VIII spouse abusers
Retzlaff & Gibertini (1987a)	49	Type III Air Force pilot trainees
Mannis et al. (1987)	25	Chronic eye disease patients
	32	No eye disease controls
Lemkau et al. (1988)	67	Family practice residents
Joffe & Regan (1988)	42	Major Depression patients in remission
Chandarana et al. (1990)	16	Morbidly obese patients, pre- & postsurgical code
Wall et al. (1990)	42	Normals with low alpha on EEG
	13	ACOAs with low alpha on EEG
Reich (1990)	16	Panic Disorder patients, treatment completers
McMahon, Malow, & Peneod (1998) – II	160	Type II inpatient drug abusers
Tisdale et al. (1990)	30	Normal volunteers
Joffe & Regan (1991)	21	Depressed, family history positive for alcoholism, code in remission
Terpylak & Schuerger (1994)	32	Undergraduate college students

(continued)

Within Normal Limits (WNL)	Sample Size	Diagnosis
Donat et al. (1991)	200	Type I inpatient alcoholics
Donat et al. (1992)	31	Type I inpatient alcoholics
Beasley & Stoltenberg (1992) – II	35	Nonabused males (control group)
King (1994) – II	82	Aviators
Matano et al. (1994)	XX	Female alcoholics (Cluster I)
Craig & Olson (1995) – II	75	Women in marital therapy
Hastings & Hamberger (1994)	48	Nonviolent community, good premorbid history
Boone et al. (1995)	135	Worker's compensation claimants
Weekes & Morison (1996)	35	Type V prison inmates
Parry, Ehlers, et al. (1996)	X	Late Luteal Phase Dysphoric Disorder females; both follicular and luteal phase had same code type
Schweitzer, Tuckwell, et al. (2001) – II	6	Major Depression *DSM* no suppressors

*73

Millon (1987) – II	94	Obsessive-Compulsive PD patients

*75

Chantry & Craig (1994b) – II	114	Type I adult rapists

*76A

Bartsch & Hoffman (1985)	19	Type I alcoholics

*8A

McMahon et al. (1989)	54	Episodic drinkers
Holliman & Guthrie (1989)	49	Depressed students
Retzlaff & Gibertini (1990b)	89	VA alcoholics
Reich (1990)	12	Panic Disorder patients, treatment dropouts
McMahon et al. (1991)	31	Episodic drinkers
Lewis & Harder (1991)	11	Psychiatric outpatients
Swirsky-Sacchetti et al. (1993)	10	Normal volunteers
Wetzler et al. (1995)	26	Bipolar PD patients

*8A3

McMahon et al. (1985b)	33	Misc. drug abusers
McMahon et al. (1985b)	96	Alcoholics

Within Normal Limits (WNL)	Sample Size	Diagnosis
McMahon et al. (1986)	43	High-functioning alcoholics
Torgersen & Alneas (1990)	272	Norwegian psychiatric outpatients
Norman et al. (1993)	58	Bulimics
*8A4		
Jay et al. (1987)	26	Chronic pain patients
*8B2		
Millon (1987) – II	66	Anxiety Disorder patients
Petrocelli, Glaser, et al. (2001) – II	28	Moderately depressed patients
*8B6B		
Haller, Miles, & Dawson (2002) – II	21	Type I female addicts
1*		
Millon (1987) – II	27	Schizoid PD patients
12*		
Retzlaff & Bromley (1991)	89	Type VI VA alcoholic inpatients ($N = 7$)
Fals-Stewart (1992) – II	45	Type III drug addicts in therapeutic community
128A*		
Blackburn (1996)	26	Type V prisoners in England
18A2*		
Hyer, Davis, et al. (1994) – II	?	Type III PTSD patients
2A*		
Widiger & Sanderson (1987)	20	Antisocial PD patients
Davis & Greenblatt (1990)	38	Young, Black paranoid schizophrenics
Millon (1987) – II	17	Bipolar Affective Disorder patients
Fink & Golinkoff (1990) – II	11	Schizophrenics
2A*13		
Fals-Stewart & Lucente (1993)	21	Obsessive-Compulsive PD patients

(continued)

Within Normal Limits (WNL)	Sample Size	Diagnosis
2A*38A		
Davis & Greenblatt (1990)	45	Old, White nonparanoid schizo-phrenics
2A1*		
Jackson et al. (1991)	X	White schizophrenics, symptom reporters
Millon (1987) – II	60	Avoidant PD patients
	101	Avoidant PD patients
2A138A		
Mayer & Scott (1988)	15	Type IV alcoholics
2A18A		
Jackson et al. (1991)	X	Black schizophrenics, symptom reporters
McMahon et al. (1993)	31	Alcoholics, detached type
Matano et al. (1994)	44	Male alcoholics (Cluster II)
2A2B8B		
Allen, Huntoon, & Evans (1999) – III	44	Women with PTSD
Schweitzer, Tuckwell, et al. (2001) – II	19	Major Depression patients
2A3*		
Bryer et al. (1987)	14	Sexually abused patients
Josiassen et al. (1988)	10	Nonpsychotic schizophrenics
Hicklin & Widiger (2000) – III	82	Psychiatric outpatients
2A31		
Chantry & Craig (1994b) – II	31	Adult rapists
2A31		
Rudd, Ellis, et al. (2000) – II	13	Type II suicidal patients
2A3P		
Jossiassen et al. (1988)	10	Psychotic schizophrenics
2A38A*		
Bryer et al. (1987)	14	Sexually abused patients
2A38A1		
Donat (1988)	44	Type V alcoholics
Ellis, Rudd, et al. (1996)	54	Type II suicidal outpatients
Derecho et al. (1996) – II	7	Atypical depression patients

Within Normal Limits (WNL)	Sample Size	Diagnosis
2A38B		
Petrocelli, Glaser, Calhoun, et al. (2001) – II	28	Type V psychiatric outpatients
2A6A3		
Schinka et al. (1999) – II	46	Female drug addicts in therapeutic community, admission code
2A6A8A		
Munley et al. (1998) – II	65	Black psychiatric inpatients
2A8A		
Widiger & Sanderson (1987)	26	Passive-Aggressive PD patients
McMahon & Davidson (1985a)	28	Alcoholics with transient depression
Murphy et al. (1990)	150	Psychiatric inpatients
Sherwood et al. (1990)	189	Vietnam vets with PTSD
Davis & Greenblatt (1990)	20	Old, Black paranoid schizophrenics
Greenblatt & Davis (1992)	66	Black nonangry psychotic psychiatric inpatients
Swirsky-Sacchetti et al. (1993)	10	Borderline PD patients (female)
Blackburn (1996)	31	Type II prisoners in England
Millon (1987) – II	?	Delusional Disorder patients
2A8A1		
Widiger & Sanderson (1987)	18	Avoidant PD patients
Davis & Greenblatt (1990)	8	Young, Black nonpsychotic inpatients
Donat et al. (1991)	200	Type III inpatient alcoholics
Hyer, Davis, et al. (1994) – I	?	Type II PTSD patients
2A8A3*		
McMahon & Davidson (1985a)	28	Alcoholics with enduring depression
Norman et al. (1993)	12	Bulimics/anorexics
2A8A6A		
Donat (1994) – II	19	Type IV polydrug-abusing inpatients

(continued)

Within Normal Limits (WNL)	Sample Size	Diagnosis
2A8A8B		
McCann & Gergelis (1990) – II	40	Suicide attempters
2A8B		
Miller et al. (1993) – II	141	Psychiatric inpatients
Dell (1998) – II	42	Dissociative Identity Disorder patients
Osuch, Noll, & Putnam (1999) – II	48	Low self-injury patients
Gunsalus & Kelly (2000) – III	147	Korean college students
2A8B*3		
Espelage et al. (2002) – II	33	Anorexics
2A8B3		
Piersma (1989a) – II	98	Psychiatric inpatients (90% with Major Depression)
Millon (1987) – II	65	Major Depression patients
2A8B38A		
Millon (1987) – II	46	Major Depression patients
2A8B8A		
Fink & Golinkoff (1990) – II	16	Multiple Personality Disorder patients
McCann & Gergelis (1990) – II	40	Patients with suicide ideation but no attempts
Ellason & Ross (1996) – II	35	Dissociative PD patients
Osuch, Noll, & Putnam (1999) – II	48	High self-injury patients
2B*3		
Piersma & Boes (1997) – III	97	Psychiatric inpatients
2B8B		
Allen, Coyne, & Console (1997)	102	Dissociative PD women
2B8BI		
Allen, Huntoon, & Evans (1999) – III	44	Women with PTSD
2B8B3		
Allen, Huntoon, & Evans (1999) – III	81	Women with PTSD
2B8B2A		
Allen, Huntoon, & Evans (1999) – III	147	Women with PTSD

Within Normal Limits (WNL)	Sample Size	Diagnosis
3*		
Hyer & Jacobson (1986)	60	Older psychiatric inpatients
Greenblatt & Davis (1992)	67	Black nonangry, nonpsychotic psychiatric inpatients
McMahon et al. (1993)	49	Alcoholics, dependent type
Del Rosario et al. (1994)	35	Schizophrenic inpatients
Barrett & Etheridge (1994)	18	College student "hallucinators"
	18	College student "hallucinators" (2nd sample)
Davis & Greenblatt (1990) – II	25	Young, White nonparanoid schizophrenics
	35	Old, White nonparanoid schizophrenics
Wetzler et al. (1995) – II	158	Unipolar PD patients (depression)
	26	Bipolar PD patients
Blais et al. (1998) – II	16	Major Depression patients post-ECT
Nadeau et al. (1999)	79	Pedophiliacs
3*2		
Donat et al. (1992)	66	Type II psychiatric inpatients
3*7		
Hamberger & Hastings (1986)	12	Type III spouse abusers
Lorr & Strack (1990) – II	31	Type III misc. psychiatric patients
3*8A		
Derecho et al. (1996) – II	14	Nonatypical depression patients
312A		
Chantry & Craig (1994b) – II	46	Type II child molesters
Blackburn (1996)	26	Type IV prisoners in England
Weekes & Morrison (1996)	13	Type II prison inmates
32A*		
Widiger & Sanderson (1987)	27	Dependent PD patients
Goldberg et al. (1989)	8	Depressed outpatients

(continued)

Within Normal Limits (WNL)	Sample Size	Diagnosis
Kennedy et al. (1990)	44	Eating Disorder patients, admission code
Greenblatt & Davis (1992)	185	White nonangry, psychotic inpatients
Craig & Olson (1995) – II	49	Type III patients in marital therapy
32A1*		
Bartsch & Hoffman (1985)	31	Type V alcoholics
Golberg et al. (1989)	8	Sociotropic depression patients
Kennedy et al. (1990)	44	Eating Disorder patients
Davis & Greenblatt (1990) – II	32	Old, White paranoid schizophrenics
Blais et al. (1998) – II	16	Major Depression patients, pre-ECT
32A18B		
Donat et al. (1992) – II	35	Type III psychiatric inpatients
32A8A		
Piersma (1986a)	151	Psychiatric inpatients (90% with Major Depression)
Joffe & Regan (1991)	20	Depressed patients, family history negative for alcoholism
Donat et al. (1991)	200	Type IV inpatient alcoholics
32A8A1		
McCann & Suess (1988)	33	Misc. psychiatric patients
32A8B		
Espelage et al. (2002) – II	62	Type II Eating Disorder patients
32A8B7		
Rubino et al. (1995) – II	62	Type I psoriasis patients
35*		
Hamberger & Hastings (1986)	11	Type VI spouse abusers
38A2		
Wetzler et al. (1989)	48	Major Depression patients
Joffe & Regan (1986b)	19	Major Depression patients, nontreatment response
Davis & Greenblatt (1990)	12	Old, Black nonpsychotic inpatients

Within Normal Limits (WNL)	Sample Size	Diagnosis
Wetzler & Marlowe (1993)	73	Depressed inpatients
Chantry & Craig (1994b) – II	40	Type III child molesters

4*

Jay et al. (1987)	20	Student control group
Stark & Campbell (1998)	31	Drug addict dropouts
Hibbard (1989)	15	ACOAs
Fals-Stewart & Lucente (1993)	29	Obsessive-Compulsive PD patients
Sinha & Watson (2001) – II	194	College females

45*

Fals-Stewart (1992)	40	Type V drug addicts in therapeutic community
Matano et al. (1994)	xx	Type III female alcoholics
Millon (1987) – II	84	Histrionic PD patients
May & Bos (2000) – III	21	ADHD with Oppositional Disorder patients

458A6B

Petrocelli, Glaser, Calhoun, et al. (2001) – II	21	Type IV psychiatric outpatients

48A8B

Millon (1987) – II	32	Bipolar Affective Disorder patients

48B

Petrocelli, Glaser, Calhoun, et al. (2001) – II	31	Type II psychiatric outpatients

5*

Retzlaff & Bromley (1991)	89	Type IV VA inpatient alcoholics ($N = 17$)
Wetzler & Marlowe (1993) – II	15	Manic patients
Boyle & Le Dean (2000) – III	38	College students

5*4

Retzlaff & Gilbertini (1987a)	138	Type II Air Force pilot trainees

5*6A

McNeil & Meyer (1990)	47	Prison inmates
Wetzler & Marlowe (1993)	21	Manic patients

(continued)

Within Normal Limits (WNL)	Sample Size	Diagnosis
54*		
Retzlaff & Gibertini (1987a)	50	Type I Air Force pilot trainees
Wetzler et al. (1990)	24	Normal controls
Wall et al. (1990)	13	ACOAs with high alpha on EEG
Retzlaff & Bromley (1991)	89	Type II inpatient alcoholics (N=18)
Millon (1987) – II	28	Narcissistic PD patients
	69	Narcissistic PD patients
Ellis, Rudd, et al. (1996)	25	Type IV suicidal outpatients
546A*		
Bartsch & Hoffman (1985)	23	Type II alcoholics
Donat (1988)	9	Type II alcoholics
Donat (1991)	200	Type II inpatient alcoholics
Fals-Stewart (1992)	52	Type II drug addicts in therapeutic community
56A		
Hamberger & Hastings (1986)	14	Type II spouse abusers
Calsyn & Saxon (1988)	45	Opiate addicts
Craig & Olson (1990)	56	Type I cocaine addicts
	26	Type I heroin addicts
Matano et al. (1994)	XX	Type III male alcoholics
Chantry & Craig (1994b) – II	50	Type II adult rapists
Weekes & Morison (1996)	27	Type III prison inmates
56A3		
Weekes & Morison (1996)	32	Type III prison inmates
56A4		
Mayer & Scott (1988)	28	Type II alcoholics
Donat et al. (1992) – II	27	Type V psychiatric inpatients
56A6B		
Cogen et al. (2002) – II	20	Pedophiles (heterosexual type)
56B3		
Craig & Olson (1995) – II	29	Type I patients in marital therapy
58A4		
DiGiuseppe, Robin, et al. (1995) – II	34	Type III Narcissistic PD outpatients

Within Normal Limits (WNL)	Sample Size	Diagnosis
58A48B		
DiGiuseppe, Robin, et al. (1995) – II	50	Type I Narcissistic PD outpatients
58A6A		
Pollock & Perry (1999) – II	14	Negatively disinterested antenatal women
6A*		
Davis & Greenblatt (1990)	21	Old, Black nonparanoid schizophrenics
Blackburn (1996)	29	Type III prisoners in England
Millon (1987) – II	19	Antisocial PD patients
Millon (1987) – II	53	Drug addicts
Lorr & Strack (1990) – II	31	Type III misc. psychiatric patients
Litman & Cernovsky (1993) – II	129	Inpatient alcoholics
Craig, Bivens, & Olson (1997) – III	46	Type I heroin/cocaine addicts
	38	Type II heroin/cocaine addicts
6A*4		
Schinka et al. (1999) – II	46	Female addicts in therapeutic community, 1 year post-treatment
6A2A*		
Fals-Stewart & Lucente (1994) – II	55	Cognitively impaired substance abusers
6A2A8A		
Munley et al. (1995) – II	39	Misc. psychiatric inpatients
6A3*		
Funari et al. (1991)	36	Vietnam vets after 140 days of treatment
6A4*5		
Turley et al. (1992) – II	19	Recent-onset Bipolar PD patients
6A5*		
Corbisiero & Reznikoff (1991)	247	Type II VA inpatient alcoholics ($N = 58$)

(continued)

Within Normal Limits (WNL)	Sample Size	Diagnosis
McMahon et al. (1993)	45	Alcoholics, independent type
Hastings & Hamberger (1994)	12	Violent batters with poor premorbid history
Blackburn (1996)	26	Type I prisoners in England
Flynn et al. (1995) – II	136	Cocaine addicts
Rudd & Orman (1996)	84	Good-functioning military personnel
Marlowe et al. (1997) – II	144	Cocaine addicts
6A56B		
Hart et al. (1991) – II	119	Inmate psychopaths
McMahon, Malow, & Peneod (1998) – II	160	Type II inpatient drug abusers
6A58A*		
Hamberger & Hastings (1986)	12	Type IV spouse abusers
6A6B		
Millon (1987) – II	25	Drug addicts
Craig, Kuncel, & Olson (1994) – II	50	Drug addicts
Flynn et al. (1995) – II	146	Heroin addicts
Flynn et al. (1997) – II	659	Drug addicts (heroin/cocaine)
6A6B8A		
Fals-Stewart (1995) – II	62	Polydrug abusers
6A8A*		
Millon (1987) – II	43	Alcoholics
Hyer, Davis, et al. (1994)	?	Type III PTSD patients
Ellis, Rudd, et al. (1996)	66	Type III suicidal outpatients
6A8A6B		
McMahon et al. (1993) – II	47	Cocaine addicts in therapeutic community, dropouts and
	50	completers
6B6A*		
Millon (1987)	36	Aggressive Sadistic PD patients
Beasley & Stoltenberg (1992)	49	Spouse abusers
6B6A5*		
DiGiuseppe, Robin, et al. (1995) – II	23	Type I Narcissistic PD outpatients

Within Normal Limits (WNL)	Sample Size	Diagnosis
6B6A8A*		
Millon (1987) – II	32	Antisocial PD patients
6B75*		
Millon (1987) – II	20	Paranoid PD patients
Millon (1987) – II	?	Delusional Disorder patients
6B8A*		
Millon (1987) – II	36	Borderline PD patients
6B8A6A		
Murphy et al. (1993) – II	24	Maritally violent spouse abusers
7*		
Piersma (1987c)	52	Seminary students
McMahon & Tyson (1990)	19	Female alcoholics with enduring depression, code after 1 month of treatment
73*		
Fals-Stewart & Lucente (1993)	39	Obsessive-Compulsive PD patients
756B4		
Rubino et al. (1995)	59	Type II psoriasis patients
76B		
Rubino et al. (1995)	192	Psoriasis patients
8A*		
Stark & Campbell (1988)	26	Drug addicts, treatment completers
Wetzler et al. (1990)	19	Panic Disorder patients
Craig & Olson (1990)	56	Type IV heroin addicts
Millon (1987) – II	90	Passive-Aggressive PD patients
Greenblatt & Davis (1992)	115	White angry, nonpsychotic psychiatric inpatients
	34	Black angry, nonpsychotic, psychiatric inpatients

(continued)

Within Normal Limits (WNL)	Sample Size	Diagnosis
Matano et al. (1994)	xx	Type II female alcoholics
Howard et al. (1995)	74	Cocaine-abusing females
8A*2A		
McMahon et al. (1986)	37	Low-functioning alcoholics
Mayer & Scott (1988)	48	Type I alcoholics
Garner et al. (1990)	19	Bulimics with poor treatment response, posttest code
McMahon et al. (1991)	94	Episodic drinkers, postcode
Schuller, Bagby, et al. (1993)	17	Depressives with SADS
8A*2A3		
Bartsch & Hoffman (1985)	35	Type III alcoholics
8A12A		
Ellis, Rudd, et al. (1996)	154	Type I suicidal outpatients
8A2A*		
McMahon & Davidson (1986a)	144	Depressed alcoholics
Robert et al. (1985)	25	PTSD patients
Goldberg et al. (1989)	8	Autonomously depressed patients
Sherwood et al. (1990)	189	Vietnam vets with PTSD
Hyer et al. (1991)	100	Vietnam vets with PTSD
Greenblatt & Davis (1992)	34	Black angry, nonpsychotic, psychiatric inpatients
Hyer, Davis, et al. (1994)	?	Type I PTSD patients
Rudd & Orman (1996)	69	Military in mental health center
Nadeau et al. (1999)	182	Male substance abusers
	73	Female substance abusers
8A2A1		
Hyer et al. (1988)	60	Vietnam vets with PTSD
Hamberger & Hastings (1986)	12	Type I spouse abusers
Funari et al. (1991)	36	Vietnam vets with PTSD
Hyer et al. (1991)	100	Vietnam vets with PTSD; 33% with this code
Corbisiero & Reznikoff (1991)	165	Type III VA inpatient alcoholics
Greenblatt & Davis (1992)	215	White angry, psychotic psychiatric inpatients
	105	Black angry, psychotic psychiatric inpatients

Within Normal Limits (WNL)	Sample Size	Diagnosis
Hyer, Davis, et al. (1992)	92	Vietnam vets with PTSD (inpatient)
8A2A13		
Hyer et al. (1991)	100	Vietnam vets with PTSD; 33% with this code
8A2A16A		
Retzlaff & Bromley (1991)	11	Type I VA inpatient alcoholics
Hyer, Davis, et al. (1992) – II	92	Vietnam vets with PTSD (inpatient)
8A2A3*		
Butters et al. (1986)	53	Air Force trainees, administratively separated
	69	Air Force trainees, discharged
Joffe & Regan (1988)	42	Major Depression patients
Joffe & Regan (1988)	42	Major Depression patients, acute phase
Joffe & Regan (1989a)	43	Major Depression patients, no suicide attempt
Libb, Stankovic, Sokol, et al. (1990)	28	Major Depression patients, admission code
Joffe & Regan (1991)	21	Depressed patients, family history negative
Lewis & Harder (1991)	27	Borderline PD outpatients
8A2A31*		
Joffe & Regan (1989a)	10	Major Depression patients, suicide attempt
8A2A36A*		
Joffe & Regan (1989b)	23	Major Depression patients, treatment responders
McMahon & Tyson (1990)	19	Female alcoholics with enduring depression, admission code
8A2A6A		
Munley et al. (1995) – II	39	Vietnam vets with PTSD (inpaient)

(continued)

Within Normal Limits (WNL)	Sample Size	Diagnosis
8A2A8B		
del Rosario et al. (1994)	35	Psychiatric inpatients
Hyer, Davis, et al. (1994) – II	?	Type II PTSD patients
Rudd, Ellis, et al. (2000) – II	61	Type I suicidal patients
8A3*		
Donat (1988)	60	Type III alcoholics
	14	Type IV alcoholics
8A32A*		
Hamberger & Hastings (1986)	10	Type V spouse abusers
Wetzler et al. (1990)	21	Major Depression patients
Weekes & Morison (1996)	23	Type I prison inmates
8A34*		
Hamberger & Hastings (1986)	11	Type VII spouse abusers
8A4		
Donat (1991)	200	Inpatient alcoholics
8A56B6A*		
Millon (1987) – II	8	Paranoid patients
8A6A		
Craig & Olson (1990)	56	Cocaine addicts
Donat (1994) – II	51	Type III polydrug-abusing inpatients
Haller, Miles, & Dawson (2002) – II	29	Type III female addicts
8A6A2A		
Dutton (1995) – II	132	Wife assaulters
8A6A2A6B+		
McMahon, Malow, et al. (1988) – II	91	Type I inpatient substance abusers
8A6A6B		
Lorr & Strack (1990) – II	41	Type I misc. psychiatric patients
8A6B		
Craig & Olson (1995) – II	44	Type II patients in marital therapy

342

Within Normal Limits (WNL)	Sample Size	Diagnosis
8A6B6A		
May & Bos (2000) – II	32	ADHD & Oppositional Disorder patients with comorbidity
8A6B46A*		
Rubino et al. (1995) – II	36	Type IV psoriasis patients
8A8B		
Fals-Stewart (1995) – II	54	Forensic patients in pretrial sentencing evaluation
8A8B2A6A		
Petrocelli, Glaser, Calhoun, et al. (2001) – II	9	Type III psychiatric outpatients
8A8B3		
Allen, Huntoon, & Evans (1999)	35	Women with PTSD-III
8A8B4		
Espelage et al. (2002) – II	90	Type II Eating Disorder patients
8A8B6A		
Donat (1994) – II	61	Type II polydrug-abusing inpatients
8A8B26A		
Hyer, Davis, et al. (1994) – II	?	Type IV PTSD patients
8B*		
Millon (1987) – II	14	Self-Defeating PD patients
8B*34		
Espelage et al. (2002) – II	91	Bulimics
8B*2A8A		
Haller, Miles, & Dawson (2002) – II	28	Type II female addicts
8B2A3		
Stankovic et al. (1993)	43	Major Depression patients, admission code
8B2A8A		
Fink & Golinkoff (1990) – II	11	Borderline PD patients

(continued)

343

Within Normal Limits (WNL)	Sample Size	Diagnosis
8B3*		
Espelage et al. (2002) – II	183	Eating Disorder patients
	59	Eating Disorder NOS patients
8B32A*		
Millon (1987) – II	49	Self-Defeating PD patients
8B8A2A		
Lorr & Strack (1990) – II	41	Type I misc. psychiatric patients
8B8A2A6A		
Donat et al. (1992) – II	35	Type IV psychiatric inpatients
8B2A8A		
Petrocelli, Glaser, et al. (2001) – II	14	Severely depressed patients
C*4		
Pollock & Perry (1999) – II	14	Negatively preoccupied antenatal cocaine-abusing pregnant women

Disorder	Sample Size	MCMI (I/II) Code
PERSONALITY DISORDERS (GENERIC)		
Divac-Jovanovic et al. (1993)	121	8A2
Aggressive Sadistic PD		
Millon (1987) – II	4	6A456B
	36	6B6A
Antisocial PD		
Widiger & Sanderson (1987)	20	2*
Millon (1987) – II	19	6A*
	32	6B6A8A
Hart, Forth, & Hare (1991) – II	199	6A56B
Avoidant PD		
Widiger & Sanderson (1987)	18	28A1
Millon (1987) – II	60	21
	101	21
Borderline PD		
Fink & Golinkoff (1990)	11	8B28A
Lewis & Harder (1991)	27	8A23
Swirsky-Sacchetti et al. (1993)	10	28A
Millon (1987) – II	4	6A456B
	36	6B8A
McCann, Flynn, et al. (1992) – II	26	8A8B2
Dependent PD		
Widiger & Sanderson (1987)	27	32
Histrionic PD		
Millon (1987) – II	21	*28
	84	45*
Narcissistic PD		
Millon (1987) – II	84	54*
	69	54*
DiGiuseppe, Robin, et al. (1995) – II		
Type I	50	58A48B*
Type II	23	6B6A5*
Type III	34	58A4*
Obsessive-Compulsive PD		
Joffe et al. (1988)	23	*2
Fals-Stewart & Lucente (1993)	48	WNL[a]
	39	73*
	29	4*
	21	2*13
Millon (1987) – II	42	*6B7
	94	*73
		(continued)

[a]WNL = Within normal limits.

Disorder	Sample Size	MCMI (I/II) Code
Paranoid PD		
Millon (1987) – II	8	8A56B6A
	20	6B75
Passive-Aggressive PD		
Widiger & Sanderson (1987)	26	28A*
Millon (1987) – II	35	*6B
	90	8A*
Schizoid PD		
Millon (1987) – II	27	1*C
Schizotypal PD	X	X
Self-Defeating PD		
Millon (1987) – II	14	8B*
CLINICAL SYNDROMES		
Alcoholism		
Craig (1985)	196	*38A
McMahon & Davidson (1985a)		
With enduring depression	28	28A3
With transient depression	31	18A
	X	28A*
Bartsch & Hoffman (1985)		
Type I	19	*76A
Type II	23	546A*
Type III	35	8A*32
Type IV	17	*6A5
Type V	31	321*
McMahon et al. (1985b)	96	*8A3
McMahon & Davidson (1986a)		
Depressed	144	8A2
Not depressed	74	*56A
McMahon et al. (1986)		
High-functioning	43	*8A3
Low-functioning	37	8A*2
Donat (1988)		
Type I	23	*7
Type II	9	546A*
Type III	60	8A3*
Type IV	14	8A3
Type V	44	238A1
Mayer & Scott (1988)		
Type I	48	8A*2
Type II	28	56A4*
Type III	21	*7
Type IV	15	2138A

Disorder	Sample Size	MCMI (I/II) Code
McMahon et al. (1989)		
Continuous drinkers	117	8A*23
Episodic drinkers	54	*8A
McMahon & Tyson (1990)		
Women with enduring depression, admission code	9	8A23
1 month later		7*
Women with transient depression, admission code	14	3*
1 month later		7*
Retzlaff & Gibertini (1990b)		
VA patients	89	*5
Air Force patients	124	*8A
McMahon et al. (1991)		
Continuous drinkers	94	8A*2
Episodic drinkers	31	*8A2
Retzlaff & Bromley (1991)		
VA inpatients	89	
Type I	11	8A216A
Type II	18	54*
Type III	21	3*8A
Type IV	17	5*
Type V	15	8A32*
Type VI	7	12*
Corbisiero & Reznikoff (1991)		
VA inpatients	257	
Type II	24	*54
Type II	58	6A5*
Type III	165	8A21*
Donat (1991)		
Type I	200	*7
Type II		546A*
Type III		28A1*
Type IV		32*8A
Type V		8A4*
McMahon et al. (1993)		
VA inpatients	125	
Dependent	49	3*
Detached	31	218A*
Independent	45	6A5*
Matano et al. (1994)		
Males, Type I	111	*54
Type II		218A*
Type III		56A*
Females, Type I	84	*7
Type II		8A*
Type III		45*

(continued)

Disorder	Sample Size	MCMI (I/II) Code
Saxby & Peniston (1995)	14	WNL
Millon (1987) – II	20	6A6B8A
	43	6A8A
Litman & Cernovsky (1993) – II		
Inpatients	129	6A*
Anxiety Disorder		
Millon (1987) – II	66	*8B2
	143	*12
Bipolar Disorder		
Wetzler & Marlowe (1993)	21	5*6A
Millon (1987) – II	17	2*
	32	48A8B*
Turley et al. (1992) – II	19	6A4*5
Wetzler & Marlowe (1993) – II	15	5*
Wetzler et al. (1995) – II	26	*8A
Child Molesters		
Barnett & McCormack (1988)	147	*3
Chantry & Craig (1994a) – II	202	*3
Chantry & Craig (1994b) – II	115	*7
	46	38A2*
	40	312*
Nadeau et al. (1999)	79	3*
Cohen et al. (2002) – II	20	57A6B*
Depression		
Joffe et al. (1988)	23	*1
Goldberg et al. (1989)		
Sociotropic	8	321*
Joffe & Regan (1991)		
Family history positive	21	8A23
Family history negative remission	20	328A
Family history positive		*7
Family history negative		*37
Schuller, Bagby, et al. (1993)		
Depressives with SADS	17	8A*2
Non-SADS Depressed	24	WNL
Wetzler & Marlowe (1993)		
Outpatients	73	38A2*
Wetzler et al. (1995) – II		*2
Unipolars	158	3*
Type IV	19	28A6A*
Type V	24	*3

Disorder	Sample Size	MCMI (I/II) Code
Fals-Stewart & Lucente (1994) – II		
Cognitively impaired	55	6B2*
Non-cognitively impaired	191	*6B8A
Fals-Stewart (1995) – II		
Polydrug abusers	62	6A6B8A
Flynn et al. (1995) – II		
Heroin addicts	146	6A6B
Cocaine addicts	136	6A5
Howard et al. (1995)		
Cocaine-abusing females	74	8A*
Marlowe et al. (1995)		
Cocaine addicts	144	6A45
Flynn et al. (1997) – II		
Heroin/cocaine addicts	659	6A68*
Craig, Bivens, & Olson (1997) – III		
Heroin/cocaine addicts, Type I	161	6A2A18A
Type II	46	6A*
Type III	38	6A*
Type IV	45	WNL
McMahon, Malow, & Penedo (1998) – II		
Inpatients, Type I	91	8A6A2A6B+
Type II	160	6A56B
Type III	40	WNL
Schinka et al. (1999) – II		
Females in therapeutic community, admission	46	2A6A3
Posttreatment (1 year)		6A*4
Pollock & Percy (1999) – II		
Negatively disinterested cocaine-abusing pregnant women	14	58A6A*
Negatively preoccupied cocaine-abusing pregnant women	24	C*4
Calsyn, Wells, et al. (2000)		
Methadone patients:		
Light drug use:	89	
Pretreatment		*6A5
Posttreatment		*6A5
Heavy drug use:	141	
Pretreatment	*56A	
Posttreatment	*6A5	
Petrocelli, Glaser, et al. (2001) – II		
Nondepressed outpatients	58	WNL
Mildly depressed	39	WNL
Moderately depressed	28	*8B2A
Severely depressed	14	8B2A8A

(continued)

349

Disorder	Sample Size	MCMI (I/II) Code
Dysthymia		
Millon (1987) – II	133	*28B
	184	*28A
Eating Disorders		
Garner et al. (1990)		
Bulimics	50	
Good treatment response:		
Pretest		*4
Posttest		*4
Poor treatment response:		
Pretest		*2
Posttest		8A*2
Kennedy et al. (1990)		
Miscellaneous, pretreatment	44	32*
Posttreatment		*3
Tisdale et al. (1990)		
Bulimics	37	3*
Derecho et al. (1996) – II		
Atypical depression	7	2A38A1
Non-atypical depression	14	3*8A
Espelage et al. (2002) – II		
Anorexics	33	2A8B*3
Bulimics	91	8B*34
Eating Disorder NOS	59	8B3
Total sample	183	8B3*
Type I		WNL
Type II		8A8B4
Type III		32A8B
Dissociative Disorder		
Ellason & Ross (1996) – II	35	2A8B8A*
Allen, Coyne, & Console (1997) – III	102	2B8B
Dell (1998) – II	42	2B8B
Drug Abusers		
Craig (1984)		
Opiate addicts:	100	
Program completers	71	*56A
Program dropouts	29	*58A
Craig (1985)		
Opiate addicts	100	*56A
Marsh et al. (1988)		
Opiate addicts	163	*56A
Calsyn & Saxon (1988)		
Opiate addicts	45	56A*

Disorder	Sample Size	MCMI (I/II) Code
McMahon et al. (1985b)		
Miscellaneous	33	*8A3
Stark & Campbell (1988)		
Miscellaneous		X
Program completers	26	8A*
Program dropouts	31	4*
Craig & Olson (1990)		
Cocaine addicts	107	6A*5
Type I	56	56A*
Type II	37	8A6A*
Heroin addicts	86	*56A
Type I	26	56A*
Type II	56	8A6A*
Yeager et al. (1992)		
Miscellaneous inpatients	144	*54
Fals-Stewart (1992)		
Therapeutic community patients	235	
Type I	55	6A*
Type II	52	546A*
Type III	45	12*
Type IV	43	*3
Type V	40	45*
Millon (1987) – II		
Miscellaneous	25	6A6B
Miscellaneous	53	6A*
McMahon et al. (1993) – II		
Cocaine addicts	97	
Program dropouts	47	6A8A6B
Program completers	50	6A8A6B
Craig, Kuncel, & Olson (1994) – II		
Drug addicts	50	6A6B
Donat (1994) – II		
Polydrug-abusing inpatients	217	
Type I	62	*45
Type II	61	8A8B6A*
Type III	51	8A6A2*
Norman et al. (1993)		
Bulimics	58	*8A3
Anorexics	17	*2
Bulimic/anorexic	12	28A3*
Haller, Miles, & Dawson (2002) – II		
Females	78	
Type I	21	8B6A8A
Type II	28	8B*2A8A
Type III	29	8A6A*4

(continued)

Disorder	Sample Size	MCMI (I/II) Code
Forensic Patients		
Fals-Stewart (1995) – II		
Pretrial sentencing	54	8A8B*
Major Depression		
Joffe & Regan (1988)		
Admission	42	8A23*
In remission		*7
Wetzler et al. (1989)	48	38A2*
Joffe & Regan (1989a)		
Suicide attempters	10	8A231
No suicide attempts	43	8A23
Joffe & Regan (1989b)		
Treatment responders	23	8A236A
Treatment nonresponders	19	38A2
Piersma (1989a)		
(90% Major Depression) Admission	98	28B3
Discharged		*32
Goldberg et al. (1989)		
Autonomous	8	8A2*
Wetzler et al. (1990)	21	8A32*
Libb et al. (1990)	28	8A23
Millon (1987) – II	46	28B38A
	65	28B3
Beasley & Stoltenberg (1992) – II		
Pretreatment	43	8B23
Posttreatment	8B*	
Piersma & Boes (1997) – III		
Psychiatric inpatients	97	2B*3
Blais et al. (1998) – II		
Pre-ECT	16	32A1*
Post-ECT		3*
Schweitzer, Tuckwell, et al. (2001) – II		
DSM suppresssors	19	2A2B8A
DMS nonsuppressors	6	*7
Panic Disorder		
Wetzler et al. (1990)	19	8A*
Reich (1990)		
Program dropouts	12	*8A
Program completers	16	*7
Pedophiles		
Nadeau et al. (1999) – I	79	3*2A
PTSD		
Robert et al. (1985)		
Vietnam vets	25	8A2*

Disorder	Sample Size	MCMI (I/II) Code
Hyer et al. (1988)		
Vietnam vets	60	8A21*
Hyer et al. (1989)		
Vietnam vets, admission	50	8A21*
35 days later		8A21*
Hyer et al. (1990)		
Vietnam vets	60	8A21
Sherwood et al. (1991)		
Vietnam vets	36	8A2
140 days later		6A3
Hyer et al. (1991)		
Vietnam vets	100	8A2
Type I	4	8A2
Type II	33	8A21
Type III	33	8A213
Type IV	30	8A216A
Hyer, Davis, et al. (1994) – II		8A216A
Vietnam vets	92	8A21
Hyer, Davis, et al. (1994) – II		
Type I	256	8A2
Type II		28A1
Type III		6A8A
Type I	113	8A6A6B
Type II		8A8B26A
Type III		18A2
Type IV		8A8B26A
Allen, Coyne, & Huntoon (1998) – III		
Females	147	2B8B2A
Allen, Huntoon, & Evans (1999) – III		
Females	227	
Type I	35	8A8B3
Type II	44	2A2B8B
Type III	81	2B8B3
Type IV	44	2B8B1
Type V	23	WNL

Rapists

Disorder	Sample Size	MCMI (I/II) Code
Chantry & Craig (1994b) – II	195	
Type I	114	*75
Type II	50	56A*
Type III	31	231*
Nadeau et al. (1999) – I	34	*2A

(continued)

	Sample Size	MCMI (I/II) Code
Disorder		
Schizophrenia		
Josiassen et al. (1988)		
Psychotic	10	23
Nonpsychotic	10	23*
Davis & Greenblatt (1990)		
Young, White paranoid schizophrenics	27	*3
Young, White, nonparanoid schizophrenics		253*
Young, Black, paranoid schizophrenics	38	2*
Young, Black, nonparanoid schizophrenics	27	*3
Old, White, paranoid schizophrenics	32	321*
Old, White, nonparanoid schizophrenics	35	3*
Old, Black, paranoid schizophrenics	20	28A
Old, Black, nonparanoid schizophrenics	21	6A
Jackson et al. (1991)		
White symptom nonreporters	84	*3
Black symptom nonreporters		*5
White symptom reporters	174	21*
Black symptom reporters		218A*
Fink & Golinkoff (1990) – II	16	2*
del Rosario et al. (1994) – II		
Inpatients	35	3*
Munley et al. (1995) – II		
Vietnam vet inpatients	39	8A2A6A
Sexually Abused		
Bryer et al. (1987)	14	23*
Sexually and physically abused	14	238A*
Sexual Dysfunction		
Nadeau et al. (1999) – I	173	WNL
Spouse Abusers		
Hamberger & Hastings (1986)		
Type I	12	8A21*
Type II	14	56A*
Type III	12	3*7
Type IV	12	6A58A*
Type V	10	8A32*
Type VI	11	35*
Type VII	11	8A34*
Type VIII	12	*7
Beasley & Stoltenberg (1992) – II		
Outpatients	49	6B6A*
Murphy et al. (1993) – II		
Outpatients	24	6B8A6A*

Disorder	Sample Size	MCMI (I/II) Code
Hastings & Hamberger (1994)		
Spouse abusers:		
Nonviolent community:		
Good premorbid history	48	*7
Poor premorbid history	23	*4
Violent community:		
Good premorbid history	20	*4
Poor premorbid history	12	6A5*
Agency batterers:		
Good premorbid history	33	*5
Poor premorbid history	66	*6A
Dutton (1995) – II		
Outpatients	132	A6A2A*
Saghara & Warner (1999) – III		
Mexican American male batterers	60	NLP
Mexican American male nonbatterers	45	*4

Substance Abusers (Misc.)

Disorder	Sample Size	MCMI (I/II) Code
Nadeau et al. (1999) – I		
Males	182	8A2A*
Females	73	8A2A*

Miscellaneous

Child Custody

Disorder	Sample Size	MCMI (I/II) Code
McCann et al. (2001)		
Males and females	259	WNL

ACOAs

Disorder	Sample Size	MCMI (I/II) Code
Wall et al. (1990)		
Low alpha	13	*7
High alpha		54*

ADHD

Disorder	Sample Size	MCMI (I/II) Code
May & Bos (2000) – III	26	*4

Marital Therapy Patients

Disorder	Sample Size	MCMI (I/II) Code
Craig & Olson (1995) – II		
Males	70	*6B
Females	75	*7
Type I	29	56B3*
Type II	44	8A6B*
Type III	49	32*
Type IV	23	*37

Multiple Personality Disorder

Disorder	Sample Size	MCMI (I/II) Code
Fink & Golinkoff (1990) – II	16	28B8A

(continued)

Disorder	Sample Size	MCMI (I/II) Code
Offenders		
McNeil & Meyer (1990)		
Forensic inpatients	11	*3
Prison inmates	47	5*6A
Chantry & Craig (1994a) – II		
Rapists	195	*3
Felons	205	*5
McKee & Klohn (1994) – I		
Prison inmates	135	
Type I	27	8A32A*
Type II	13	312A*
Type III	27	56A*
Type IV	32	56A3*
Type V	35	*7
Blackburn (1996) – I		
Prisoners in England	138	
Type I	26	6A5*
Type II	31	28A*
Type III	29	6A*
Type IV	26	312*
Type V	26	128A*
Schwartz et al. (2004) – III		
Male inmates	366	WNL
Self-Injury		
Osuch, Noll, & Putnam (1999) – II		
High self-injury	48	2A8AB8A
Low self-injury	48	2A8B
Suicide		
McCann & Gergelis (1990) – II		
Suicide attempters	40	28A8B
Suicide ideation but no attempts	40	28B8A
Ellis, Rudd, et al. (1996)		
Psychiatric outpatients	299	
Type I	154	8A12*
Type II	54	238A1*
Type III	66	6A8A*
Type IV	25	54*
Rudd, Ellis, et al. (2000) – II		
Type I	61	8A2A8B
Type II	13	2A31
Type III	9	8A6A2A

Millon Clinical Multiaxial Inventory Bibliography

Robert J. Craig

FOLLOWING ARE primary resource references pertaining to the MCMI since its inception through June 2004. These citations are primarily from English-speaking references and journals. They are organized by manuals, books, reviews, journal articles, monographs, book chapters, cross-cultural research, and conference proceedings. At the end of journal citations, we use the designation (**II**) when the paper pertains to the MCMI-II and (**III**) when the citation pertains to the MCMI-III. If there is no citation at the end of the reference, that article pertains to the MCMI-I.

MANUALS

Millon, T. (1983). *Millon Clinical Multiaxial Inventory Manual* (3rd ed.). New York: Holt, Rinehart and Winston.

Millon, T. (1987). *Millon Clinical Multiaxial Inventory-II: Manual for the MCMI-II.* Minneapolis: Pearson Assessments.

Millon, T. (1994). *Millon Clinical Multiaxial Inventory-III: Manual.* Minneapolis: Pearson Assessments.

Millon, T. (1997). *Millon Clinical Multiaxial Inventory-III: Manual* (2nd ed.). Minneapolis: Pearson Assessments.

BOOKS

Choca, J. P. (2004). *Interpretive guide to the Millon Clinical Multiaxial Inventory* (3rd ed.). Washington, DC: American Psychological Association.

Craig, R. J. (1993a). *Psychological assessment with the Millon Clinical Multiaxial Inventory-II: An interpretive guide.* Odessa, FL: Psychological Assessment Resources.

Craig, R. J. (Ed.). (1993b). *The Millon Clinical Multiaxial Inventory: A clinical and research information synthesis.* Hillsdale, NJ: Erlbaum.

Craig, R. J. (Ed.). (2005). *New directions in interpreting the Millon Clinical Multiaxial Inventory-III: Essays on current issues.* New York: Wiley.

Jankowski, D. (2002). *A beginner's guide to the MCMI-III.* Washington, DC: American Psychological Association.

McCann, J., & Dyer, F. J. (1996). *Forensic assessment with the Millon inventories.* New York: Guilford Press.

Millon, T. (Ed.). (1997). *The Millon inventories: Clinical and personality assessment.* New York: Guilford Press.

Retzlaff, P. D. (Ed.). (1995). *Tactical psychotherapy of the personality disorders: An MCMI-III-based approach.* Needham Heights, MA: Allyn & Bacon.

Strack, S. (1999). *Essentials of Millon inventories assessment.* New York: Wiley.

Strack, S. (in press). *Handbook of personology and psychopathology: Essays in honor of Theodore Millon.* Hoboken, NJ: Wiley.

REVIEWS

Choca, J. (2001). Review of the Millon Clinical Multiaxial Inventory-III Manual (2nd ed.). In J. C. Impara & B. S. Plake (Eds.), *Fourteenth mental measurements yearbook* (pp. 765–767). Lincoln, NE: Buros Institute of Mental Measurements.

Craig, R. J. (1999). Overview and current status of the Millon Clinical Multiaxial Inventory. *Journal of Personality Assessment, 72,* 390–406.

Dana, R., & Cantrell, J. (1988). An update on the Millon Clinical Multiaxial Inventory (MCMI). *Journal of Clinical Psychology, 44,* 760–763.

Fleishauer, A. (1987). The MCMI-II: A reflection of current knowledge. *Noteworthy Response, 3,* 7.

Greer, S. (1984). Testing the test: A review of the Millon Multiaxial Inventory. *Journal of Counseling and Development, 63,* 262–263.

Haladyna, T. M. (1992). Review of the Millon Clinical Multiaxial Inventory-II. In J. J. Kramer & J. C. Conoley (Eds.), *Eleventh mental measurement yearbook* (pp. 532–533). Lincoln, NE: University of Nebraska Press.

Hess, A. K. (1985). Review of Millon Clinical Multiaxial Inventory. In J. Mitchell Jr. (Ed.), *Ninth mental measurements yearbook* (Vol. 1, pp. 984–986). Lincoln, NE: University of Nebraska Press.

Hess, A. K. (1990). Review of the Millon Clinical Multiaxial Inventory-III. In S. Mitchell Jr. (Ed.), *Mental Measurements Yearbook.* Lincoln, NE: University of Nebraska Press.

Lanyon, R. (1984). Personality assessment. *Annual Review of Psychology, 35,* 667–701.

McCabe, S. (1984). Millon Clinical Multiaxial Inventory. In D. Keyser & R. Sweetland (Eds.), *Test critiques* (Vol. 1, pp. 455–456). Kansas City, KS: Westport.

Reynolds, C. R. (1992). Review of the Millon Clinical Multi-axial Inventory-II. In J. J. Kramer & J. C. Conoley (Eds.), *Eleventh mental measurement yearbook* (pp. 533–535). Lincoln, NE: University of Nebraska Press.

Wetzler, S. (1990). The Millon Clinical Multiaxial Inventory: A review. *Journal of Personality Assessment, 55,* 445–464.

Widiger, T. A. (1985). Review of the Millon Clinical Multiaxial Inventory. In J. Mitchell Jr. (Ed.), *Ninth mental measurements yearbook* (Vol. 1, pp. 986–988). Lincoln, NE: University of Nebraska Press.

JOURNAL ARTICLES

Adams, W. E., & Clopton, J. R. (1990). Personality and dissonance among Mormon missionaries. *Journal of Personality Assessment, 54,* 684–693.

Ahlmeyer, S., Kleinsasser, D., Stoner, J., & Retzlaff, P. (2003). Psychopathology of incarcerated sex offenders. *Journal of Personality Disorders, 17,* 306–318. (**III**)

Ahrens, J. A., & Evans, R. G. (1990). Factors related to dropping out of school in an incarcerated population. *Educational and Psychological Measurement, 50,* 610–617.

Alden, L. (1989). Short-term structured treatment for avoidant personality disorder. *Journal of Consulting and Clinical Psychology, 57,* 756–764.

Alexander, P. C. (1993). The differential effects of abuse characteristics and attachment in the prediction of long-term effects of sexual abuse. [Special issue: Research on treatment of adults sexually abused in childhood]. *Journal of Interpersonal Violence, 8,* 346–362. (**II**)

Alexander, P. C., Anderson, C. L., Brand, B., Schaffer, C. M., Grelling, B. Z., & Kretz, L. (1998). Adult attachment and long-term effects in survivors of incest. *Child Abuse and Neglect, 22,* 45–61. (**II**)

Allen, J. G., Coyne, L., & Console, D. A. (1997). Dissociative detachment relates to psychotic symptoms and personality decompensation. *Comprehensive Psychiatry, 38,* 327–334. (**III**)

Allen, J. G., Coyne, L., & Huntoon, J. (1998). Complex posttraumatic stress disorder in women from a psychometric perspective. *Journal of Personality Assessment, 70,* 277–298. (**III**)

Allen, J. G., Huntoon, J., & Evans, R. B. (1999). Complexities in complex posttraumatic stress disorder in inpatient women: Evidence from cluster analysis of MCMI-III personality disorder scales. *Journal of Personality Disorders, 73,* 449–471. (**III**)

Alnaes, R., & Torgersen, S. (1990). MCMI personality disorders among patients with major depression with and without anxiety disorders. *Journal of Personality Disorders, 64,* 141–149.

Alnaes, R., & Torgersen, S. (1991). Personality and personality disorders among patients with various affective disorders. *Journal of Personality Disorders, 5,* 107–121.

Antoni, M., Levine, J., Tischer, P., Green, C., & Millon, T. (1986). Refining personality instruments by combining MCMI high-point profiles and MMPI codes. Part IV: MMPI code 89/98. *Journal of Personality Assessment, 50,* 65–72.

Antoni, M., Levine, J., Tischer, P., Green, C., & Millon, T. (1987). Refining personality assessments by combining MCMI high point profiles and MMPI codes: V. MMPI 78/87. *Journal of Personality Assessment, 51,* 375–387.

Antoni, M., Tischer, P., Levine, J., Green, C., & Millon, T. (1985a). Refining personality assessments by combining MCMI high point profiles and MMPI codes. Part I: MMPI code 28/82. *Journal of Personality Assessment, 49,* 392–398.

Antoni, M., Tischer, P., Levine, J., Green, C., & Millon, T. (1985b). Refining personality assessments by combining MCMI high point profiles and MMPI codes. Part III: MMPI code 24/42. *Journal of Personality Assessment, 49,* 508–515.

Auerback, J. S. (1984). Validation of two scales for narcissistic personality disorder. *Journal of Personality Assessment, 48,* 649–653.

Bagby, R. M., Gillis, J. R., & Dickens, S. (1990). Detection of dissimulation with the new generation of objective personality measures. *Behavioral Sciences and the Law, 8,* 93–102. **(II)**

Bagby, R. M., Gillis, J. R., & Rogers, R. (1991). Effectiveness of the Millon Clinical Multiaxial Inventory Validity Index in the detection of random responding. *Psychological Assessment, 3,* 285–287. **(II)**

Bagby, R. M., Gillis, J. R., Toner, B. B., & Goldberg, J. (1991). Detecting fake-good and fake-bad responding on the Millon Clinical Multiaxial Inventory-II. *Psychological Assessment, 3,* 496–498. **(II)**

Bagby, R. M., Joffe, R. T., Parker, J. D., & Schuller, D. R. (1993). Re-examination of the evidence for the *DSM-III* personality disorder clusters. *Journal of Personality Disorders, 7,* 320–328.

Baggi, L., Rubino, I. A., Zanna, V., & Martignoni, M. (1995). Personality disorders and regulative styles of patients with tempero-mandibular joint pain dysfunction syndrome. *Perceptual and Motor Skills, 80,* 267–273. **(II)**

Baile, W. F., Gibertini, M., Scott, L., & Endicott, J. (1993). Prebiopsy assessment of patients with suspected head and neck cancer. *Journal of Psychosocial Oncology, 10,* 79–91.

Baker, J. D., Capron, E. W., & Azorlosa, J. (1996). Family environment characteristics of persons with histrionic and dependent personalities. *Journal of Personality Disorders, 10,* 82–87.

Barnett, R. W., & McCormack, J. K. (1988). MCMI child molester profiles. *Corrective and Social Psychiatry and Journal of Behavior Technology Methods and Therapy, 34,* 14–16.

Barrett, T., & Etheridge, J. R. (1994). Verbal hallucinations in normals: III. Dysfunctional personality correlates. *Personality and Individual Differences, 16,* 57–62.

Barrington, W. W., Angle, C. R., Willcockson, N. K., Padula, M. A., & Korn, T. (1998). Autonomic functioning in manganese alloy workers. *Environmental Research, 50–58.* **(III)**

Bartsch, T., & Hoffman, J. (1985). A cluster analysis of Millon Clinical Multiaxial Inventory (MCMI) profiles: More about a taxonomy of alcoholic subtypes. *Journal of Clinical Psychology, 41,* 707–713.

Bayon, C., Hill, K., Svrakic, D. M., Przybeck, T. R., & Cloninger, C. R. (1996). Dimensional assessment of personality in an outpatient sample: Relations of the systems of Millon and Cloninger. *Journal of Psychiatric Research, 30,* 341–352. **(II)**

Beasley, R., & Stoltenberg, C. D. (1992). Personality characteristics of male spouse abusers. *Professional Psychology: Research and Practice, 23*, 310–317.

Beckwith, L., Howard, J., Espinoza, M., & Tyler, R. (1999). Psychopathology, mother-child interactions, and infant development: Substance-abusing mothers and their offspring. *Development and Psychopathology, 11*, 715–725.

Berman, S. M., & McCann, J. T. (1995). Defense mechanisms and personality disorders: An empirical test of Millon's theory. *Journal of Personality Assessment, 64*, 132–144.

Birtchnell, J. (1991). The measurement of dependence by questionnaire. *Journal of Personality Disorders, 5*, 281–295.

Bishop, D. R. (1993). Validity issues in using the Millon-II with substance abusers. *Psychological Reports, 73*, 27–33. (**II**)

Blackburn, R. (1987). Two scales for the assessment of personality disorders in antisocial populations. *Personality and Individual Differences, 8*, 81–93.

Blackburn, R. (1996). Replicated personality disorder clusters among mentally disordered offenders and their relation to dimensions of personality. *Journal of Personality Disorders, 10*, 68–81.

Blackburn, R. (1998). Relationship of personality disorders to observer ratings of interpersonal style in forensic psychiatric patients. *Journal of Personality Disorders, 12*, 77–85.

Blais, M. A. (1995). MCMI-II personality traits associated with the MMPI-2 masculinity-femininity scale. *Assessment, 2* 131–136. (**II**)

Blais, M. A., Benedict, K., & Norman, D. (1994). Associations among MCMI-II clinical syndrome scales and the MMPI-2 clinical scales. *Assessment, 1*, 407–413. (**II**)

Blais, M. A., Benedict, K., & Norman, D. (1995). Concurrent validity of the MCMI-II modifier indices. *Journal of Clinical Psychology, 51*, 783–789. (**II**)

Blais, M. A., Holdwick, D. J., McLean, R. Y., Otto, M. W., Pollack, M. H., & Hilsenroth, M. J. (2003). Exploring the psychometric properties and construct validity of the MCMI-III Anxiety and Avoidant personality scales. *Journal of Personality Assessment, 81*, 237–241. (**III**)

Blais, M. A., Matthews, J., Schouten, R., O'Keefe, S. M., & Summergrad, P. (1998). Stability and predictive value of self-report personality traits pre-and-post-electroconvulsive therapy: A preliminary study. *Comprehensive Psychiatry, 39*, 231–235. (**II**)

Blount, C., Evans, C., Birch, S., Warren, F., & Norton, K. (2002). The properties of self-report research measures: Beyond psychometrics. *Psychology and Psychotherapy: Theory, Research and Practice, 75*, 151–164. (**III**)

Bonato, D., Cyr, J., Kalpin, R., Predergast, P., & Sanhueza, P. (1988). The utility of the MCMI as a *DSM-III* Axis I diagnostic tool. *Journal of Clinical Psychology, 44*, 867–875.

Boone, K. B., Savodnik, I., Ghaffarian, S., Lee, A., Freeman, D., & Berman, N. G. (1995). Rey 15-item memorization and DOT Counting scores in a "stress" claim worker's compensation population: Relationship to personality (MCMI) scores. *Journal of Clinical Psychology, 51*, 457–463.

Borchgrevink, G. E., Stiles, T. C., Borchgrevink, P. C., & Lereim, I. (1997). Personality profile among symptomatic and recovered patients with neck sprain injury, measured by MCMI-I acutely and 6 months after car accidents. *Journal of Psychosomatic Research, 42,* 357–367.

Bornstein, R. F. (1995). Sex differences in objective and projective dependency tests: A meta-analytic review. *Assessment, 2,* 319–331.

Boswell, P. C., & Murray, E. J. (1981). Depression, schizophrenia and social attraction. *Journal of Consulting and Clinical Psychology, 49,* 641–647.

Boyle, G. J., & Le Dean, L. (2000). Discriminant validity of the illness behavior questionnaire and Millon Clinical Multiaxial Inventory-III in a heterogeneous sample of psychiatric outpatients. *Journal of Clinical Psychology, 56,* 779–791. **(III)**

Braver, M., Bumberry, J., Green, K., & Rawson, R. (1992). Childhood abuse and current psychological functioning in a university counseling center population. *Journal of Counseling Psychology, 39,* 252–257.

Briner, W., Risey, J., Guth, P., & Norris, C. (1990). Use of the Millon Clinical Multiaxial Inventory in evaluating patients with severe tinnitus. *American Journal of Otology, ll,* 334–337.

Broday, S. E. (1988). Perfectionism and the Millon basic personality patterns. *Psychological Reports, 63,* 791–794.

Bryer, J. B. (1990). Inpatient psychiatric outcome: A research program and initial findings. *The Psychiatric Hospital, 21,* 79–88.

Bryer, J. B., Nelson, B. A., Miller, J. B., & Krol, P. A. (1987). Childhood sexual and physical abuse as factors in adult psychiatric illness. *American Journal of Psychiatry, 144,* 1426–1430.

Bryer, J. B., Martines, K. A., & Dignan, M. A. (1990). Millon Clinical Multiaxial Inventory Alcohol Abuse and Drug Abuse Scales and the identification of substance-abuse patients. *Psychological Assessment: A Journal of Clinical and Consulting Psychology, 4,* 438–441.

Busby, D. M., Glenn, E., Steggel, G. L., & Adamson, D. W. (1993). Treatment issues for survivors of physical and sexual abuse. *Journal of Marital and Family Therapy, 19,* 377–392.

Butler, S. F., Gaulier, B., & Haller, D. (1991). Assessment of Axis II personality disorders among female substance abusers. *Psychological Reports, 68,* 1344–1346. **(II)**

Butters, M., Retzlaff, P., & Gibertini, M. (1986). Non-adaptability to basic training and the Millon Clinical Multiaxial Inventory. *Military Medicine, 151,* 574–576.

Calsyn, D. A., Flaming, C., Wells, E. A., & Saxon, A. J. (1996). Personality disorder subtypes among opiate addicts in methadone maintenance. *Psychology of Addictive Behaviors, 10,* 3–8. **(III)**

Calsyn, D. A., & Saxon, A. J. (1988). Identification of personality disorder subtypes among drug abusers using the Millon Clinical Multiaxial Inventory. 49th Annual Scientific Meeting of the Committee on Problems of Drug Dependence. *National Institute on Drug Abuse: Research Monograph Series.*

Calsyn, D. A., & Saxon, A. J. (1990). Personality disorder subtypes among cocaine and opioid addicts using the Millon Clinical Multiaxial Inventory. *International Journal of the Addictions, 25,* 1037–1049.

Calsyn, D. A., Saxon, A. J., & Daisy, F. (1990). Validity of the MCMI drug abuse scale with drug abusing and psychiatric samples. *Journal of Clinical Psychology, 46,* 244–246.

Calsyn, D. A., Saxon, A. J., & Daisy, F. (1991). Validity of the MCMI Drug Abuse Scale varies as a function of drug choice, race, and Axis II subtypes. *American Journal of Drug and Alcohol Abuse, 17,* 153–159.

Calsyn, D. A., Wells, E. A., Fleming, C., & Saxon, A. J. (2000). Changes in Millon Clinical Multiaxial Inventory scores among opiate addicts as a function of retention in methadone maintenance treatment and recent drug use. *American Journal of Drug and Alcohol Abuse, 26,* 297–309.

Campbell, N. B., Franco, K., & Jurs, S. (1988). Abortion in adolescence. *Adolescence, 23,* 813–823.

Campbell, B. K., & Stark, M. J. (1991). Psychopathology and personality characteristics in different forms of substance abuse. *International Journal of the Addictions, 25,* 1467–1474.

Cantrell, J., & Dana, R. (1987). Use of the Millon Clinical Multiaxial Inventory (MCMI) as a screening instrument at a community mental health center. *Journal of Clinical Psychology, 43,* 366–375.

Carpenter, D. R., Peed, S. F., & Eastman, B. (1995). Personality characteristics of adolescent sexual offenders: A pilot study. *Sexual Abuse: A Journal of Research and Treatment, 7,* 195–202.

Cash, T., Mikulka, P., & Brown, T. (1989). Validity of Millon's computerized interpretation system for the MCMI: Comment on Moreland and Onstad. *Journal of Consulting and Clinical Psychology, 57,* 311–312.

Chambless, D. L., Renneberg, B., Goldstein, A., & Gracely, E. J. (1992). MCMI diagnosed personality disorders among agoraphobic outpatients: Prevalence and relationship to severity and treatment outcome. *Journal of Anxiety Disorders, 6,* 193–211. **(II)**

Chandarana, P. C., Conlon, P., Holliday, M. D., Deslippe, T., & Field, V. A. (1990). A prospective study of psychosocial aspects of gastric stapling surgery. *Psychiatric Journal of the University of Ottawa, 15,* 32–35.

Chandarana, P. C., Cooper, A. J., Goldbach, M. M., Coles, J. C., & Vesely, M. A. (1988). Perceptual and cognitive deficit following coronary artery bypass surgery. *Stress Medicine, 4,* 163–171.

Chandarana, P. C., Holliday, R., Conlon, P., & Deslippe, T. (1988). Psychosocial considerations in gastric stapling surgery. *Journal of Psychosomatic Research, 32,* 85–92.

Chantry, K., & Craig, R. J. (1994a). MCMI typologies of criminal sexual offenders. *Sexual Addiction and Compulsivity, 1,* 215–226.

Chantry, K., & Craig, R. J. (1994b). Psychological screening of sexually violent offenders with the MCMI. *Journal of Clinical Psychology, 50,* 430–435.

Charter, R. A. (2000). Random responding to objective tests. *Journal of Psychoeducational Assessment, 18,* 308–315.

Charter, R. A., & Lopez, M. N. (2002). Millon Clinical Multiaxial Inventory (MCMI-III): The inability of the validity conditions to detect random responding. *Journal of Clinical Psychology, 58,* 1615–1617. **(III)**

Chatham, P. M., Tibbals, C. J., & Harrington, M. E. (1993). The MMPI and the MCMI in the evaluation of narcissism in a clinical sample. *Journal of Personality Assessment, 60,* 239–251.

Chick, D., Martin, S. K., Nevels, R., & Cotton, C. R. (1994). Relationship between personality disorders and clinical symptoms in psychiatric inpatients as measured by the Millon Clinical Multiaxial Inventory. *Psychological Reports, 74,* 331–336.

Chick, D., Sheaffer, C. I., & Goggin, W. C. (1993). The relationship between MCMI personality scales and clinician-generated *DSM-III-R* personality disorder diagnoses. *Journal of Personality Assessment, 61,* 264–276.

Choca, J. P., Bresolin, L., Okonek, A., & Ostrow, D. (1988). Validity of the MCMI in the assessment of affective disorders. *Journal of Personality Assessment, 52,* 96–105.

Choca, J. P., Peterson, C. S., & Shanley, L. S. (1986). Factor analysis of the Millon Clinical Multiaxial Inventory. *Journal of Consulting and Clinical Psychology, 54,* 253–255.

Choca, J., Retzlaff, P., Strack, S., Mouton, A., & Vandenburg, E. (1996). Factorial elements in Millon's personality theory. *Journal of Personality Disorders, 10,* 377–383. **(II)**

Choca, J. P., Shanley, L. A., Peterson, C. A., & Vandenburg, E. (1990). Racial bias and the MCMI. *Journal of Personality Assessment, 54,* 479–490.

Choca, J. P., Shanley, L. A., Vandenburg, E., Agresti, A., Mouton, A., & Vidger, L. (1992). Personality disorder or personality style: That is the question. *Journal of Counseling and Development, 70,* 429–431.

Clark, J. W., Schneider, H. G., & Cox, R. L. (1998). Initial evidence for reliability and validity of a brief screening inventory for personality traits. *Psychological Reports, 82,* 1115–1120. **(III)**

Cohen, L. J., Gans, S. W., McGeoch, P. G., Poznansky, O., Itskovich, Y., Murphy, S., et al. (2002). Impulsive personality traits in male pedophiles versus healthy controls: Is pedophilia an impulsive-aggressive disorder? *Comprehensive Psychiatry, 43,* 127–134. **(II)**

Cohen, L. J., McGeoch, P. G., Eatras-Gans, S., Acker, S., Poznansky, O., Cullen, K., et al. (2002). Personality impairment in male pedophiles. *Journal of Clinical Psychiatry, 63,* 912–919. **(II)**

Coolidge, F. L., & Merwin, M. M. (1992). Reliability and validity of the Coolidge Axis II Inventory: A new inventory for the assessment of personality disorders. *Journal of Personality Assessment, 59,* 233–238.

Corbisiero, J. R., & Reznikoff, M. (1991). The relationship between personality type and style of alcohol use. *Journal of Clinical Psychology, 47,* 291–298.

Costa, P. T., & McCrae, R. R. (1990). Personality disorders and the five-factor model of personality. *Journal of Personality Disorders, 4,* 362–371.

Craig, R. J. (1984). Can personality tests predict treatment dropouts? *International Journal of the Addictions, 19,* 665–674.

Craig, R. J. (1988). A psychometric study of the prevalence of *DSM-III* personality disorders among treated opiate addicts. *International Journal of the Addictions, 23,* 115–124.

Craig, R. J. (1995). Clinical diagnoses and MCMI code types. *Journal of Clinical Psychology, 51,* 352–360.

Craig, R. J. (1997). Sensitivity of MCMI-III Scales T (Drugs) and B (Alcohol) in detecting substance abuse. *Substance Use and Misuse, 32,* 1385–1393. (**III**)

Craig, R. J. (1999). Testimony based on the Millon Clinical Multiaxial Inventory: Review, commentary, and guidelines. *Journal of Personality Assessment, 73,* 290–316.

Craig, R. J. (2000). Prevalence of personality disorders among cocaine and heroin addicts. *Substance Abuse, 21,* 87–94. (**III**)

Craig, R. J. (2003). Use of the Millon Clinical Multiaxial Inventory in the psychological assessment of domestic violence: A review. *Aggression and Violent Behavior, 8,* 235–243.

Craig, R. J., & Bivens, A. (1998). Factor structure of the MCMI-III. *Journal of Personality Assessment, 70,* 190–196. (**III**)

Craig, R. J., & Bivens, A. (2000). MCMI-III scores on substance abusers with and without histories of suicide attempts. *Substance Abuse, 21,* 155–161. (**III**)

Craig, R. J., Bivens, A., & Olson, R. (1997). MCMI-III-derived typological analysis of cocaine and heroin addicts. *Journal of Personality Assessment, 69,* 583–595. (**III**)

Craig, R. J., & Horowitz, M. (1990). Current utilization of psychologist tests at diagnostic practicum sites. *The Clinical Psychologist, 43,* 29–36.

Craig, R. J., Kuncel, R., & Olson, R. E. (1994). Ability of drug addicts to avoid detection of substance abuse on the MCMI-II. *Journal of Social Behavior and Personality, 9,* 95–106. (**II**)

Craig, R. J., & Olson, R. (1992). Relationship between MCMI-II scales and normal personality traits. *Psychological Reports, 71,* 699–705. (**II**)

Craig, R. J., & Olson, R. (1995). MCMI-II profiles and typologies for patients seen in marital therapy. *Psychological Reports, 76,* 163–170. (**II**)

Craig, R. J., & Olson, R. (1997). Assessing PTSD with the Millon Clinical Multiaxial Inventory-III. *Journal of Clinical Psychology, 53,* 943–952.

Craig, R. J., & Olson, R. (1998). Stability of the MCMI-III in a substance-abusing inpatient sample. *Psychological Reports, 83,* 1273–1274. (**III**)

Craig, R. J., & Olson, R. (2001). Adjectival descriptions of personality disorders: A convergent validity study of the MCMI-III. *Journal of Personality Assessment, 77,* 259–271. (**III**)

Craig, R. J., Verinis, J., & Wexler, S. (1985). Personality characteristics of drug addicts and alcoholics on the Millon Clinical Multiaxial Inventory. *Journal of Personality Assessment, 49,* 156–160.

Craig, R. J., & Weinberg, D. (1992a). Assessing alcoholics with the Millon Clinical Multiaxial Inventory: A review. *Psychology of Addictive Behaviors, 6,* 200–208.

Craig, R. J., & Weinberg, D. (1992b). Assessing drug abusers with the Millon Clinical Multiaxial Inventory: A review. *Journal of Substance Abuse Treatment, 9,* 249–255.

Curtis, J. M., & Cowell, D. R. (1993). Relation of birth order and scores on measures of pathological narcissism. *Psychological Reports, 72,* 311–315.

Dalton, J. E., Garte, S. H., Lips, O. J., & Ryan, J. J. (1986). Psychological assessment instruments in PTSD treatment programs. *VA Practitioner, 3,* 41–51.

Dagan, Y., Sela, H., Omer, H., Hallis, D., & Dar, R. (1996). High prevalence of personality disorders among circadian rhythm sleep disorders (CRSD) patients. *Journal of Psychosomatic Research, 41,* 357–363.

Daubert, S. D., & Metzler, A. E. (2000). The detection of fake-bad and fake-good responding on the Millon Clinical Multiaxial Inventory III. *Psychological Assessment, 12,* 418–424. **(III)**

Davis, S. E., & Hays, L. W. (1997). An examination of the clinical validity of the MCMI-III depressive personality scale. *Journal of Clinical Psychology, 53,* 15–23.

Davis, W. E., & Greenblatt, R. L. (1990). Age differences among psychiatric inpatients on the MCMI. *Journal of Clinical Psychology, 46,* 770–774.

Davis, W. E., Greenblatt, R. L., & Pochyly, J. M. (1990). Test of MCMI black norms for five scales. *Journal of Clinical Psychology, 46,* 175–178.

De Groot, M. H., Franken, I. H., van der Meer, C. W., & Hendriks, V. M. (2003). Stability and change in dimensional ratings of personality disorders in drug abuse patients during treatment. *Journal of Substance Abuse Treatment, 24,* 115–120. **(II)**

del Rosario, P. M., McCann, J. T., & Navarra, J. W. (1994). The MCMI-II diagnosis of schizophrenia: Operating characteristics and profile analysis. *Journal of Personality Assessment, 63,* 438–452. **(II)**

Dell, J. J., Ruzicka, M. F., & Palsi, A. T. (1981). Personality and other factors associated with gambling addiction. *International Journal of the Addictions, 16,* 149–156.

Dell, P. F. (1998). Axis II pathology in outpatients with dissociative identity disorder. *Journal of Nervous and Mental Diseases, 186,* 352–356. **(II)**

Derecho, C. N., Wetzler, S., McGinn, L. K., Sanderson, W. C., & Asnis, G. M. (1996). Atypical depression among psychiatric inpatients: Clinical features and personality traits. *Journal of Affective Disorders, 39,* 55–59. **(II)**

DeWolfe, A., Larsen, J., & Ryan, J. (1985). Diagnostic accuracy of the Millon test computer reports for bipolar affective disorder. *Journal of Psychopathology and Behavioral Assessment, 7,* 185 189.

DiGiuseppe, R., Robin, M., Szeszko, P. R., & Primavera, L. H. (1995). Cluster analysis of narcissistic personality disorders on the MCMI-II. *Journal of Personality Disorders, 9,* 304–317. **(II)**

Dillon, S. K. (1988). Narcissism and embellishments of signature. *Psychological Reports, 62,* 152–154.

Divac-Jovanovic, M., Svrakic, D., & Lecic-Tosevskli, D. (1993). Personality disorders: Model for conceptual approach and classification. *American Journal of Psychotherapy, 47,* 558–571.

Donat, D. C. (1988). Millon Clinical Multiaxial Inventory (MCMI) clusters for alcohol abusers: Further evidence of validity and implications for medical psychotherapy. *Medical Psychotherapy, 1,* 41–50.

Donat, D. C. (1994). Empirical groupings of perceptions of alcohol use among alcohol dependent persons: A cluster analysis of the alcohol use inventory (AUI) scales. *Assessment, 1*, 103–110. **(II)**

Donat, D. C. (1997). Personality traits and psychiatric rehospitalization: A two-year follow-up. *Journal of Personality Assessment, 68*, 703–711. **(II)**

Donat, D. C., Geczy, B., Helmrich, J., & LeMay, M. (1992). Empirically derived personality subtypes of public psychiatric patients: Effect on self-reported symptoms, coping inclinations, and evaluation of expressed emotion in caregivers. *Journal of Personality Assessment, 58*, 36–50. **(II)**

Donat, D. C., Walters, J., & Hume, A. (1991). Personality characteristics of alcohol dependent inpatients: Relationship of MCMI subtypes to self-reported drinking behavior. *Journal of Personality Assessment, 57*, 335–344.

Donat, D. C., Walters, J., & Hume, A. (1992). MCMI differences between alcoholics and cocaine abusers: Effects of age, sex, and race. *Journal of Personality Assessment, 58*, 96–104.

Dougherty, R. J., & Lesswing, N. J. (1989). Inpatient cocaine abusers: An analysis of psychological and demographic variables. *Journal of Substance Abuse Treatment, 6*, 45–47.

Dubro, A. F., & Wetzler, S. (1989). An external validity study of the MMPI personality disorder scales. *Journal of Clinical Psychology, 45*, 570–575.

Dutton, D. G. (1994). The origin and structure of the abusive personality. *Journal of Personality Disorders, 8*, 181–191.

Dutton, D. G. (1995). Trauma symptoms and PTSD-like profiles in perpetrators of intimate abuse. *Journal of Traumatic Stress, 8*, 299–316. **(II)**

Dutton, D. G. (2002). Personality dynamics of intimate abusiveness. *Journal of Psychiatric Practice, 8*, 216–228. **(II)**

Dutton, D. G. (2003). MCMI Results for Batterers: A response to Gondolf. *Journal of Family Violence, 18*, 253. **(III)**

Dyce, J. A., O'Connor, B. P., Parkins, S. Y., & Janzen, H. L. (1997). Correlational structure of the MCMI-III personality disorder scales and comparisons with other data sets. *Journal of Abnormal Psychology, 69*, 568–582. **(III)**

Dyer, F. J. (1994). Factorial trait variance and response bias in MCMI-II personality disorder scale scores. *Journal of Personality Disorders, 8*, 121–130. **(II)**

Dyer, F. J., & McCann, J. T. (2000). The Millon clinical inventories, research critical of their application, and *Daubert* criteria. *Law and Human Behavior, 24*, 487–497. **(III)**

Eckblad, M., & Chapman, L. J. (1986). Development and validation of a scale for hypomanic personality. *Journal of Abnormal Psychology, 95*, 214–222.

Ellason, J. W., & Ross, C. A. (1996). Millon Clinical Multiaxial Inventory-II: Follow-up of patients with dissociative identity disorder. *Psychological Reports, 78*, 707–716. **(II)**

Ellason, J. W., Ross, C. A., & Fuchs, D. L. (1995). Assessment of dissociative identity disorder with the Millon Clinical Multiaxial Inventory-II. *Psychological Reports, 76*, 895–905.

Ellis, T. E., Rudd, M. D., Rajab, M. H., & Wehrly, T. E. (1996). Cluster analysis of MCMI scores of suicidal psychiatric patients: Four personality profiles. *Journal of Clinical Psychology, 52*, 411–422.

Emmons, R. A. (1987). Narcissism: Theory and measurement. *Journal of Personality and Social Psychology, 52*, 11–17.

Espelage, D. L., Mazzeo, S. E., Aggen, S. H., Quittner, A. L., Sherman, R., & Thompson, R. (2003). Examining the construction validity of the Eating Disorder Inventory. *Psychological Assessment, 15*, 71–80. (**II**)

Espelage, D. L., Mazzeo, S. E., Sherman, R., & Thompson, R. (2002). MCMI-II profiles of women with eating disorders: A cluster analytic investigation. *Journal of Personality Disorders, 16*, 453–463. (**II**)

Evered, L., Ruff, R., Baldo, J., & Isomura, A. (2003). Emotional risk factors and postconcussional disorder. *Assessment, 10*, 420–427. (**III**)

Fals-Stewart, W. (1992). Personality characteristics of substance abusers: An MCMI cluster typology of recreational drug users treated in a therapeutic community and its relationship to length of stay and outcome. *Journal of Personality Assessment, 59*, 515–527.

Fals-Stewart, W., & Lucente, S. (1993). An MCMI cluster typology of obsessive-compulsives: A measure of personality characteristics and its relationship to treatment participation, compliance and outcome in behavior therapy. *Journal of Psychiatric Research, 27*, 139–154.

Fals-Stewart, W., & Lucente, S. (1994). Effect of neuro-cognitive status and personality functioning on length of stay in residential substance abuse treatment: An integrative study. *Psychology of Addictive Behaviors, 8*, 179–190. (**II**)

Fals-Stewart, W. (1995). The effect of defensive responding by substance-abusing patients on the Millon Clinical Multiaxial Inventory. *Journal of Personality Assessment, 64*, 540–551. (**II**)

Fink, D. L., & Golinkoff, M. (1991). MPD, borderline personality disorder and schizophrenia: A comparative study of clinical features. *Dissociation: Progress in the Dissociative Disorders, 3*, 127–134.

Flett, G. L., & Hewitt, P. L. (1995). Criterion validity and psychometric properties of the affect intensity measure in a psychiatric sample. *Personality of Individual Differences, 19*, 585–591.

Flynn, P. M., Luckey, J. W., Brown, B. S., Hoffman, J. A., Dunteman, G. H., Theisen, A. C., et al. (1995). Relationship between drug preference and indicators of psychiatric impairment. *American Journal of Drug and Alcohol Abuse, 21*, 153–166.

Flynn, P. M., McCann, J. T., & Fairbank, J. A. (1995). Issues in the assessment of personality disorder and substance abuse using the Millon Clinical Multiaxial Inventory (MCMI-II). *Journal of Clinical Psychology, 51*, 415–421.

Flynn, P. M., McCann, J. T., Luckey, J. W., Rounds-Bryant, J. L., Theisen, A. C., Hoffman, J. A., et al. (1997). Drug dependence scale of the Millon Clinical Multiaxial Inventory. *Substance Use and Misuse, 32*, 733–741. (**II**)

Flynn, P., & McMahon, R. C. (1983a). Indicators of depression and suicidal ideation among drug abusers. *Psychological Reports, 52*, 784–786.

Flynn, P., & McMahon, R. C. (1983b). Stability of the drug misuse scale of the Millon Clinical Multiaxial Inventory. *Psychological Reports, 52,* 536–538.

Flynn, P., & McMahon, R. C. (1984a). An examination of the drug abuse scale of the Millon Clinical Multiaxial Inventory. *International Journal of the Addictions, 19,* 459–468.

Flynn, P., & McMahon, R. C. (1984b). An examination of the factor structure of the Millon Clinical Multiaxial Inventory. *Journal of Personality Assessment, 48,* 308–311.

Foster, L. M. (1978). Psychopathology and employment in a VA psychiatric outpatient population. *Psychological Reports, 41,* 1294.

Franco, K., Campbell, N., Tamburrino, M., & Jurs, S. (1989). Anniversary reactions and due date responses following abortion. *Psychotherapy and Psychosomatics, 52,* 151–154.

Franco, K. N., Tamburrino, M. B., Campbell, N. B., Pentz, J. E., & Jurs, S. G. (1989). Psychological profile of dysphoric postabortion. *Journal of the American Medical Women's Association, 44,* 113–115.

Freeman, A. M., Kablinger, A. S., Rolland, P. D., & Brannon, G. E. (1999). Millon Multiaxial personality patterns differentiate depressed and anxious outpatients. *Depression and Anxiety, 10,* 73–76. (**III**)

Frost, R. O., Krause, M. S., & Steketee, G. (1996). Hoarding and obsessive-compulsive symptoms. *Behavior Modification, 20,* 116–132.

Funari, D. J., Piekarski, A. M., & Sherwood, R. J. (1991). Treatment outcomes of Vietnam veterans with post-traumatic stress disorder. *Psychological Reports, 68,* 571–578.

Funtowicz, M. N., & Widiger, T. A. (1995). Sex bias in the diagnosis of personality disorders: A different approach. *Journal of Psychopathology and Behavioral Assessment, 17,* 145–165. (**II**)

Gabrys, J. B., Schump, D., & Utendale, K. A. (1987). Short-term memory for two meaningful stories and self report on the adult Eysenck Personality Questionnaire. *Psychological Reports, 61,* 51–59.

Gabrys, J. B., Utendale, K. A., Schump, D., Phillips, N., Peters, K., Robertson, G., et al. (1988). Two inventories for the measurement of psychopathology: Dimensions and common factorial space on Millon's clinical and Eysenck's general personality scales. *Psychological Reports, 62,* 591–601.

Gallucci, N. T. (1990). On the synthesis of information from psychological tests. *Psychological Reports, 67,* 1243–1260.

Ganellen, R. J. (1996). Comparing the diagnostic efficiency of the MMPI, MCMI-II, and the Rorschach. *Journal of Personality Assessment, 67,* 219–243. (**II**)

Garner, D. M., Olmsted, M. R., Davis, R., Rocket, W., Goldbloom, D., & Eagle, M. (1990). The association between bulimic symptoms and reported psychopathology. *International Journal of Eating Disorders, 9,* 1–15.

Gayford, J. J., & Jungalwa, H. N. (1986). Personality disorder according to *ICD-9* and the *DSM-III* and their value in court reporting. *Medicine Science and the Law, 26,* 113–124.

Gibertini, M., Brandenberg, N., & Retzlaff, P. (1986). The operating characteristics of the Millon Clinical Multiaxial Inventory. *Journal of Personality Assessment, 50,* 554–567.

Gibertini, M., & Retzlaff, P. (1988). Factor invariance of the Millon Clinical Multiaxial Inventory. *Journal of Psychopathology and Behavioral Assessment, 10,* 65–74.

Gilbride, T., & Hebert, J. (1980). Pathological characteristics of good and poor interpersonal problem-solvers among psychiatric outpatients. *Journal of Clinical Psychology, 36,* 121–127.

Glass, M. H., Bieber, S. L., & Tkachuk, M. J. (1996). Personality styles and dynamics of Alaska native and nonnative incarcerated men. *Journal of Personality Assessment, 66,* 583–603. **(II)**

Goldberg, J. O., Segal, Z. V., Vella, D. D., & Shaw, B. F. (1989). Depressive personality: Millon Clinical Multiaxial Inventory profiles of sociotropic and autonomous subtypes. *Journal of Personality Disorders, 3,* 193–198.

Goldberg, J. O., Shaw, B., & Segal, Z. V. (1987). Concurrent validity of the MCMI depression scales. *Journal of Consulting and Clinical Psychology, 55,* 785–787.

Gondolf, E. W. (1999). MCMI-III results for batterer program participants in four cities: Less "pathological" than expected. *Journal of Family Violence, 14,* 1–17. **(III)**

Green, C. (1982). The diagnostic accuracy and utility of MMPI and MCMI computer interpretive reports. *Journal of Personality Assessment, 46,* 359–365.

Greenblatt, R. L., & Davis, W. E. (1992). Accuracy of MCMI classification of angry and psychotic black and white patients. *Journal of Clinical Psychology, 48,* 59–63.

Greer, S. (1985). Scoring of the MCMI: Effects on validity—A reply to Millon and Moreland. *Journal of Counseling and Development, 63,* 632.

Grillo, J., Brown, R. S., & Hilsabeck, R. (1994). Raising doubts about claims of malingering: Implications of relationships between MCMI-II and MMPI-2 performances. *Journal of Clinical Psychology, 50,* 651–655. **(II)**

Guisado, J. A., Vaz, F. J., Alarcon, J., Lopez-Ibor, J. J., Rubio, M. A., & Gaite, L. (2002). Psychopathological status and interpersonal functioning following weight loss in morbidly obese patients undergoing bariatric surgery. *Obesity Surgery, 12,* 835–840. **(II)**

Guthrie, P. C., & Mobley, B. D. (1994). A comparison of the differential diagnostic efficiency of three personality disorder inventories. *Journal of Clinical Psychology, 50,* 656–665. **(II)**

Haller, D. L., & Miles, D. R. (2004). Personality disturbances in drug-dependent women: Relationship to childhood abuse. *American Journal of Drug and Alcohol Abuse, 30,* 269–286.

Haller, D. L., & Miles, D. R. (2003). Victimization and perpetration among perinatal substance abusers. *Journal of Interpersonal Violence, 18,* 760–780. **(III)**

Haller, D. L., Miles, D. R., & Dawson, K. S. (2002). Psychopathology influences treatment retention among drug-dependent women. *Journal of Substance Abuse Treatment, 23,* 431–436. **(II)**

Halon, R. L. (2001). The Millon Clinical Multiaxial Inventory-III: The normal quartet in child custody cases. *American Journal of Forensic Psychology, 19,* 57–75. **(III)**

Hamberger, L. K., & Hastings, J. E. (1986). Personality correlates of men who abuse their partners: A cross-validational study. *Journal of Family Violence, l*, 323–341.

Hamberger, L. K., & Hastings, J. E. (1988). Characteristics of male spouse abusers consistent with personality disorders. *Hospital and Community Psychiatry, 39*, 763–770.

Hamberger, L. K., & Hastings, J. E. (1989). Counseling male spouse abusers: Characteristics of treatment completers and dropouts. *Violence and Victims, 4*, 275–286.

Hamberger, L. K., & Hastings, J. E. (1992). Racial differences on the MCMI in an outpatient clinical sample. *Journal of Personality Assessment, 58*, 90–95.

Hastings, J. E., & Hamberger, L. K. (1994). Psychosocial modifiers of psychopathology for domestically violent and nonviolent men. *Psychological Reports, 74*, 112–114.

Hart, S. D., Dutton, D. G., & Newlove, T. (1993). The prevalence of personality disorder among wife assaulters. *Journal of Personality Disorders, 7*, 329–341. (**II**)

Hart, S. D., Forth, A. E., & Hare, R. D. (1991). The MCMI-II and psychopathy. *Journal of Personality Disorders, 5*, 318–327. (**II**)

Head, S. B., Baker, J. D., & Williamson, D. A. (1991). Family environment characteristics and dependent personality disorder. *Journal of Personality Disorders, 5*, 253–263.

Head, S. B., & Williamson, D. A. (1991). Association of family environment and personality disturbances in bulimia nervosa. *International Journal of Eating Disorders, 9*, 667–674.

Helmes, E. (1989). Stability of the internal structure of the Millon Clinical Multiaxial Inventory. *Journal of Psychopathology and Behavioral Assessment, II*, 327–338.

Helmes, E., & Barilko, O. (1988). Comparison of three multiscale inventories in identifying the presence of psychopathological symptoms. *Journal of Personality Assessment, 52*, 74–80.

Henning, K., Jones, A., & Holdford, R. (2003). Treatment needs of women arrested for domestic violence: A comparison with male offenders. *Journal of Interpersonal Violence, 18*, 839–856. (**III**)

Herrick, S. M., & Elliot, T. R. (2001). Social problem-solving abilities and personality disorder characteristics among dual-diagnosed persons in substance abuse treatment. *Journal of Clinical Psychology, 57*, 75–92. (**II**)

Herron, L., Turner, J., & Weiner, P. (1986). A comparison of the Millon Clinical Multiaxial Inventory and the Minnesota Multiphasic Personality Inventory as predictors of successful treatment by lumbar laminectomy. *Clinical Orthopaedics and Related Research, 203*, 232–238.

Hibbard, S. (1989). Personality and object relational pathology in young adult children of alcoholics. *Psychotherapy, 26*, 504–509.

Hibbard, S., Hilsenroth, M. J., Hibbard, J. K., & Nash, M. R. (1995). A validity study of two projective object representation measures. *Psychological Assessment, 7*, 432–439. (**II**)

Hicklin, J., & Widiger, T. A. (2000). Convergent validity of alternative MMPI-2 personality disorder scale. *Journal of Personality Assessment, 75*, 502–518. (**III**)

Hiller, M. L., Knight, K., & Simpson, D. D. (1996). An assessment of comorbid psychological problems in a residential criminal justice drug treatment program. *Psychology of Addictive Behaviors, 10,* 181–189.

Hills, H. A. (1995). Diagnosing personality disorders: An examination of the MMPI-2 and MCMI-II. *Journal of Personality Assessment, 65,* 21–34.

Hogg, B., Jackson, H. J., Rudd, R. P., & Edwards, J. (1990). Diagnosing personality disorders in recent-onset schizophrenia. *Journal of Nervous and Mental Diseases, 179,* 194–199.

Holliman, N., & Guthrie, P. (1989). A comparison of the MCMI and the CPI in assessment of a nonclinical population. *Journal of Clinical Psychology, 45,* 373–382.

Holt, S. E., Meloy, J. R., & Strack, S. (1999). Sadism and psychopathy in violent and sexually violent offenders. *Journal of the American Academy of Psychiatry and Law, 27,* 23–32. **(II)**

Howard, J., Beckwith, L., Espinosa, M., & Tyler, R. (1995). Development of infants born to cocaine-abusing women: Biologic/maternal influences. *Neurotoxicology and Teratology, 17,* 403–411.

Hsu, L. M. (2002). Diagnostic validity statistics and the MCMI-III. *Psychological Assessment, 14,* 410–422. **(III)**

Hsu, L. M. (1994). Item overlap correlations: Definitions, interpretations, and implications. *Multivariate Behavioral Research, 29,* 127–140.

Hull, J. S., Range, L. M., & Goggin, W. C. (1992). Suicide ideas: Relationship to personality disorders on the MCMI. *Death Studies, 16,* 371–375.

Hunsley, J. (1988). The intrapersonal and systemic ramifications of symptom prescription. *Psychotherapy, 25,* 273–279.

Hyer, L. A., Albrecht, J. W., Boudewyns, P. A., Woods, M. G., & Brandsma, J. (1993). Dissociative experiences of Vietnam veterans with chronic posttraumatic stress disorder. *Psychological Reports, 73,* 519–530.

Hyer, L., & Boudewyns, P. (1985). The 8–2 MCMI personality profile among Vietnam veterans with PTSD. *PTSD Newsletter, 4,* 2.

Hyer, L., Boyd, S., Stanger, E., Davis, H., & Walters, P. (1997). Validation of the MCMI-III PTSD scale among combat veterans. *Psychological Reports, 80,* 720–722. **(III)**

Hyer, L., Braswell, L., Albrecht, B., Boyd, S., Boudewyns, P., & Talbert, S. (1994). Relationship of NEO-PI to personality styles and severity of trauma in chronic PTSD victims. *Journal of Clinical Psychology, 50,* 699–707.

Hyer, L., Carson, M., Nixon, D., Tamkin, A., & Saucer, R. T. (1987). Depression among alcoholics. *International Journal of the Addictions, 22,* 1235–1241.

Hyer, L., Davis, H., Albrecht, W., Boudewyns, P., & Woods, G. (1994). Cluster analysis of MCMI and MCMI-II of chronic PTSD victims. *Journal of Clinical Psychology, 50,* 502–515. **(II)**

Hyer, L., Davis, H., Woods, G., Albrecht, W., Boudewyns, P. A., & Brandsma, J. (1994). Relationship between the Millon Clinical Multiaxial Inventory and the Millon-II: Value of scales for aggressive and self-defeating personalities in posttraumatic stress disorder. *Psychological Reports, 71,* 867–879. **(II)**

Hyer, L., & Harrison, W. R. (1986). Later life personality model: Diagnosis and treatment. *Clinical Gerontologist* (3/4), 399–416.

Hyer, L., Harrison, W. R., & Jacobsen, R. H. (1987). Later-life depression: Influences of irrational thinking and cognitive impairment. *Journal of Rational-Emotive Therapy, 5,* 43–48.

Hyer, L., O'Leary, W. C., Elkins, R., & Arena, J. (1985). PTSD: Additional criteria for evaluation. *VA Practitioner, 2,* 67–75.

Hyer, L., Woods, M. G., & Boudewyns, P. A. (1991). A three tier evaluation of PTSD among Vietnam combat veterans. *Journal of Traumatic Stress, 4,* 165–194.

Hyer, L., Woods, M. G., Boudewyns, P. A., Bruno, R., & O'Leary, W. C. (1988). Concurrent validation of the Millon Clinical Multiaxial Inventory among Vietnam veterans with posttraumatic stress disorder. *Psychological Reports, 63,* 271–278.

Hyer, L., Woods, M. G., Boudewyns, P. A., Harrison, W. R., & Tamkin, A. S. (1990). MCMI and 16PF with Vietnam veterans: Profiles and concurrent validation of MCMI. *Journal of Personality Disorders, 4,* 391–401.

Hyer, L., Woods, M. G., Bruno, R., & Boudewyns, P. (1989). Treatment outcomes of Vietnam veterans with PTSD and consistency of the MCMI. *Journal of Clinical Psychology, 45,* 547–552.

Hyer, L., Woods, M. G., Summers, M. N., Boudewyns, P., & Harrison, W. R. (1990). Alexithymia among Vietnam veterans with posttraumatic stress disorder. *Journal of Clinical Psychiatry, 51,* 243–247.

Inch, R., & Crossley, M. (1993). Diagnostic utility of the MCMI-I and MCMI-II with psychiatric outpatients. *Journal of Clinical Psychology, 49,* 358–366. (**II**)

Jackson, J. L., Greenblatt, R. L., Davis, W. E., Murphy, T. T., & Trimakas, K. (1991). Assessment of schizophrenic inpatients with the MCMI. *Journal of Personality Assessment, 51,* 243–253.

Jaffe, L., & Archer, R. (1987). The prediction of drug use among college students from the MMPI, MCMI and Sensation Seeking Scales. *Journal of Personality Assessment, 51,* 243–253.

Jay, G. W., Grove, R. N., & Grove, K. S. (1987). Differentiation of chronic headache from non-headache pain patients using the Millon Clinical Multiaxial Inventory (MCMI). *Headache, 27,* 124–129.

Joffe, R. T., & Regan, J. J. (1988). Personality and depression. *Journal of Psychiatric Research, 22,* 279–286.

Joffe, R. T., & Regan, J. J. (1989a). Personality and response to tricyclic antidepressants in depressed patients. *Journal of Nervous and Mental Diseases, 177,* 745–749.

Joffe, R. T., & Regan, J. J. (1989b). Personality and suicidal behavior in depressed patients. *Comprehensive Psychiatry, 30,* 157–160.

Joffe, R. T., & Regan, J. J. (1991). Personality and family history of depression in patients with affective illness. *Journal of Psychiatric Research, 25,* 67–71.

Joffe, R. T., Swinson, R. P., & Regan, J. J. (1988). Personality features of obsessive-compulsive disorder. *American Journal of Psychiatry, 145,* 1127–1129.

Joiner, T. E., & Rudd, M. D. (2002). The incremental validity of passive-aggressive personality symptoms rivals or exceeds that of other personality symptoms in suicidal outpatients. *Journal of Personality Assessment, 79,* 161–170.

Jones, A. (2000). An examination of the MMPI-2 Wiener-Harmon subtle subscales for, D., & Hy: Implications for parent scale and neurotic triad. *Journal of Personality Assessment, 77,* 105–121. (**II**)

Jones, R. A., & Wells, M. (1996). An empirical study of parentification and personality. *American Journal of Family Therapy, 24,* 1435–1452.

Josiassen, R. C., Shagass, C., & Roemer, R. A. (1988). Somato-sensory evoked potential correlates of schizophrenic subtypes identified by the Millon Clinical Multiaxial Inventory. *Psychiatry Research, 23,* 209–219.

Josiassen, R. C., Shagass, C., Roemer, R. A., & Straumanis, J. (1987). The attention-related somatosensory patients. *Psychiatry Research, 5,* 147–155.

Karlin, N. J., & Retzlaff, P. D. (1995). Psychopathology in caregivers of the chronically ill: Personality and clinical syndromes. *Hospice Journal, 10,* 55–61. (**II**)

Kaszniak, A. K., Nussbaum, P. D., Berren, M. R., & Santiago, J. (1988). Amnesia as a consequence of male rape: A case report. *Journal of Abnormal Psychology, 97,* 100–104.

Kelln, B. R., Dozois, D. J., & McKenzie, I. E. (1998). An MCMI-III discriminant function analysis of incarcerated felons: Prediction of subsequent institutional misconduct. *Criminal Justice and Behavior, 25,* 177–189. (**III**)

Kennedy, S. H., Katz, R., Rockert, W., Mendlowitz, S., Ralevski, E., & Clewes, C. J. (1995). Assessment of personality disorders in anorexia nervosa and bulimia nervosa: A comparison of self-report and structured interview methods. *Journal of Nervous and Mental Diseases, 183,* 358–364. (**II**)

Kennedy, S. H., McVey, G., & Katz, R. (1990). Personality disorders in anorexia nervosa and bulimia nervosa. *Journal of Psychiatric Research, 24,* 259–269.

King, A. R. (1998). Relations between MCMI-II personality variables and measures of academic performance. *Journal of Personality Assessment, 71,* 253–268. (**II**)

King, R. E. (1994, March). Assessing aviators for personality pathology with the Millon Clinical Multiaxial Inventory (MCMI). *Aviation, Space, and Environmental Medicine,* 227–231.

Klein, M. H., Benjamin, L. S., Rosenfeld, R., Treece, C., Husted, J., & Greist, J. H. (1993). The Wisconsin Personality Disorders Inventory: Development, reliability, and validity. *Journal of Personality Disorders, 7,* 285–303.

Korchin, S., & Schuldberg, D. (1981). The future of clinical assessment. *American Psychologist, 36,* 1147–1158.

Kreiner, S., Simonsen, E., & Mogensen, J. (1991). Validation of a Personality Inventory Scale: The MCMI-P scale. *Journal of Personality Disorders, 4,* 303–311.

Kringlen, E., & Cramer, G. (1989). Offspring of monozygotic twins discordant for schizophrenia. *Archives of General Psychiatry, 46,* 873–877.

Kristensen, H., & Torgersen, S. (2001). MCMI-II personality traits and symptom traits in parents of children with selective mutism: A case-controlled study. *Journal of Abnormal Psychology, 110,* 648–652. (**II**)

Lally, S. J. (2003). What tests are acceptable for use in forensic evaluations? A survey of experts. *Professional Psychology: Research and Practice, 26,* 54–60. (**II/III**)

Lampel, A. K. (1999). Use of the Millon Clinical Multiaxial Inventory-III in evaluating child custody litigants. *American Journal of Forensic Psychology, 17,* 19–31. (**III**)

Langevin, R., Lang, R., Reynolds, R., Wright, P., Garrels, D., Marchese, V., et al. (1988). Personality and sexual anomalies: An examination of the Millon Clinical Multiaxial Inventory. *Annals of Sex Research, 1,* 13–32.

Langevin, R., Paitich, D., Freeman, R., Mann, K., & Handy, L. (1979). Personality characteristics and sexual anomalies in males. *Canadian Journal of Behavioral Science, 10,* 222–238.

Lapan, R., & Patton, M. J. (1986). Self psychology and the adolescent process: Measures of pseudoautonomy and peer group dependence. *Journal of Counseling Psychology, 33,* 136–142.

Lazowski, L. E., Miller, F. G., Boyc, M. W., & Miller, G. A. (1998). Efficacy of the Substance Abuse Subtle Screening Inventory-3 (SASSI-3) in identifying substance dependence disorders in clinical settings. *Journal of Personality Assessment, 71,* 114–128. **(II)**

Leaf, R. C., Alington, D. E., Mass, R., DiGiuseppe, R., & Ellis, A. (1991). Personality disorders, life events, and clinical syndromes. *Journal of Personality Disorders, 5,* 264–280.

Leaf, R. C., Alington, D. E., Ellis, A., DiGiuseppe, R., & Mass, R. (1992). Personality disorders, underlying traits, social problems, and clinical syndromes. *Journal of Personality Disorders, 6,* 134–152.

Leaf, R. C., DiGiuseppe, R., Ellis, A., Mass, R., BackX, W., Wolf, J., et al. (1990). "Healthy" correlates of MCMI scales 4, 5, 6, and 7. *Journal of Personality Disorders, 4,* 312–328.

Leaf, R. C., Ellis, A., DiGiuseppe, R., & Mass, R. (1991). Rationality, self-regard and the "healthiness" of personality disorders. *Journal of Rational Emotive and Cognitive Behavior Therapy, 9,* 3–37.

Lecic-Tosevski, D., Gavrilovic, J., Knezevic, G., & Priebe, S. (2003). Personality factors and posttraumatic stress: Associations in civilians one year after air attacks. *Journal of Personality Disorders, 17,* 537–549.

Lees-Haley, P. R. (1992). Efficacy of MMPI-2 validity scales and MCMI-II modifier scales for detecting spurious PTSD claims: F, F-K, Fake Bad scale, Ego Strength, Subtle-Obvious subscales, D. I. S., & DEB. *Journal of Clinical Psychology, 48,* 681–688. **(II)**

Lemkau, J. P., Purdy, R. R., Rafferty, J. P., & Rudisill, J. R. (1988). Correlates of burnout among family practice residents. *Journal of Medical Education, 63,* 682–691.

Lenzenweger, M. F. (1999). Stability and change in personality disorder features. *Archives of General Psychiatry, 56,* 1009–1018. **(III)**

Leroux, M. D., Vincent, K. R., McPherson, R. H., & Williams, W. (1990). Construct validity of the Diagnostic Inventory of Personality and symptoms: External correlates. *Journal of Clinical Psychology, 46,* 285–291.

Lesswing, N. J., & Dougherty, R. J. (1993). Psychopathology and alcohol-and-cocaine-dependent patients: A comparison of findings from psychological testing. *Journal of Substance Abuse Treatment, 10,* 53–57.

Levine, J. B., Tischer, P., Antoni, M., Green, C., & Millon, T. (1985). Refining personality assessments by combining MCMI high point profiles and MMPI codes. Part, I. I. MMPI code 27/72. *Journal of Personality Assessment, 49,* 501–507.

Levine, S. B., Althof, S. E., & Risen, C. B. (1999). The sexual struggles of 23 clergymen: A follow-up study. *Journal of Sex and Marital Therapy, 25,* 183–195. **(III)**

Lewis, S. J., & Harder, D. W. (1990). Factor structure of the MCMI among personality disordered outpatients and in other populations. *Journal of Clinical Psychology, 46,* 613–617.

Lewis, S. J., & Harder, D. W. (1991). A comparison of four measures to diagnose *DSM-III-R* borderline personality disorder in outpatients. *Journal of Nervous and Mental Diseases, 179,* 320–337.

Libb, J. W., Murray, J., Thurstin, H., & Alarcon, R. D. (1992). Concordance of the MCMI-II, the MMPI, and Axis I discharge diagnosis in psychiatric inpatients. *Journal of Personality Assessment, 58,* 580–590. **(II)**

Libb, J. W., Stankovic, S., Freeman, A., Sokol, R., Switzer, P., & Houck, C. (1990). Personality disorders among depressed outpatients as identified by the MCMI. *Journal of Clinical Psychology, 46,* 277–284.

Libb, J. W., Stankovic, S., Sokol, A., Houck, C., & Switzer, P. (1990). Stability of the MCMI among depressed psychiatric outpatients. *Journal of Personality Assessment, 55,* 209–218.

Lindsay, K. A., Sankis, L. M., & Widiger, T. A. (2000). Gender bias in self-report personality disorder inventories. *Journal of Personality Disorders, 14,* 218–232. **(III)**

Lindsay, K. A., & Widiger, T. A. (1995). Sex and gender bias in self-report personality disorder inventories: Item analysis of the MCMI-II, MMPI, and PDQ.-R. *Journal of Personality Assessment, 65,* 1–20.

Litman, L. C., & Cernovsky, Z. Z. (1993). An MCMI-II taxonomy of substance abusers. *Research Communications in Psychology, Psychiatry and Behavior, 18,* 67–72.

Livesley, W. J., West, M., & Tanney, A. (1985). Historical comment on *DSM-III* schizoid and avoidant personality disorders. *American Journal of Psychiatry, 142,* 1344–1347.

Llorente, M. D., Currier, M. B., & Norman, S. E. (1992). Night terrors in adults: Phenomenology and relationship to psychopathology. *Journal of Clinical Psychiatry, 53,* 392–394. **(II)**

Locke, K. D. (2000). Circumplex scales of interpersonal values: Reliability, validity, and applicability to interpersonal problems and personality disorders. *Journal of Personality Assessment, 75,* 244–267.

Lohr, J. M., Hamberger, L. K., & Bonge, D. (1988). The nature of irrational beliefs in different personality clusters of spouse abusers. *Journal of Rational-Emotive and Cognitive Behavior Therapy, 6,* 273–285.

Lorr, M., Retzlaff, P. D., & Tarr, H. C. (1989). An analysis of the MCMI-1 at the item level. *Journal of Clinical Psychology, 45,* 884–890.

Lorr, M., & Strack, S. (1990). Profile clusters of the MCMI-II personality disorder scales. *Journal of Clinical Psychology, 46,* 606–612. **(II)**

Lorr, M., Strack, S., Campbell, L., & Lamnin, A. (1990). Personality and symptom dimensions of the MCMI-II: An item factor analysis. *Journal of Clinical Psychology, 46,* 749–754. **(II)**

Lundholm, J. K. (1989). Alcohol use among university females: Relationship to eating disordered behavior. *Addictive Behaviors, 14,* 181–185.

Lundholm, J. K., Pelegreno, D. D., Wolins, L., & Graham, S. L. (1989). Predicting eating disorders in women: A preliminary measurement study. *Measurement and Evaluation in Counseling and Development, 22,* 23–30.

Luty, D., & Thackery, M. (1993). Graphomotor interpretation of the MMPI-2. *Journal of Personality Assessment, 60,* 604. (**II**)

Maddi, S. R., Khoshaba, D. M., Perisco, M., Lu, J., Harvey, R., & Bleecker, F. (2002). The personality construct of hardiness II: Relationships with comprehensive tests of personality and psychopathology. *Journal of Research in Personality, 36,* 72–85. (**III**)

Malec, J. F., Romsaas, E., & Trump, D. (1985). Psychological and personality disturbance among patients with testicular cancer. *Journal of Psychosocial Oncology, 3,* 55–64.

Malec, J., Wolberg, W., Romsaas, E., Trump, D., & Turner, M. (1988). Millon Clinical Multiaxial Inventory (MCMI) findings among breast clinic patients after initial evaluation and at 4- or-8 month follow-up. *Journal of Clinical Psychology, 44,* 175–180.

Mannis, M. J., Morrison, T. L., Holland, E. J., & Krachmer, J. H. (1987). Personality trends in keratoconus: An analysis. *Archives of Opthamology, 105,* 798–800.

Marlowe, D. B., Husband, S. D., Bonieskie, L. M., Kirby, K. C., & Platt, J. J. (1997). Structured interview versus self-report test vantages for the assessment of personality pathology in cocaine dependence. *Journal of Personality Disorders, 11,* 177–190. (**II**)

Marlowe, D. B., Festinger, D. S., Kirby, K. C., Rubenstein, D. F., & Platt, J. J. (1998). Congruence of the MCMI-II and MCMI-III in cocaine dependence. *Journal of Personality Assessment, 71,* 15–28. (**II/III**)

Marlowe, D. B., & Wetzler, S. (1994). Contributions of discriminant analysis to differential diagnosis by self-report. *Journal of Personality Assessment, 62,* 320–331.

Marsh, D. T., Stile, S. A., Stoughton, N. L., & Trout-Landen, B. L. (1988). Psychopathology among opiate addiction: Comparative data from the MMPI and MCMI. *American Journal of Drug and Alcohol Abuse, 14,* 17–27.

Marshall, M., Helmes, E., & Deathe, A. (1992). A comparison of psychosocial functioning and personality in amputee and chronic pain populations. *The Clinical Journal of Pain, 8,* 351–357.

Matano, R. A., & Locke, K. D. (1995). Personality disorder scales as predictors of interpersonal problems of alcoholics. *Journal of Personality Disorders, 9,* 62–67.

Matano, R. A., Locke, K. D., & Schwartz, K. (1994). MCMI personality subtypes for male and female alcoholics. *Journal of Personality Assessment, 63,* 250–264.

May, B., & Bos, J. (2000). Personality characteristics of ADHD adults assessed with the Millon Clinical Personality Inventory-II: Evidence of four distinct subtypes. *Journal of Personality Assessment, 75,* 237–246. (**II**)

Mayer, G. S., & Scott, K. J. (1988). An exploration of heterogeneity in an inpatient male alcoholic population. *Journal of Personality Disorders, 2,* 243–255.

McAllister, H. A., Baker, J. D., Mannes, C., Stewart, H., & Sutherland, A. (2002). The optimal margin of illusion hypothesis: Evidence from the self-serving bias and personality disorders. *Journal of Social and Clinical Psychology, 21,* 414–426. (**II**)

McCann, J. T. (1989). MMPI personality disorder scales and the MCMI: Concurrent validity. *Journal of Clinical Psychology, 45,* 365–369.

McCann, J. T. (1990a). A multitrait-multimethod analysis of the MCMI-II clinical syndrome scales. *Journal of Personality Assessment, 55,* 465–476. (**II**)

McCann, J. T. (1990b). Bias and Millon Clinical Multiaxial Inventory (MCMI-II) diagnosis. *Journal of Psychopathology and Behavioral Assessment, 12,* 17–26. **(II)**

McCann, J. T. (1991). Convergent and discriminant validity of the MCMI-II and MMPI personality disorder scales. *Psychological Assessment: A Journal of Consulting and Clinical Psychology, 3,* 9–18. **(II)**

McCann, J. T. (1992). A comparison of two measures for obsessive-compulsive personality disorder. *Journal of Personality Disorders, 6,* 18–23. **(II)**

McCann, J. T. (2002). Guidelines for forensic application of the MCMI-III. *Journal of Forensic Psychology Practice, 2,* 55–69. **(III)**

McCann, J. T., Flens, J. R., Campagna, V., Collman, P., Lazarro, T., & Connor, E. (2001). The MCMI-III in child custody evaluations: A normative study. *Journal of Forensic Psychology Practice, 1,* 27–44. **(III)**

McCann, J. T., Flynn, P. M., & Gersh, D. M. (1992). MCMI-II diagnosis of borderline personality disorders: Base rates versus prototypic items. *Journal of Personality Assessment, 58,* 105–114. **(II)**

McCann, J. T., & Gergelis, R. E. (1990). Utility of the MCMI-II in assessing suicide risk. *Journal of Clinical Psychology, 46,* 764–770. **(II)**

McCann, J. T., & Suess, J. (1988). Clinical applications of the MCMI: The 1-2-3-8 code type. *Journal of Clinical Psychology, 44,* 181–191.

McConnaughy, E. A., DiClemente, C. C., Prochaska, J. O., & Velicer, W. F. (1989). Stages of change in psychotherapy: A followup report. *Psychotherapy, 26,* 494–503.

McCormack, J. K., Barnett, R. W., & Wallbrown, F. H. (1989). Factor structure of the Millon Clinical Multiaxial Inventory with an offender sample. *Journal of Personality Assessment, 53,* 442–448.

McCormick, R. A., Taber, J. I., & Kruedelback, N. (1989). The relationship between attributional style and post-traumatic stress disorder in addicted patients. *Journal of Traumatic Stress, 2,* 477–487.

McCrae, R. R. (1991). The five factor model and its assessment in clinical settings. *Journal of Personality Assessment, 57,* 399–414.

McCray, J. A., & King, A. R. (2003). Personality disorder attributes as supplemental goals for change in interpersonal psychotherapy. *Journal of Contemporary Psychotherapy, 33,* 79–92.

McKee, G. R., & Klohn, L. S. (1994). MCMI profiles of pretrial defendants. *Psychological Reports, 74,* 1346.

McMahon, R. C. (2001). Personality, stress, and social support in cocaine relapse prediction. *Journal of Substance Abuse Treatment, 21,* 77–87. **(II)**

McMahon, R. C., & Davidson, R. S. (1985a). An examination of the relationship between personality patterns and symptom/mood patterns. *Journal of Personality Assessment, 49,* 552–556.

McMahon, R. C., & Davidson, R. S. (1985b). Transient versus enduring depression among alcoholics in inpatient treatment. *Journal of Psychopathology and Behavioral Assessment, 7,* 317–328.

McMahon, R. C., & Davidson, R. S. (1986a). An examination of depressed and non-depressed alcoholics in inpatient treatment. *Journal of Clinical Psychology, 42,* 177–184.

McMahon, R. C., & Davidson, R. S. (1986b). Concurrent validity of the clinical symptom syndrome scales of the Millon Clinical Multiaxial Inventory. *Journal of Clinical Psychology, 42,* 908–912.

McMahon, R. C., Davidson, R. S., Gersh, D., & Flynn, P. (1991). A comparison of continuous and episodic drinkers using the MCMI, MMPI, and Alceval-R. *Journal of Clinical Psychology, 47,* 148–159.

McMahon, R. C., Davidson, R. S., & Flynn, P. M. (1986). Psychological correlates and treatment outcomes for high and low social functioning alcoholics. *International Journal of the Addictions, 21,* 819–835.

McMahon, R. C., Davidson, R. S., Flynn, P., & Gersh, D. (1991). A comparison of continuous and episodic drinkers using the MCMI. *Journal of Clinical Psychology, 47,* 148–159.

McMahon, R. C., Flynn, P. M., & Davidson, R. S. (1985a). Stability of the personality and symptom scales of the Millon Clinical Multiaxial Inventory. *Journal of Personality Assessment, 49,* 231–234.

McMahon, R. C., Flynn, P. M., & Davidson, R. S. (1985b). The personality and symptom scales of the Millon Clinical Multiaxial Inventory: Sensitivity to posttreatment outcomes. *Journal of Clinical Psychology, 41,* 862–866.

McMahon, R. C., Gersh, D., & Davidson, R. S. (1989). Personality and symptom characteristics of continuous vs. episodic drinkers. *Journal of Clinical Psychology, 45,* 161–168.

McMahon, R. C., Kelley, A., & Kouzakanani, K. (1993). Personality and coping styles in the prediction of dropout from treatment of cocaine abuse. *Journal of Personality Assessment, 61,* 147–155. **(II)**

McMahon, R. C., Malow, R. M., & Penedo, F. J. (1998). Substance abuse problems, psychiatric severity, and HIV risk in Millon Clinical Multiaxial Inventory-II personality subgroups. *Psychology of Addictive Behaviors, 12,* 3–13.

McMahon, R. C., & Richards, S. K. (1996). Profile patterns, consistency, and change in the Millon Clinical Multiaxial Inventory-II in cocaine abusers. *Journal of Clinical Psychology, 52,* 75–79. **(II)**

McMahon, R. C., Schram, L. L., & Davidson, R. S. (1993). Negative life events, social support, and depression in three personality types. *Journal of Personality Disorders, 7,* 241–254.

McMahon, R. C., & Tyson, D. (1990). Personality factors in transient versus enduring depression among inpatient alcoholic women: A preliminary analysis. *Journal of Personality Disorders, 4,* 150–160.

McNeil, K., & Meyer, R. G. (1990). Detection of deception on the Millon Clinical Multiaxial Inventory (MCMI). *Journal of Clinical Psychology, 46,* 755–764.

Medalia, A., Merriam, A., & Sandberg, M. (1989). Neuropsychological deficits in choreoacanthosytosis. *Archives of Neurology, 46,* 573–575.

Meehan, J. C., Holtzworth-Munroe, A., & Herron, K. (2001). Maritally violent men's heart rate reactivity to marital interactions: A failure to replicate the Gottman et al. (1995). Typology. *Journal of Family Psychology, 15,* 394–408. **(III)**

Messina, N., Wish, E., Hoffman, J., & Nemes, S. (2001). Diagnosing antisocial personality disorder among substance abusers: The SCID versus the MCMI-II. *American Journal of Drug and Alcohol Abuse, 27,* 699–2001. **(II)**

Messina, N., Wish, E., Hoffman, J., & Nemes, S. (2002). Antisocial personality disorder and TC treatment outcomes. *American Journal of Drug and Alcohol Abuse, 28,* 197–212. (**II**)

Meyer, G., Riethmiller, R. J., Brooks, R. D., Benoit, W. A., & Handler, L. (2000). A replication of Rorschach and MMPI-2 convergent validity. *Journal of Personality Assessment, 74,* 175–215. (**II**)

Meyer, M. H. (1985). A new look at mothers of incest victims. *Journal of Social Work and Human Sexuality, 3,* 47–58.

Michalek, J. E., Barrett, D. H., Morris, R. D., Jackson, W. G., & Stat, M. (2003). Serum dioxin and psychological functioning in U.S. Air Force veterans of the Vietnam war. *Military Medicine, 168,* 153–159.

Michel, D. M. (2002). Psychological assessment as a therapeutic intervention in patients hospitalized with eating disorders. *Professional Psychology: Research and Practice, 33,* 470–477. (**III**)

Miller, T. W., Martin, W., & Spiro, K. (1991). Traumatic stress disorder: Diagnostic and clinical issues in former prisoners of war. *Comprehensive Psychiatry, 30,* 139–148.

Miller, H. R., Goldberg, J. O., & Streiner, D. L. (1993). The effects of the modifier and correction indices on MCMI-II profiles. *Journal of Personality Assessment, 60,* 477–485. (**II**)

Miller, H. R., & Streiner, D. L. (1990). Using the Millon Clinical Multiaxial Inventory's Scale, B., & the MacAndrew's Alcoholism Scale to identify alcoholics with concurrent psychiatric diagnosis. *Journal of Personality Assessment, 54,* 736–746.

Miller, H. R., Streiner, D. L., & Parkinson, A. (1992). Maximum likelihood estimates of the ability of the MMPI and MCMI personality disorder scales and the SIDP to identify personality disorders. *Journal of Personality Assessment, 59,* 1–13.

Millon, C., Salvato, F., Blaney, N., Morgan, R., Mantero-Atienza, E., Klimas, N., et al. (1989). A psychological assessment of chronic fatigue syndrome/chronic Epstein-Barr virus patients. *Psychology and Health, 3,* 131–141.

Millon, T. (1984). On the renaissance of personality assessment and personality theory. *Journal of Personality Assessment, 48,* 450–466.

Millon, T. (1985a). The MCMI provides a good assessment of *DSM-III* disorders: The MCMI-II will prove even better. *Journal of Personality Assessment, 49,* 379–391.

Millon, T. (1985b). Response to Greer's review of the MCMI. *Journal of Counseling and Development, 63,* 631–632.

Millon, T. (1986c). The MCMI and *DSM-III:* Further commentaries. *Journal of Personality Assessment, 50,* 205–207.

Millon, T. (1988). Personologic psychotherapy: 10 commandments for a post eclectic approach to integrative treatment. *Psychotherapy, 25,* 209–219. (**II**)

Millon, T. (1992a). An appreciative rejoiner. *Journal of Counseling and Development, 70,* 432–433. (**II**)

Millon, T. (1992b). Tests and assessments: Millon Clinical Multiaxial Inventory I & II. *Journal of Counseling and Development, 70,* 421–426. (**II**)

Millon, T., & Davis, R. D. (1997). The MCMI-III. Present and future directions. *Journal of Personality Assessment, 68,* 69–85.

Montag, I., & Comrey, A. L. (1987). Millon MCMI scales factor analyzed and correlated with MMPI and CPS scales. *Multivariate Behavioral Research, 22,* 401–413.

Moravic, J. D., & Munley, P. H. (1983). Psychological test findings on the pathological gamblers in treatment. *International Journal of the Addictions, 18,* 1003–1009.

Moreland, K. L. (1985). Scoring of the MCMI: Effects on utility—Further response to Greer. *Journal of Counseling and Development, 63,* 632.

Moreland, K. L., & Godfrey, J. O. (1989). Yes, our study could have been better: Reply to Cash, Mikulka, and Brown. *Journal of Consulting and Clinical Psychology, 57,* 313–314.

Moreland, K. L., & Onstad, J. (1987). Validity of Millon's computerized interpretation system for the MCMI: A controlled study. *Journal of Consulting and Clinical Psychology, 55,* 113–114.

Morey, L. C. (1985). An empirical approach of interpersonal and *DSM-III* approaches to classification of personality disorders. *Psychiatry, 48,* 358–364.

Morey, L. C. (1986). A comparison of three personality disorder assessment approaches. *Journal of Psychopathology and Behavior Assessment, 8,* 25–30.

Morey, L. C. (1988). Personality disorders in *DSM-III* and *DSM-III-R:* Convergence, coverage, and internal consistency. *American Journal of Psychiatry, 145,* 573–577.

Morey, L. C., & Levine, D. J. (1988). A multitrait-multimethod examination of Minnesota Multiphasic Personality Inventory (MMPI) and Millon Clinical Multiaxial Inventory (MCMI). *Journal of Psychopathology and Behavioral Assessment, 10,* 333–344.

Morgan, C. D., Schoenberg, M. R., Dorr, D., & Burke, M. J. (2002). Overreport on the MCMI-III: Concurrent validation with the MMPI-2 using a psychiatric inpatient sample. *Journal of Personality Assessment, 78,* 288–300. (**III**)

Mullins, L. S., & Kopelman, R. E. (1988). Toward an assessment of the construct validity of 4 measures of narcissism. *Journal of Personality Assessment, 52,* 610–625.

Munley, P. H., Bains, D. S., Bloem, W. D., Busby, R. M., & Pendziszewski, S. (1995). Posttraumatic stress disorder and the MCMI-II. *Psychological Reports, 76,* 939–944. (**II**)

Munley, P. H., Bains, D. S., Frazee, J., & Schwartz, L. T. (1994). Inpatient PTSD treatment: A study of pretreatment measures, treatment dropout, and therapist ratings of response to treatment. *Journal of Traumatic Stress, 7,* 319–325.

Munley, P. H., Vacha-Haase, T., Busby, R. M., & Paul, B. D. (1998). The MCMI-II and race. *Journal of Personality Assessment, 70,* 183–189. (**II**)

Muran, E. M., & Motta, R. W. (1993). Cognitive distortion and irrational beliefs in Post-Traumatic stress, anxiety, and depressive disorders. *Journal of Clinical Psychology, 49,* 166–176. (**II**)

Muran, J. C., Segal, Z. V., Samstag, L. W., & Crawfrod, C. E. (1994). Patient pre-treatment interpersonal problems and therapeutic alliance in short-term cognitive therapy. *Journal of Consulting and Clinical Psychology, 62,* 185–190.

Murphy, C. M., Meyer, S. L., & O'Leary, K. D. (1993). Family of origin violence and MCMI-II psychopathology among partner assaultive men. *Violence and Victims, 8,* 165–176. **(II)**

Murphy, T. J., Greenblatt, R. L., Modzierz, G. J., & Trimakas, K. A. (1991). Stability of the Millon Clinical Multiaxial Inventory among psychiatric inpatients. *Journal of Psychopathology and Behavioral Assessment, 12,* 143–150.

Nadeau, L., Landry, M., & Racine, S. (1999). Prevalence of personality disorders among clients in treatment for addiction. *Canadian Journal of Psychiatry, 44,* 592–596.

Nelson-Gray, R. O., Johnson, D., Foyle, L. W., Daniel, S. C., & Harmon, R. (1996). The effectiveness of cognitive therapy tailored to depressives with personality disorders. *Journal of Personality Disorders, 10,* 132–152.

Norman, D., Blais, M. A., & Herzog, D. (1993). Personality characteristics of eating-disordered patients as identified by the Millon Clinical Multiaxial Inventory. *Journal of Personality Disorders, 7,* 1–9.

O'Connor, B. P. (2002). The search for dimensional structure differences between normality and abnormality: A statistical review of published data on personality and psychopathology. *Journal of Personality and Psychopathology, 83,* 962–982. (all).

O'Connor, B. P., & Dyce, J. A. (2001). Rigid and extreme: A geometric representation of personality disorders in five-factor model space. *Journal of Personality and Social Psychology, 81,* 1119–1130. **(III)**

Osuch, E. A., Noll, J. G., & Putnam, F. W. (1999). The motivators for self-injury in psychiatric inpatients. *Psychiatry, 62,* 334–336. **(II)**

Organista, P. B., & Miranda, J. (1991). Psychosomatic symptoms in medical outpatients: An investigation of self-handicapping theory. *Health Psychology, 10,* 427–431.

Oronato, V. A. (1987). The conditioned neurologic syndrome. *International Journal of Clinical Neuropsychology, 9,* 125–131.

Overholser, J. C. (1990). Retest reliability of the Millon Clinical Multiaxial Inventory. *Journal of Personality Assessment, 55,* 202–208.

Overholser, J. C. (1991). Categorical assessment of the dependent personality disorder in depressed inpatients. *Journal of Personality Disorders, 5,* 243–255.

Overholser, J. C. (1992). Aggregation of personality measures: Implications for personality research. *Journal of Personality Disorders, 6,* 267–277.

Overholser, J. C., & Freiheit, S. R. (1994). Assessment of interpersonal dependency using the Millon Clinical Multiaxial Inventory-II (MCMI-II) and the Depressive Experiences Questionnaire. *Psychology of Individual Differences, 17,* 71–78. **(II)**

Overholser, J. C., Kabakoff, R., & Norman, W. H. (1989). The assessment of personality characteristics in depressed and dependent psychiatric inpatients. *Journal of Personality Assessment, 53,* 40–50.

Ownby, R. L., Wallbrown, F. H., Carmin, C. N., & Barnett, R. W. (1990). A combined factor analysis of the Millon Clinical Multiaxial Inventory and the MMPI in an offender population. *Journal of Clinical Psychology, 46,* 89–96.

Palacios, W. R., Urmann, C. F., Newel, R., & Hamilton, N. (1999). Developing a sociological framework for dually diagnosed women. *Journal of Substance Abuse Treatment, 17,* 91–102. **(II)**

Papciak, A. S., & Fuererstein, M. (1991). Psychological factors affecting isoki netic trunk strength testing in patients with work-related chronic low back pain. *Journal of Occupational Rehabilitation, 1,* 95–104. **(II)**

Parry, B. L., Ehlers, C. L., Mostofi, N., & Phillips, E. (1996). Personality traits in LLPDD and normal controls during follicular and luteal menstrual-cycle phases. *Psychological Medicine, 26,* 197–202.

Patrick, J. (1988). Concordance of the MCMI and the MMPI in the diagnosis of three *DSM-III* Axis I disorders. *Journal of Clinical Psychology, 44,* 186–190.

Patrick, J. (1993). Validation of the MCMI-1 borderline personality disorder scale with a well-defined criterion sample. *Journal of Clinical Psychology, 49,* 29–32.

Petrocelli, J. V., Glaser, B. A., Calhoun, G. B., & Campbell, L. F. (2001). Personality and affect characteristics of outpatients with depression. *Journal of Personality Assessment, 77,* 162–175. **(II)**

Petrocelli, J. V., Glaser, B. A., Calhoun, G. B., & Campbell, L. F. (2001). Early maladaptive schemes of personality disorder subtypes. *Journal of Personality Disorders, 15,* 546–559.

Pertrovic, M., Vandierendonck, A., Mariman, A., van Maele, G., Afschrift, M., & Pevernagie, D. (2002). Personality traits and socio-epidemiological status of hospitalized elderly benzodiazepine users. *International Journal of Geriatric Psychiatry, 17,* 733–738.

Pettem, O., West, M., Mahoney, A., & Keller, A. (1993). Depression and attachment problems. *Journal of Psychiatric Neuroscience, 18,* 78–81.

Petzel, T. P., & Rado, E. D. (1990). Divergent validity evidence for Eckblad and Chapman's Hypomanic Personality Scale. *Journal of Clinical Psychology, 46,* 43–46.

Piersma, H. L. (1986a). The factor structure of the Millon Clinical Multiaxial Inventory for psychiatric inpatients. *Journal of Personality Assessment, 50,* 578–584.

Piersma, H. L. (1986b). The Millon Clinical Multiaxial Inventory (MCMI) as a treatment outcome measure for psychiatric inpatients. *Journal of Clinical Psychology, 42,* 493–499.

Piersma, H. L. (1986c). The stability of the Millon Clinical Multiaxial Inventory for psychiatric inpatients. *Journal of Personality Assessment, 50,* 193–197.

Piersma, H. L. (1987a). MCMI computer generated diagnosis How do they compare to clinical judgment? *Journal of Psychopathology and Behavior Assessment, 9,* 305–312.

Piersma, H. L. (1987b). The MCMI as a measure of *DSM-III* Axis II diagnosis: An empirical comparison. *Journal of Clinical Psychology, 43,* 478–483.

Piersma, H. L. (1987c). The use of the Millon Clinical Multiaxial Inventory in the evaluation of seminary students. *Journal of Psychology and Theology, 15,* 227–233.

Piersma, H. L. (1989a). The MCMI-II as a treatment outcome measure for psychiatric inpatients. *Journal of Clinical Psychology, 45,* 87–93. (**II**)

Piersma, H. L. (1989b). The stability of the MCMI-II for psychiatric inpatients. *Journal of Clinical Psychology, 45,* 781–785. (**II**)

Piersma, H. L. (1991). The MCMI-II depression scales: Do they assist in the differential prediction of depressive disorders? *Journal of Personality Assessment, 56,* 478–486. (**II**)

Piersma, H. L., & Boes, J. L. (1997). MCMI-III as a treatment outcome measure for psychiatric inpatients. *Journal of Clinical Psychology, 53,* 825–831. (**III**)

Piersma, H. L., Ohnishi, H., Lee, J., & Metcalfe, W. E. (2002). An empirical evaluation of Millon's dimensional polarities. *Journal of Psychopathology and Behavioral Assessment, 24,* 151–158. (**III**)

Piersma, H. L., & Smith, A. Y. (1991). Individual variability in self-reported improvement for depressed psychiatric inpatients on the MCMI-II. *Journal of Clinical Psychology, 47,* 227–232. (**II**)

Piersma, H. L., & Boes, J. L. (1997). The relationship between length of stay to MCMI-II and MCMI-III change scores. *Journal of Clinical Psychology, 53,* 535–542. (**III**)

Piersma, H. L., & Boes, J. L. (1997). Comparison of psychiatric day hospital patient and inpatient scores on the MCMI-III. *Journal of Clinical Psychology, 53,* 629–634. (**III**)

Piotrowski, C. (1997). Use of the Millon Clinical Multiaxial Inventory in clinical practice. *Perceptual and Motor Skills, 84,* 1185–1186.

Piotrowski, N. A., Trusel, D. J., Sees, K. L., Banys, P., & Hall, S. M. (1995). Psychopathy and antisocial personality in men and women with primary opiate dependence. *Issues in Criminology and Legal Psychology, 24,* 123–126. (**II?**)

Pollock, P. H. (1996). Clinical issues in the cognitive analytic therapy of sexually abused women who commit violent offenses against their partners. *British Journal of Medical Psychology, 69,* 117–127. (**II**)

Pollock, P. H., & Percy, A. (1999). Maternal antenatal attachment style and potential fetal abuse. *Child Abuse and Neglect, 23,* 1345–1357. (**II**)

Porcerelli, J. H., Cogan, R., & Hibbard, S. (1998). Cognitive and affective representations of people and MCMI-II personality pathology. *Journal of Personality Assessment, 70,* 535–540. (**II**)

Powell, R. A., & Howell, A. J. (1998). Effectiveness of treatment for dissociative identity disorder. *Psychological Reports, 83,* 483–490. (**II**)

Prifitera, A., & Ryan, J. J. (1984). Validity of the Narcissistic Personality Inventory (NPI) in a psychiatric sample. *Journal of Clinical Psychology, 40,* 140–142.

Pryor, T., Wiederman, M. W., & McGilley, B. (1995). Laxative abuse among women with eating disorders: An indication of psychopathology? *International Journal of Eating Disorders, 20,* 13–18.

Raskin, R., & Terry, H. (1988). A principal component analysis of the narcissistic personality inventory and further evidence of its construct validity. *Journal of Personality and Social Psychology, 54,* 890–902.

Rathus, J. H., Anderson, W. C., Miler, A. L., & Wetzler, S. (1995). Impact of personality functioning on cognitive behavioral treatment of panic disorder: A preliminary report. *Journal of Personality Disorders, 9,* 160–168. (**II**)

Rebillot, J. (1985). Scoring of the MCMI: Effects on utility. *Journal of Counseling and Development, 63,* 631.

Reich, J. (1987a). Prevalence of *DSM-III-R* self-defeating (masochistic) personality disorder in normal and outpatient populations. *Journal of Nervous and Mental Diseases, 175,* 52–54.

Reich, J. (1987b). Sex distribution of *DSM-III* personality disorders in psychiatric outpatients. *American Journal of Psychiatry, 144,* 485–488.

Reich, J. (1988). *DSM-III* personality disorders and the family history of mental illness. *Journal of Nervous and Mental Diseases, 176,* 45–49.

Reich, J. (1991). The effect of personality on placebo response in panic patients. *Journal of Nervous and Mental Diseases, 178,* 699–702.

Reich, J. H., & Noyes, R. (1987). A comparison of *DSM-III* personality disorders in acutely ill panic and depressed patients. *Journal of Anxiety Disorders, 1,* 123–131.

Reich, J. H., Noyes, R., & Troughton, E. (1987). Dependent personality disorder associated with phobic avoidance in patients with panic disorder. *American Journal of Psychiatry, 144,* 323–326.

Reich, J. H., Noyes, R., & Troughton, E. (1988). Frequency of *DSM-III* personality disorders in patients with panic disorder: Comparison with psychiatric and normal control subjects. *Psychiatry Research, 26,* 89–100.

Reich, J. H., & Troughton, E. (1988). Comparison of *DSM-III* personality disorders in recovered depressed and panic disorder patients. *Journal of Nervous and Mental Diseases, 176,* 300–304.

Renneberg, B., Chambless, D. L., Dowdall, D. J., Fauerbach, J. A., & Gracely, E. J. (1992). The Structured Clinical Interview for *DSM-III-R,* Axis-II and the Millon Clinical Multiaxial Inventory: A concurrent validity study of personality disorders among anxious patients. *Journal of Personality Disorders, 6,* 117–124. (**II**)

Repko, G. R., & Cooper, R. (1985). The diagnosis of personality disorder: A comparison of MMPI profile, Millon inventory, and clinical judgment in a Worker's Compensation population. *Journal of Clinical Psychology, 41,* 867–881.

Retzlaff, P. D. (1996). MCMI-III diagnostic validity: Bad test or bad validity study. *Journal of Personality Assessment, 66,* 431–437. (**III**).

Retzlaff, P. D. (2000). Comment on the validity of the MCMI-III. *Law and Human Behavior, 24,* 499–500. (**III**)

Retzlaff, P. D., & Bromley, S. (1991). A multi-test alcoholic taxonomy: Canonical coefficient clusters. *Journal of Clinical Psychology, 47,* 299–309.

Retzlaff, P., & Cicerello, A. (1995). Compensation and pension evaluations: Psychotic, neurotic, and post-traumatic stress disorder. *Military Medicine, 160,* 493–496. (**II**)

Retzlaff, P., & Deatherage, T. (1993). Air Force mental health consultation: A six-year retention follow-up. *Military Medicine, 158,* 338–340.

Retzlaff, P. D., & Gibertini, M. (1987a). Air Force pilot personality: Hard data on "The Right Stuff." *Multivariate Behavioral Research, 22,* 383–399.

Retzlaff, P. D., & Gibertini, M. (1987b). Factor structure of the MCMI basic personality scales and common-item artifact. *Journal of Personality Assessment, 51,* 588–594.

Retzlaff, P. D., & Gibertini, M. (1988, July). Objective psychological testing of U.S. Air Force officers in pilot training. *Aviation, Space, and Environmental Medicine,* 661–663.

Retzlaff, P. D., & Gibertini, M. (1990a). Active-duty and veteran alcoholics: Differences in psychopathology presentation. *Military Medicine, 155,* 334–336.

Retzlaff, P. D., & Gibertini, M. (1990b). Factor-based special scales for the MCMI. *Journal of Clinical Psychology, 46,* 47–52.

Retzlaff, P. D., Lorr, M., Hyer, L., & Ofman, P. (1991). An MCMI-II item-level component analysis: Personality and clinical factors. *Journal of Personality Assessment, 57,* 323–334. **(II)**

Retzlaff, P. D., Ofman, P., Hyer, L., & Matheson, S. (1994). MCMI-II high-point codes: Severe personality disorder and clinical syndrome extensions. *Journal of Clinical Psychology, 50,* 228–234. **(II)**

Retzlaff, P. D., Sheehan, E. P., & Fiel, A. (1991). MCMI-II report style and bias: Profile and validity scales analyses. *Journal of Personality Assessment, 56,* 466–477. **(II)**

Retzlaff, P. D., Sheehan, E. P., & Lorr, M. (1990). MCMI-II scoring: Weighted and unweighted algorithms. *Journal of Personality Assessment, 55,* 219–223. **(II)**

Retzlaff, P., Stoner, J., & Kleinasser, D. (2002). The use of the MCMI-III in the screening and triage of offenders. *International Journal of Offender Therapy and Comparative Criminology, 46,* 319–332. **(III)**

Richman, H., & Nelson-Gray, R. (1994). Nonclinical panicker personality: Profile and discriminative ability. *Journal of Anxiety Disorders, 8,* 33–47.

Robbins, S. B. (1989). Validity of the Superiority and Goal Instability scales as measures of defects in the self. *Journal of Personality Assessment, 53,* 122–132.

Robbins, S. B., & Patton, M. J. (1985). Self psychology and career development: Construction of the superiority and goal instability scales. *Journal of Counseling and Development, 32,* 221–231.

Robbins, S. B., & Patton, M. J. (1986). Procedures for construction of scales for rating counselor outcomes. *Measurement and Evaluation in Counseling and Development, 19,* 131–140.

Robert, J. A., Ryan, J. J., McEntyre, W. L., McFarland, R. S., Lips, O. J., & Rosenberg, S. J. (1985). MCMI characteristics of *DSM-III* posttraumatic stress disorder in Vietnam veterans. *Journal of Personality Assessment, 49,* 226–230.

Roehling-P. V., & Gaumond, E. (1996). Reliability and validity of the codependent questionnaire. *Alcoholism Treatment Quarterly, 14,* 85–95.

Rogers, R. (2003). Forensic use and abuse of psychological tests: Multiscale inventories. *Journal of Psychiatric Practice, 9,* 316–320. **(III)**

Rogers, R., Salekin, R. T., & Sewell, K. W. (1999). Validation of the Millon Clinical Multiaxial Inventory for Axis II disorders: Does it meet the Daubert standard? *Law and Human Behavior, 23,* 425–443.

Rogers, R., Salekin, R. T., & Sewell, K. W. (2000). The MCMI-III and the. *Daubert* standard: Separating rhetoric from reality. *Law and Human Behavior, 24,* 501–506. (**III**)

Ronningstam, E. (1996). Pathological narcissism and narcissistic personality disorder in Axis I disorders. *Harvard Review of Psychiatry, 3,* 326–340. (**I/II**)

Rossi, G., Hauben, C., Van den Brande, I., & Sloore, H. (2003). Empirical evaluation of the MCMI-III personality disorder scales. *Psychological Reports, 92,* 627–642. (**III**)

Rossi, G., Van den Brande, I., Tobac, A., Sloore, H., & Hauben, C. (2003). Convergent validity of the MCMI-III personality disorder scales and the MMPI-2 scales. *Journal of Personality Disorders, 17,* 330–340. (**III**)

Rubino, I. A., Saya, A., & Pezzarossa, B. (1992). Percept-genetic signs of repression in histrionic personality disorder. *Perceptual and Motor Skills, 74,* 451–464. (**II**)

Rubino, I. A., Sonnino, A., Pezzarossa, B., Ciani, N., & Basi, R. (1995). Personality disorders and psychiatric symptoms in psoriasis. *Psychological Reports, 77,* 547–553. (**II**)

Rudd, M. D., Ellis, T. E., Rajab, M. H., & Wehrly, T. (2000). Personality types and suicidal behavior: An exploratory study. *Suicide and Life-Threatening Behavior, 30,* 199–212. (**II**)

Rudd, M. D., & Orman, D. T. (1996). Millon Clinical Multiaxial Inventory profiles and maladjustment in the military: Preliminary findings. *Military Medicine, 161,* 349–351.

Safran, J. D., Segal, Z. V., Vallis, T. M., Shaw, B. F., & Samstag, L. W. (1993). Assessing patient suitability for short-term cognitive therapy with an interpersonal focus. *Cognitive Therapy and Research, 17,* 23–38.

Safran, J. D., & Wallner, L. K. (1991). The relative predictive validity of two therapeutic alliance measures in cognitive therapy. *Psychological Assessment: A Journal of Consulting and Clinical Psychology, 3,* 188–195.

Sansone, R. A., Fine, M. A., Seuferer, S., & Bovenzi, J. (1989). The prevalence of borderline personality symptomotology among women with eating disorders. *Journal of Clinical Psychology, 45,* 603–610.

Sansone, R. A., & Fine, M. A. (1992). Borderline personality disorder as a predictor of outcome in women with eating disorders. *Journal of Personality Disorders, 6,* 176–186.

Saxby, E., & Peniston, E. G. (1995). Alpha-theta brainwave neurofeedback training: An effective treatment for male and female alcoholics with depressive symptoms. *Journal of Clinical Psychology, 51,* 685–693.

Schinka, J. A., & Borum, R. (1994). Readability of adult psychopathology inventories. *Psychological Assessment, 5,* 384–386. (**II**)

Schinka, J. A., Hughes, P. H., Coletti, S. D., Hamilton, N. L., & Urmann, C. F. (1999). Changes in personality characteristics in women treated in a therapeutic community. *Journal of Substance Abuse Treatment, 16,* 137–142. (**II**)

Schoenberg, M. R., Dorr, D., & Morgan, C. D. (2003). The ability of the Millon Clinical Multiaxial Inventory—third edition to detect malingering. *Psychological Assessment, 15,* 198–204.

Schoenberg, M. R., Dorr, D., Morgan, C. D., & Burke, M. (2004). A comparison of the MCMI-III personality disorder and modifier indices with the MMPI-2 clinical and validity scales. *Journal of Personality Assessment, 82,* 273–280. **(III)**

Schuler, C. E., Snibbe, J. R., & Buckwalter, J. G. (1994). Validity of the MMPI personality disorder scales (MMPI-Pd). *Journal of Clinical Psychology, 50,* 220–227.

Schuller, D. R., Bagby, R. M., Levitt, A. J., & Joffe, R. T. (1993). A comparison of personality characteristics of seasonal and nonseasonal major depression. *Comprehensive Psychiatry, 34,* 360–362.

Schutte, J. W. (2001). Using the MCMI-III in forensic evaluations. *American Journal of Forensic Psychology, 19,* 5–20. **(III)**

Schwartz, J. P., Seemann, E., Buboltz, W. C., & Flye, A. (2004). Personality styles: Predictors of masculine gender role conflict in male prison inmates. *Psychology of Men and Masculinity, 5,* 59–64. **(III)**

Schweitzer, I., Tuckwell, V., Maguire, K., & Tiller, J. (2001). Personality pathology, depression and HPA Axis functioning. *Human Psychopharmacology: Clinical and Experimental, 16,* 303–308. **(II)**

Segal, D. L., Hersen, M., Van Hasselt, V. B., Silberman, C. S., & Roth, L. (1996). Diagnosis and assessment of personality disorders in older adults: A critical review. *Journal of Personality Disorders, 10,* 384–399. **(I/II)**

Selzer, M. A., Kernberg, P., Fibel, B., Cherbuli, T., & Morati, S. G. (1987). The personality assessment interview preliminary report. *Psychiatry, 50,* 142–153.

Sexton, D., McIwraith, R., Barnes, G., & Dunn, R. (1987). Comparison of the MCMI and MMPI-168 as psychiatric inpatient screening inventories. *Journal of Personality Assessment, 51,* 388–398.

Shafi, M., Carrigan, S., Whillinghill, J. R., & Derrick, A. (1985). Psychological autopsy of completed suicide in children and adolescents. *American Journal of Psychiatry, 142,* 1061–1064.

Shafi, M., Steltz-Lenarsky, J., Derrick, A., Bechner, C., & Whillinghill, Jr., R. (1988). Morbidity of mental disorders in the post mortem diagnosis of completed suicide in children and adolescents. *Journal of Affective Disorders, 15,* 227–233.

Sherwood, R. J., Funari, D. J., & Piekarski, A. M. (1990). Adapted character styles of Vietnam veterans with posttraumatic stress disorder. *Psychological Reports, 66,* 623–631.

Shinka, J. A., Hughes, P. H., Coletti, S. D., Hamilton, N. L., Renard, C., Urmann, C. F., et al. (1999). Changes in personality characteristics in women treated in a therapeutic community. *Journal of Substance Abuse Treatment, 16,* 137–142. **(II)**

Sidall, J. W. (1986). Use of the MCMI with substance abusers. *Noteworthy Responses, 2,* 1–3.

Sidall, J. W., & Keogh, N. J. (1993). Utility of computer reports based on counselor's ratings of the Diagnostic Inventory of Personality and Symptoms. *Psychological Report, 72,* 347–350.

Silberman, C. S., Roth, L., Segal, D. L., & Burns, W. J. (1997). Relationship between the Millon Clinical Multiaxial Inventory-II and Coolidge Axis II Inventory in chronically mentally ill older adults: A pilot study. *Journal of Clinical Psychology, 53,* 559–566. **(II)**

Silverman, J. S., & Loychik, S. G. (1990). Brain-mapping abnormalities in a family with three obsessive compulsive children. *Journal of Neuropsychiatry and Clinical Neurosciences, 2*, 319–322. (**II**)

Silverstein, M. L., & McDonald, C. (1988). Personality trait characteristics in relation to neuropsychological dysfunction in schizophrenia and depression. *Journal of Personality Assessment, 52*, 288–296.

Sim, J. P., & Romney, D. M. (1990). The relationship between a circumplex model of interpersonal behaviors and personality disorders. *Journal of Personality Disorders, 4*, 329–341.

Sinha, B. K., & Watson, D. C. (1999). Predicting personality disorder traits with the Defense Style Questionnaire in a normal sample. *Journal of Personality Disorders, 13*, 281–286. (**II**)

Sinha, B. K., & Watson, D. C. (2001). Personality disorder in university students: A multitrait-multimethod matrix study. *Journal of Personality Disorders, 15*, 235–244.

Sinha, B. K., & Watson, D. C. (2004). Personality disorder clusters and the Defense Style Questionnaire. *Psychology and Psychotherapy: Theory, Research, and Practice, 77*, 55–66.

Smalley, S., Smith, M., & Tanguay, P. (1991). Autism and psychiatric disorders in tuberous sclerosis. *Annuals of the New York Academy of Science, 615*, 382–383.

Smith, D., Carroll, J. L., & Fuller, G. (1988). The relationship between the Millon Clinical Multiaxial Inventory and the MMPI in a private outpatient mental health clinic population. *Journal of Clinical Psychology, 44*, 165–174.

Snibbe, J. R., Peterson, P. J., & Sosner, B. (1980). Study of psychological characteristics of a Worker's Compensation sample using the MMPI and the Millon Clinical Multiaxial Inventory. *Psychological Reports, 47*, 959–966.

Soldz, S., Budman, S., Demby, A., & Merry, J. (1993a). Diagnostic agreement between the Personality Disorder Examination and the MCMI-II. *Journal of Personality Assessment, 60*, 486–499. (**II**)

Soldz, S., Budman, S., Demby, A., & Merry, J. (1993b). Representation of personality disorders in circumplex and five-factor space: Explorations with a clinical sample. *Psychological Assessment, 5*, 41–52. (**II**)

Sperling, M. B., Sharp, J. L., & Fisher, P. H. (1991). On the nature of attachment in a borderline population: A preliminary investigation. *Psychological Reports, 68*, 543–546. (**II**)

Stankovic, S. R., Libb, J. W., Freeman, A. M., & Roseman, J. M. (1992). Posttreatment stability of the MCMI-II personality scales in depressed outpatients. *Journal of Personality Disorders, 6*, 82–89. (**II**)

Stark, M. J., & Campbell, B. K. (1988). Personality, drug use, and early attrition from substance abuse treatment. *American Journal of Drug and Alcohol Abuse, 14*, 475–485.

Staudenmayer, H., & Kramer, R. E. (1999). Psychogenic chemical sensitivity: Psychogenic psuedoseizures elicited by provocation challenges with fragrances. *Journal of Psychosomatic Research, 47*, 185–190. (**II**)

Strack, S. (1987). Development and validation of an adjective checklist to assess the Millon personality types in a normal population. *Journal of Personality Assessment, 51,* 572–587.

Strack, S. (1991). Factor analysis of MCMI-II and PACL basic personality scales in a college sample. *Journal of Personality Assessment, 57,* 345–355. **(II)**

Strack, S., Choca, J. P., & Gurtman, M. B. (2001). Circular structure of the MCMI-III personality disorder scales. *Journal of Personality Disorders, 15,* 263–274. **(III)**

Strack, S., & Lorr, M. (1991). Item factor structure of the Personality Adjective Check List. *Journal of Personality Assessment, 55,* 86–94.

Strack, S., Lorr, M., & Campbell, L. (1990). An evaluation of Millon's circular model of personality disorders. *Journal of Personality Disorders, 4,* 353–361. **(II)**

Strack, S., Lorr, M., Campbell, L., & Lamnin, A. (1992). Personality disorder and clinical syndrome factors of MCMI-II scales. *Journal of Personality Disorders, 6,* 40–52. **(II)**

Streiner, D. L., Goldberg, J. O., & Miller, H. R. (1993). MCMI-II item weights: Their lack of effectiveness. *Journal of Personality Assessment, 60,* 471–476. **(II)**

Streiner, D. L., & Miller, H. R. (1989). The MCMI-II: How much better than the MCMI? *Journal of Personality Assessment, 55,* 81–84. **(II)**

Streiner, D. L., & Miller, H. R. (1991). Maximum likelihood estimates of the accuracy of four diagnostic techniques. *Educational and Psychological Measurement, 50,* 653–662.

Sugihara, Y., & Warner, J. A. (1999). Mexican-American male batterers on the MCMI-III. *Psychological Reports, 85,* 163–169. **(III)**

Sweeny, J. A., Clarkin, J. F., & Fitzgibb, M. L. (1987). Current practice of psychological assessment. *Professional Psychology: Research and Practice, 18,* 377–380.

Swirsky-Sacchetti, T., Gorton, G., Samuel, S., Sobel, R., Ganetta-Wadley, A., & Burleigh, B. (1993). Neuropsychological function in borderline personality disorder. *Journal of Clinical Psychology, 49,* 385–396.

Taber, J. I., McCormick, R. A., & Ramirez, L. F. (1987). The prevalence and impact of major stressors among pathological gamblers. *International Journal of the Addictions, 22,* 71–79.

Tamburrino, M. B., Franco, K. N., Campbell, N. B., Pentz, J. E., Evans, C. L., & Jurs, S. G. (1990). Postabortion dysphoria and religion. *Southern Medical Journal, 83,* 736–738.

Tamkin, A. S., Carson, M. F., Nixon, D. H., & Hyer, L. A. (1987). A comparison of some measures in male alcoholics. *Journal of Studies on Alcohol, 48,* 176–178.

Tango, R. A., & Dziuban, C. D. (1984). The use of personality components in the interpretation of career indecision. *Journal of College Student Personnel, 25,* 509–512.

Terpylak, O., & Schuerger, J. M. (1994). Broad factor scales of the 16PF 5th ed. and Millon personality disorder scales: A replication. *Psychological Reports, 74,* 124–126.

Thompson-Pope, S. K., & Turkat, I. O. (1988). Reactions to ambiguous stimuli among paranoid personalities. *Journal of Psychopathology and Behavioral Assessment, 10,* 21–32.

Tisdale, M. J., Pendelton, L., & Marler, M. (1990). MCMI characteristics of *DSM-III-R* bulimics. *Journal of Personality Assessment, 55,* 477–483.

Torgersen, S., & Alnaes, R. (1990). The relationship between the MCMI personality scales and *DSM III,* Axis II. *Journal of Personality Assessment, 55,* 698–707.

Trull, T. J., Widiger, T. A., & Frances, A. (1987). Covariation of criteria sets for avoidant, schizoid, and dependent personality disorders. *American Journal of Psychiatry, 144,* 767–771.

Tuokko, H., Vernon-Wilkinson, R., & Robinson, E. (1991). The use of the MCMI in the personality assessment of head-injured adults. *Brain Injury, 5,* 287–293.

Turley, B., Bates, G. W., Edwards, J., & Jackson, H. J. (1992). MCMI-II personality disorders in recent-onset bipolar disorders. *Journal of Clinical Psychology, 48,* 320–329. **(II)**

Turner, R. J. (1988). The parent-adult-child projective drawing task: A therapeutic tool in, T. A. *Transactional Analysis Journal, 18,* 60–67.

Tweed, R. G., & Dutton, D. G. (1999). A comparison of impulsive and instrumental subgroups of batterers. *Violence and Victims, 13,* 217–230. **(II)**

Uomoto, J. M., Turner, J. A., & Herron, L. D. (1988). Use of the MMPI and MCMI in predicting outcome of lumbar laminectomy. *Journal of Clinical Psychology, 44,* 191–197.

Van Gorp, W. G., & Meyer, R. G. (1986). The detection of faking on the Millon Clinical Multiaxial Inventory (MCMI). *Journal of Clinical Psychology, 42,* 742–747.

Veraldi, D. M. (1992). Assessing PTSD in personal injury cases. *American Journal of Forensic Psychology, 10,* 5–13. **(II)**

Vereycken, J., Vertommen, H., & Corveleyn, J. (2002). Authority conflicts and personality disorders. *Journal of Personality Disorders, 16,* 41–51.

Vollrath, M., Alnaes, R., & Torgersen, S. (1994a). Coping and MCMI-II personality disorders. *Journal of Personality Disorders, 8,* 53–63. **(II)**

Vollrath, M., Alnaes, R., & Torgersen, S. (1994b). Coping and MCMI-II symptom scales. *Journal of Clinical Psychology, 50,* 727–736.

Vollrath, M., Alnaes, P. R., & Torgersen, S. (1995). Coping styles predict change in personality disorders. *Journal of Personality Disorders, 9,* 371–385.

Vollrath, M., Alnaes, P. R., & Torgersen, S. (1998). Coping styles predict change in personality disorders. *Journal of Personality Disorders, 12,* 198–209. **(II)**

Wakefield, H., & Underwager, R. (1993). Misuse of psychological tests in forensic settings: Some horrible examples. American College of Forensic Psychology 8th Annual Symposium in Forensic Psychology. *American Journal of Forensic Psychology, 11,* 55–75.

Wall, T. L., Schuckit, M. A., Mungas, D., & Ehlers, C. L. (1990). EEG alpha activity and personality traits. *Alcohol, 7,* 461–464.

Waltz, J., Babcock, J. C., Jacobson, N. S., & Gottman, J. M. (2000). Testing a typology of batterers. *Journal of Consulting and Clinical Psychology, 68,* 658–669. **(II)**

Watson, D. C., & Sinha, B. K. (1995). Dimensional structure of personality disorder inventories: A comparison of normal and clinical populations. *Personality Individual Differences, 19,* 817–826. (**II**)

Weekes, J. R., & Morison, S. J. (1993). Offender typologies: Identifying treatment-relevant personality characteristics. *Forum on Corrections Research, 5,* 10–12.

Weissman, H. N. (1984). Psychological assessment and psycholegal formulations in psychiatric traumatology. *Psychiatric Annals, 14,* 517.

Wetzler, S., & Dubro, A. (1990). Diagnosis of personality disorders by the Millon Clinical Multiaxial Inventory. *Journal of Nervous and Mental Diseases, 178,* 261–263.

Wetzler, S., Khadivi, A., & Oppenheim, S. (1995). The psychological assessment of depression: Unipolars versus bipolars. *Journal of Personality Assessment, 65,* 557–566.

Wetzler, S., Kahn, R. S., Cahn, W., Van Praag, H. M., & Asnis, G. M. (1990). Psychological test characteristics of depressed and panic patients. *Psychiatry Research, 31,* 179–192.

Wetzler, S., Kahn, R. S., Strauman, T. J., & Dubro, A. (1989). Diagnosis of major depression by self-report. *Journal of Personality Assessment, 53,* 22–30.

Wetzler, S., & Marlowe, D. (1990). "Faking Bad" on the MMPI, MMPI-2, and Millon-II. *Psychological Reports, 67,* 1117–1118. (**II**)

Wetzler, S., & Marlowe, D. (1992). What they don't tell you in the test manual: A response to Millon. *Journal of Counseling and Development, 70,* 427–428. (**II**)

Wetzler, S., & Marlowe, D. B. (1993). The diagnosis and assessment of depression, mania, and psychosis by self-report. *Journal of Personality Assessment, 60,* 1–31. (**II**)

Wheeler, D. S., & Schwartz, J. C. (1989). Millon Clinical Inventory (MCMI) scores with a collegiate sample: Long term stability and self-other agreement. *Journal of Psychopathology and Behavioral Assessment, 11,* 339–352.

White, R. J., Ackerman, R. J., & Caraveo, L. E. (2001). Self-identified alcohol abusers in a low-security federal prison: Characteristics and treatment implications. *International Journal of Offender Therapy and Comparative Criminology, 45,* 214–227.

Widiger, T. A., & Frances, A. (1987). Interviews and inventories for the measure of personality disorders. *Clinical Psychology Review, 7,* 49–75.

Widiger, T., & Sanderson, C. (1987). The convergent and discriminant validity of the MCMI as a measure of the *DSM-III* personality disorders. *Journal of Personality Assessment, 51,* 228–242.

Widiger, T., Williams, J., Spitzer, R., & Frances, A. (1985). The MCMI as a measure of *DSM-III. Journal of Personality Assessment, 49,* 366–380.

Widiger, T., Williams, J., Spitzer, R., & Frances, A. (1986). The MCMI and *DSM-III:* A brief rejoinder to Millon, 1985. *Journal of Personality Assessment, 50,* 198–204.

Wiederman, M. W., & Pryor, T. L. (1997). MCMI-II personality scale scores among women with anorexia nervosa or bulimia nervosa. *Journal of Personality Assessment, 69,* 508–516. (**II**)

Wierzbicki, M. (1993a). The relationship between MCMI subtlety and severity. *Journal of Personality Assessment, 61,* 259–263.

Wierzbicki, M. (1993b). Use the MCMI subtle and obvious subscales to detect faking. *Journal of Clinical Psychology, 49,* 809–814.

Wierzbicki, M. (1997). Use of subtle and obvious scales to detect faking on the MCMI-II. *Journal of Clinical Psychology, 53,* 421–426. (**II**)

Wierzbicki, M., & Daleiden, E. L. (1993). The differential responding of college students to subtle and obvious MCMI subscales. *Journal of Clinical Psychology, 49,* 204–208.

Wierzbicki, M., & Gorman, J. L. (1995). Correspondence between students' scores on the Millon Clinical Multiaxial Inventory-II and Personality Diagnostic Questionnaire-Revised. *Psychological Reports, 77,* 1079–1082. (**II**)

Wierzbicki, M., & Golade, P. (1993). Sex-typing of the Millon Clinical Multiaxial Inventory. *Psychological Reports, 72,* 1115–1121.

Wierzbicki, M., & Howard, B. J. (1992). The differential responding of male prisoners to subtle and obvious MCMI subscales. *Journal of Personality Assessment, 58,* 115–126.

Williams, W., Coker, R. R., Vincent, K. R., Duthie, B., McLaughlin, E. S., & Overall, J. E. (1988). *DSM-III* diagnosis and code types of the diagnostic inventory of personality and symptoms. *Journal of Clinical Psychology, 44,* 326–335.

Williams, W., Weiss, T. W., Edens, A., Johnson, M., & Thornby, J. I. (1998). Hospitalization utilization and personality characteristics of veterans with psychiatric problems. *Psychiatric Services, 49,* 370–375.

Wise, E. A. (1994a). Managed care and the psychometric validity of the MMPI and MCMI personality disorder scales. *Psychotherapy in Private Practice, 13,* 81–97.

Wise, E. A. (1994b). Personality style codetype concordance between the MCMI and MBHI. *Journal of Clinical Psychology, 50,* 367–380.

Wise, E. A. (1995a). Personality disorder correspondence among the MMPI, MBHI, and MCMI. *Journal of Clinical Psychology, 51,* 790–798.

Wise, E. A. (1995b). Personality disorder correspondence between the MMPI, MBHI, and MCMI. *Journal of Clinical Psychology, 51,* 367–380.

Wise, E. A. (1996). Comparative validity of MMPI-2 and MCMI-II personality disorder classifications. *Journal of Personality Assessment, 66,* 569–582.

Wise, E. A. (2001). The comparative validity of MCMI-II and MMPI-2 personality disorder scales with forensic examinees. *Journal of Personality Disorders, 15,* 275–279. (**II**)

Wise, E. A. (2002). Relationships of personality disorders with MMPI-2 malingering, defensiveness, and inconsistent response scales among forensic examinees. *Psychological Reports, 90,* 760–766. (**II**)

Wolberg, W. H., Tanner, M. A., Romsaas, E. P., Trump, D. L., & Malec, J. F. (1987). Factors influencing options in primary breast cancer treatment. *Journal of Clinical Oncology, 5,* 68–74.

Yeager, R. J., DiGiuseppe, R., Resweber, P. J., & Leaf, R. (1992). Comparison of Millon personality profiles of chronic residential substance abusers and a general outpatient population. *Psychological Reports, 71,* 71–79.

Zarrella, K. L., Schuerger, J. M., & Ritz, G. H. (1990). Estimation of MCMI *DSM-III* Axis II constructs from MMPI scales and subscales. *Journal of Personality Assessment, 55*(1/2),195–201.

MONOGRAPHS

Hsu, L. M., & Maruish, M. E. (1992). *Conducting publishable research with the MCMI-II: Psychometric and statistical issues.* Minneapolis: National Computer Systems.

BOOK CHAPTERS

Antoni, M. (1993). The combined use of the MCMI and MMPI. In R. J. Craig (Ed.), *The Millon Clinical Multiaxial Inventory: A clinical and research information synthesis.* (pp. 279–302). Hillsdale, NJ: Erlbaum.

Antoni, M. (1997). Integrating the MCMI and the MMPI. In T. Millon (Ed.), *The Millon inventories: Clinical and personality assessment* (pp. 106–123). New York: Guilford Press.

Choca, J., & Bresolin, L. (1993). Affective disorders and the MCMI. In R. J. Craig (Ed.), *The Millon Clinical Multiaxial Inventory: A clinical and research information synthesis.* (pp. 111–124). Hillsdale, NJ: Erlbaum.

Craig, R. J. (1995). Interpersonal psychotherapy and MCMI-III-based assessment. In P. Retzlaff (Ed.), *Tactical psychotherapy of the personality disorders: An MCMI-III-based approach* (pp. 66–88). Boston: Allyn & Bacon.

Craig, R. J. (1993). The MCMI/MCMI-II with substance abusers. In R. J. Craig (Ed.), *The Millon Clinical Multiaxial Inventory: A clinical and research information synthesis* (pp. 125–146). Hillsdale, NJ: Erlbaum.

Craig, R. J. (1997). A selected review of the MCMI empirical literature. In T. Millon (Ed.), *The Millon inventories: Clinical and personality assessment* (pp. 303–326). New York: Guilford Press.

Craig, R. J. (1999, 2002). Essentials of MCMI-III interpretation. In S. Strack (Ed.), *Essentials of Millon inventories assessment* (2nd ed., pp. 1–51). New York: Wiley.

Craig, R. J. (1999). Millon Clinical Multiaxial Inventory-III. In *Interpreting personality tests: A clinical manual for the MMPI-2, MCMI-III, CPI-R, and 16 PF* (pp. 101–192). New York: Wiley.

Craig, R. J. (2001). MCMI-III. In W. Dorfman & M. Hersen (Eds.), *Understanding psychological assessment: A manual for counselors and clinicians* (pp. 173–186). New York: Plenum Press.

Craig, R. J., & Weinberg, D. (1993). MCMI: Review of the literature. In R. J. Craig (Ed.), *The Millon Clinical Multiaxial Inventory: A clinical research information synthesis.* (pp. 23–70). Hillsdale, NJ: Erlbaum.

Davis, R. D., Meagher, S. E., Goncalves, M., Woodward, M., & Millon, T. (1999). Treatment planning and outcome in adults: The Millon Clinical Multiaxial

Inventory-III. In M. E. Maruish (Ed.), *The use of psychological testing for treatment planning and outcomes assessment* (2nd ed.). Mahwah, NJ: Erlbaum.

Davis, R. D., & Millon, T. (1993). Putting Humpty Dumpty back together again: The MCMI in personality assessment. In L. Beutler (Ed.), *Integrative personality assessment* (pp. 240–279). New York: Guilford Press.

Davis, R. D., & Millon, T. (1997). Teaching and learning assessment with the Millon Clinical Multiaxial Inventory (MCMI-III). In L. Handler & M. Hilsenroth (Eds.), *Teaching and learning personality assessment*. Hillsdale, NJ: Erlbaum.

Davis, R. D., & Millon, T. (1997). MCMI assessment: An integrated case study. In T. Millon (Ed.), *The Millon inventories: Clinical and personality assessment* (pp. 59–74). New York: Guilford Press.

Davis, R. D., & Millon, T. (1997). The Millon inventories: Present and future directions. In T. Millon (Ed.), *The Millon inventories: Clinical and personality assessment* (pp. 525–538). New York: Guilford Press.

Davis, R. D., Wenger, A., & Guzman, A. (1997). Validation of the MCMI-III. In T. Millon (Ed.), *The Millon inventories: Clinical and personality assessment* (pp. 327–362). New York: Guilford Press.

Donat, D. (1995). Use of the MCMI-III in behavior therapy. In P. Retzlaff (Ed.), *Tactical psychotherapy of the personality disorders: An MCMI-III-based approach* (pp. 40–62). Boston: Allyn & Bacon.

Dorr, D. (1995). Psychoanalytic psychotherapy of the personality disorders toward morphologic change. In P. Retzlaff (Ed.), *Tactical psychotherapy of the personality disorders: An MCMI-III-based approach* (pp. 186–209). Boston: Allyn & Bacon.

Dorr, D. (1997). Clinical integration of the MCMI-III and the Comprehensive System Rorschach. In T. Millon (Ed.), *The Millon inventories: Clinical and personality assessment* (pp. 75–105). New York: Guilford Press.

Dyer, F. J. (1997). Application of the Millon inventories in forensic psychology. In T. Millon (Ed.), *The Millon inventories: Clinical and personality assessment* (pp. 124–139). New York: Guilford Press.

Escovar, L. A. (1997). The Millon inventories: Sociocultural considerations. In T. Millon (Ed.), *The Millon inventories: Clinical and personality assessment* (pp. 264–285). New York: Guilford Press.

Everly, G. S. (1995). Domain-oriented personality theory. In P. Retzlaff (Ed.), *Tactical psychotherapy of the personality disorders: An MCMI-III-based approach* (pp. 24–32). Boston: Allyn & Bacon.

Flynn, P. M., & McMahon, R. C. (1997). MCMI applications in substance abuse. In T. Millon (Ed.), *The Millon inventories: Clinical and personality assessment* (pp. 173–190). New York: Guilford Press.

Gibertini, M. (1993). Factors affecting the operating characteristics of the MCMI-II. In R. J. Craig (Ed.), *The Millon Clinical Multiaxial Inventory: A clinical and research information synthesis* (pp. 71–80). Hillsdale, NJ: Erlbaum.

Gonclaves, A. A., Woodward, M. J., & Millon, T. (1994). Millon Clinical Multiaxial Inventory-II. In M. E. Maruish (Ed.), *The use of psychological testing for treatment planning and outcome assessment.* (pp. 161–184). Hillsdale, NJ: Erlbaum.

Greenblatt, R. L., & Davis, W. E. (1993). The MCMI in the diagnosis and assessment of schizophrenia. In R. J. Craig (Ed.), *The Millon Clinical Multiaxial Inventory: A clinical and research information synthesis* (pp. 93–110). Hillsdale, NJ: Erlbaum.

Groth-Marnatt, G. (1997). Millon Clinical Multiaxial Inventory. *Handbook of psychological assessment.* (pp. 301–342). New York: Wiley.

Hall, G. C., & Phung, A. H. (2001). The Minnesota Multiphasic Personality Inventory and Millon Clinical Multiaxial Inventory. In L. A. Suzuki & J. G. Pontero (Eds.), *Handbook of multicultural assessment: Clinical, psychological, and educational applications* (2nd ed., pp. 307–330). San Francisco: Jossey-Bass.

Hyer, L., Brandsma, J., & Boyd, S. (1992). The MCMIs and posttraumatic stress disorder. In T. Millon (Ed.), *The Millon inventories: Clinical and personality assessment* (pp. 191–216). New York: Guilford Press.

Hyer, L., Brandsma, J., & Shealy, L. (1995). Experiential mood therapy with the MCMI-III. In P. Retzlaff (Ed.), *Tactical psychotherapy of the personality disorders: An MCMI-III-based approach* (pp. 210–232). Boston: Allyn & Bacon.

Hyer, L., Melton, M., & Gratton, C. (1993). Post-traumatic stress disorders and MCMI-based assessment. In R. J. Craig (Ed.), *The Millon Clinical Multiaxial Inventory: A clinical and research information synthesis* (pp. 159–172). Hillsdale, NJ: Erlbaum.

Josiassen, R. C., Shagass, C., Roemer, R. A., & Straumanis, J. (1986). Attention-related effects in non-psychotic dysphoric psychiatric patients. In C. Shagass & R. A. Roemer (Eds.) (1988). *Brain electrical potentials and psychopathology* (pp. 259–277). London, England: Elsevier Publishing Company.

Kubacki, S. R., & Smith, P. R. (1995). An intersubjective approach to assessing and treating ego defenses using the MCMI-III. In P. Retzlaff (Ed.), *Tactical psychotherapy of the personality disorders: An MCMI-III-based approach* (pp. 158–183). Boston: Allyn & Bacon.

Lehne, G. K. (1994). The NEO-PI and the MCMI in the forensic evaluation of sex offenders. In P. T. Costa & T. A. Widiger (Eds.), *Personality disorders and the five-factor model of personality* (pp. 175–188). Washington, DC: American Psychological Association.

Lehne, G. K. (2002). The NEO Personality Inventory and the Millon Clinical Multiaxial Inventory in the forensic evaluation of sex offenders. In P. T. Costa & T. A. Widiger (Eds.), *Personality disorders and the five-factor model of personality* (2nd ed., pp. 269–282). Washington, DC: American Psychological Association.

Lorr, M. (1993). Dimensional structure of the Millon Clinical Multiaxial Inventory. In R. J. Craig (Ed.), *The Millon Clinical Multiaxial Inventory: A clinical and research information synthesis* (pp. 81–89). Hillsdale, NJ: Erlbaum.

McCann, J. T. (1995). The MCMI-III and the treatment of the self. In P. Retzlaff (Ed.), *Tactical psychotherapy of the personality disorders: An MCMI-III-based approach* (pp. 137–156). Boston: Allyn & Bacon.

McMahon, R. C. (1993). The Millon Clinical Multiaxial Inventory: An introduction to theory, development, and interpretation. In R. J. Craig (Ed.), *The*

Millon Clinical Multiaxial Inventory: A clinical and research information synthesis (pp. 3–22). Hillsdale, NJ: Erlbaum.

Millon, T. (1984). Interpretive guide to the Millon Clinical Multiaxial Inventory. In P. McReynolds & G. J. Chelune (Eds.), *Advances in personality assessment (Vol. 6, pp. 1–41).* San Francisco: Jossey-Bass.

Millon, T., & Davis, R. (1994). Millon's evolutionary model of normal and abnormal personality: Theory and measures. In S. Strack (Ed.), *Differentiating normal and abnormal personality* (pp. 79–113). New York: Springer.

Millon, T., & Davis, R. D. (1995). Putting humpty dumpty together again: Using the MCMI in psychological assessment. In L. E. Beutler & M. R. Berren (Eds.), *Integrative assessment of adult personality* (pp. 240–279). New York: Guilford Press.

Millon, T., & Davis, R. (1996). The Millon Clinical Multiaxial Inventory-III. (MCMI-III). In C. Newmark (Ed.), *Major psychological assessment instruments* (2nd ed., pp. 108–147). Boston: Allyn & Bacon.

Millon, T., & Davis, R. D. (1997). The place of assessment in clinical science. In T. Millon (Ed.), *The Millon inventories: Clinical and personality assessment* (pp. 3–22). New York: Guilford Press.

Millon, C., & Millon, T. (1997). Using the MCMI in correctional settings. In T. Millon (Ed.), *The Millon inventories: Clinical and personality assessment* (pp. 140–153). New York: Guilford Press.

Millon, T., & Meagher, S. E. (2003). The Millon Clinical Multiaxial Inventory (MCMI-III). In D. L. Segal & M. J. Hilsenroth (Eds.), *Comprehensive handbook of psychological assessment: Vol. 2. Personality Assessment* (pp. 108–121). New York: Wiley.

Millon, T., & Millon, C. (1997). History, theory, and validation of the MCMI. In T. Millon (Ed.), *The Millon inventories: Clinical and personality assessment* (pp. 23–40). New York: Guilford Press.

Millon, T., & Davis, R. D. (1998). Millon Clinical Multiaxial Inventory (MCMI-III). In G. Koocher, J. Norcross, & S. Hill (Eds.), *Psychologists' desk reference* (pp. 142–148). New York: Oxford University Press.

Moreland, K. (1993). Computer-assisted interpretation of the MCMI-II. In R. J. Craig (Ed.), *The Millon Clinical Multiaxial Inventory: A clinical and research information synthesis* (pp. 213–234). Hillsdale, NJ: Erlbaum.

Nurse, A. R. (1999). The MCMI: Assessing personality styles or disorders in marital partners. In A. R. Nurse (Ed.), *Family assessment: Effective uses of personality tests with couples and families* (pp. 34–61). New York: Wiley. **(III)**

Nurse, A. R. (1997). Using the MCMI in treating couples. In T. Millon (Ed.), *The Millon inventories: Clinical and personality assessment* (pp. 245–263). New York: Guilford Press.

Piersma, H. L. (1993). The MCMI as a predictor of *DSM-III* diagnostic categories: A review of empirical research. In R. J. Craig (Ed.), *The Millon Clinical Multiaxial Inventory: A clinical and research information synthesis* (pp. 203–212). Hillsdale, NJ: Erlbaum.

Retzlaff, P. (1995). Clinical application of the MCMI-III. In P. Retzlaff (Ed.), *Tactical psychotherapy of the personality disorders: An MCMI-III-based approach* (pp. 1–21). Boston: Allyn & Bacon.

Retzlaff, P. (1993). Special scales for the MCMI: Theory, development, and utility. In R. J. Craig (Ed.), *The Millon Clinical Multiaxial Inventory: A clinical and research information synthesis* (pp. 237–252). Hillsdale, NJ: Erlbaum.

Retzlaff, P. (1997). The MCMI as a treatment planning tool. In T. Millon (Ed.), *The Millon inventories: Clinical and personality assessment* (pp. 217–244). New York: Guilford Press.

Reich, J. (1993). The MCMI and *DSM-III* anxiety disorders. In R. J. Craig (Ed.), *The Millon Clinical Multiaxial Inventory: A clinical and research information synthesis* (pp. 173–178). Hillsdale, NJ: Erlbaum.

Russell, S. L., & Russell, E. W. (1997). Using the MCMI in neurological evaluations. In T. Millon (Ed.), *The Millon inventories: Clinical and personality assessment* (pp. 154–172). New York: Guilford Press.

Sloore, H. V., & Derksen, J. L. (1997). Issues and procedures in MCMI translations. In T. Millon (Ed.), *The Millon inventories: Clinical and personality assessment* (pp. 286–302). New York: Guilford Press.

Strack, S. (1993). Measuring Millon's personality styles in normal adults. In R. J. Craig (Ed.), *The Millon Clinical Multiaxial Inventory: A clinical and research information synthesis.* (pp. 253–278). Hillsdale, NJ: Erlbaum.

Tisdale, M., & Pendleton, L. (1993). The use of the MCMI with eating disorders. In R. J. Craig (Ed.), *The Millon Clinical Multiaxial Inventory: A clinical and research information synthesis* (pp. 147–158). Hillsdale, NJ: Erlbaum.

Van Denburg, E. J. (1995). Object relations theory and the MCMI-III. In P. Retzlaff (Ed.), *Tactical psychotherapy of the personality disorders: An MCMI-III-based approach* (pp. 111–132). Boston: Allyn & Bacon.

Van Denburg, E. J., & Choca, J. P. (1997). Interpretation of the MCMI-III. In T. Millon (Ed.), *The Millon inventories: Clinical and personality assessment* (pp. 41–58). New York: Guilford Press.

Widiger, T. A., & Corbitt, E. M. (1993). The MCMI-II personality disorder scales and their relationship to *DSM-III-R* diagnosis. In R. J. Craig (Ed.), *The Millon Clinical Multiaxial Inventory: A clinical and research information synthesis* (pp. 181–202). Hillsdale, NJ: Erlbaum.

Will, T. E. (1995). Cognitive therapy and the MCMI-III. In P. Retzlaff (Ed.), *Tactical psychotherapy of the personality disorders: An MCMI-III-based approach* (pp. 90–106). Boston: Allyn & Bacon.

CROSS-CULTURAL RESEARCH

Gunsalus, A. J., & Kelly, K. R. (2001). Korean cultural influences on the Millon Clinical Multiaxial Inventory III. *Journal of Mental Health Counseling, 23,* 151–161. **(III)**

Jackson, H. J. R., Gazis, J., & Edwards, J. (1991). Using the MCMI to diagnose personality disorders in inpatients: Axis I/Axis II associations and sex differences. *Australian Psychologist, 26,* 37–41.

Luteijn, F. (1991). The MCMI in the Netherlands: First Findings. *Journal of Personality Disorders, 4,* 297–303.

Mortensen, E. L., & Simonsen, E. (1991). Psychometric properties of the Danish MCMI-I translation. *Scandinavian Journal of Psychology, 31,* 149–153.

Nazikian, H. R. P., Edwards, J., & Jackson, H. J. (1990). Personality disorder assessment for psychiatric inpatients. *Australian—New Zealand Journal of Psychiatry, 24,* 166.

O'Callaghan, T., Bates, G. W., Jackson, H. J., Rudd, R. P., & Edwards, J. (1990). The clinical utility of the Millon Clinical Multiaxial depression subscales. *Australian Psychologist, 25,* 45–61.

Overholser, J. C. (1989). Differentiation between schizoid and avoidant personalities: An empirical test. *Canadian Journal of Psychiatry, 34,* 785–790.

Ravndal, E., & Vaglum, P. (1991). Psychopathology and substance abuse as predictors of program completion in a therapeutic community for drug abusers: A prospective study. *Acta Psychiatrics Scandinavia, 83,* 217–222.

Simonsen, E., & Mellegard, M. (1986). The MCMI—Millon Clinical Multiaxial Inventory: Clinical experiences with a new questionnaire for assessing psychiatric patients. *Ugeskrift for Laeger, 148,* 2872–2875.

Simonsen, E., & Mortenstein, E. L. (1991). Difficulties in translation of personality scales. First International Congress of the Society for the Study of Personality Disorders. *Journal of Personality Disorders, 4,* 290–296.

CONFERENCE PROCEEDINGS

Auerback, J. S. (1987). Schizotypy, narcissism and psychopathology: Correlates of psychosis-proneness and MCMI scales. In C. Green (Ed.), *Conference on the Millon Inventories (MCMI, MBHI, MAPI)* (pp. 235–241). Minneapolis: National Computer Systems.

Bard, L., & Knight, R. (1987). Sex offender subtyping and the MCMI. In C. Green (Ed.), *Conference on the Millon Inventories (MCMI, MBHI, MAPI)* (pp. 133–137). Minneapolis: National Computer Systems.

Beck, M. (1987). Absenteeism in industry: A bio-psychosocial profile of the chronic absentee. In C. Green (Ed.), *Conference on the Millon Inventories (MCMI, MBHI, MAPI)* (pp. 273–284). Minneapolis: National Computer Systems.

Benjamin, L. S. (1987). Combined use of the MCMI and the SASB Intrex questionnaires to document and facilitate personality change during long-term psychotherapy. In C. Green (Ed.), *Conference on the Millon Inventories (MCMI, MBHI, MAPI)* (pp. 305–323). Minneapolis: National Computer Systems.

Bresolin, L., Choca, J., Okonek, A., & Ostrow, D. (1987). The validity of the Millon Clinical Multiaxial Inventory in the assessment of affective disorders. In C. Green (Ed.), *Conference on the Millon Inventories (MCMI, MBHI, MAPI)* (pp. 33–39). Minneapolis: National Computer Systems.

Everly, G. S., Shapiro, S., Levine, S., Newman, E. C., & Sherman, M. (1987). An investigation into the relationships between personality disorders and clinical syndromes (*DSM-III,* Axis I). In C. Green (Ed.), *Conference of the Millon clinical inventories (MCMI, MBHI, MAPI)* (pp. 295–303). Minneapolis: National Computer Systems.

C. Green (Ed.). (1987). Conference on the Millon clinical inventories (MCMI, MBHI, MAPI). Minneapolis: National Computer Systems.

Greenblatt, R. L. (1987). Nonmetric multidimensional scale of the MCMI. In C. Green (Ed.), *Conference on the Millon clinical inventories (MCMI, MBHI, MAPI)* (pp. 145–154). Minneapolis: National Computer Systems.

Greenblatt, R. L., Mozdzier, G. J., Murphy, T. J., & Kestutis, T. (1987). Pathological personality style and symptom diversity of 28/82 psychiatric patients. In C. Green (Ed.), *Conference on the Millon clinical inventories (MCMI, MBHI, MAPI)* (pp. 243–247). Minneapolis: National Computer Systems.

Gualtieri, J., Gonzales, E., & Baldwin, N. (1987). The accuracy of MCMI computer narratives for alcoholics. In C. Green (Ed.), *Conference on the Millon Clinical inventories (MCMI, MBHI, MAPI)* (pp. 263–268). Minneapolis: National Computer Systems.

Hyer, L. (1987). "Personologic Primacy" of later-life patients. In C. Green (Ed.), *Conference on the Millon Clinical inventories (MCMI, MBHI, MAPI)* (pp. 13–19). Minneapolis: National Computer Systems.

Leaf, R. C., DiGuiseppe, R., Ellis, A., Wolfe, J., Yeager, R., & Alington, D. (1987). Treatment intake status and the MCMI's "Axis II" scale scores. In C. Green (Ed.), *Conference on the Millon clinical inventories (MCMI, MBHI, MAPI)* (pp. 21–29). Minneapolis: National Computer Systems.

Lepkowsky, C. M. (1987). Personality pathology in eating disorders. In C. Green (Ed.), *Conference on the Millon clinical inventories (MCMI, MBHI, MAPI)* (pp. 215–220). Minneapolis: National Computer Systems.

Lumsden, E. A. (1987a). A signal-detection analysis of the external-criterion validation of the MCMI. In C. Green (Ed.), *Conference on the Millon clinical inventories (MCMI, MBHI, MAPI)* (pp. 141–143). Minneapolis: National Computer Systems.

Lumsden, E. A. (1987b). The impact of shared items on the internal-structural validity of the MCMI. In C. Green (Ed.), *Conference on the Millon clinical inventories (MCMI, MBHI, MAPI)* (pp. 325–333). Minneapolis: National Computer Systems.

McDermott, W. F. (1987). The diagnosis of post-traumatic stress disorder using the Millon Clinical Multiaxial Inventory. In C. Green (Ed.), *Conference on the Millon clinical inventories (MCMI, MBHI, MAPI)* (pp. 257–262). Minneapolis: National Computer Systems.

Reich, J. H., Noyes, R., & Trougton, E. (1987). Lack of agreement between instruments assessing *DSM-III* personality disorders. In C. Green (Ed.), *Conference on the Millon clinical inventories (MCMI, MBHI, MAPI)* (pp. 223–234). Minneapolis: National Computer Systems.

Sandberg, M. (1987). Is the ostensive accuracy of computer interpretive reports a result of the Barnum Effect? A study of the MCMI. In C. Green (Ed.), *Conference on the Millon clinical inventories (MCMI, MBHI, MAPI)* (pp. 155–164). Minneapolis: National Computer Systems.

Sugrue, D. P. (1987). Applications of the MCMI in the evaluation of sexual dysfunctions. In C. Green (Ed.), *Conference on the Millon Clinical inventories (MCMI, MBHI, MAPI)* (pp. 287–292). Minneapolis: National Computer Systems.

Tracy, H., Norman, D., & Weisberg, L. (1987). Anorexia and bulimia: A comparison of MCMI results. In C. Green (Ed.), *Conference on the Millon clinical inventories (MCMI, MBHI, MAPI)* (pp. 195–197). Minneapolis: National Computer Systems.

Warner, J. S. (1987). Use of the Millon Clinical Multiaxial Inventory (MCMI) in an alcoholism halfway house program. In C. Green (Ed.), *Conference on the Millon clinical inventories (MCMI, MBHI, MAPI)* (pp. 269–272). Minneapolis: National Computer Systems.

About the Editor

Robert J. Craig, Ph.D., ABPP, is a Fellow in the American Psychological Association and a Fellow in the Society for Personality Assessment. He has served as consulting editor to the *Journal of Personality Assessment* for 33 years and is the recipient of the Martin Mayman Award for Distinguished Contributions to the Literature of Personality Assessment, awarded by the Society for Personality Assessment. He is board certified in Clinical Psychology and in Administrative Psychology, directs the Drug Abuse Treatment Program at the Jesse Brown VA Medical Center, Chicago, and is adjunct professor at Roosevelt University, where he teaches courses in personality assessment and in chemical dependence. He has extensively researched the MCMI. This is his tenth book, his third on the MCMI.

Author Index

Subject Index

Printed and bound by CPI Group (UK) Ltd, Croydon, CR0 4YY

16/04/2025

14658524-0002